CW01333694

1

European Food History

European Food History

A Research Review

Edited by Hans J. Teuteberg

Leicester University Press
Leicester, London and New York

distributed exclusively in the USA and Canada by ST. MARTIN'S PRESS

© Editor and contributors, 1992

First published in Great Britain in 1992 by Leicester University Press
(a division of Pinter Publishers Limited)

All rights reserved. No part of this publication may be
reproduced, stored in a retrieval system, or transmitted
in any other form or by any means, electronic, mechanical,
photocopying, recording or otherwise, without the prior
permission of the Leicester University Press.

Editorial offices
Fielding Johnson Building, University of Leicester,
Leicester, LE1 7RH, England

Trade and other enquiries
25 Floral Street, London, WC2E 9DS, UK
and Room 400, 175 Fifth Avenue, New York, NY 10010, USA

Distributed exclusively in the USA
and Canada by St. Martin's Press, Inc.,
175 Fifth Avenue, New York, NY 10010, USA

British Library Cataloguing in Publication Data
A CIP catalogue record for this book is available from the British Library

ISBN 0 7185 1383 5

Library of Congress Cataloging in Publication Data
European food history / edited by Hans J. Teuteberg
　　　p.　cm.
　　Proceedings of a conference held at the University of Münster, May 16–19, 1989.
　　Includes bibliographical references and index.
　　ISBN 0-7185-1383-5
　　1. Diet—Europe—History—Congresses. I. Teuteberg, Hans Jürgen.
TX360.E8H57　1992
363.8'094—dc20　　91-29780
　　　　　　　　CIP

Printed and bound in Great Britain by SRP Ltd, Exeter

Contents

List of tables	vii
List of figures	viii
List of contributors	ix
Preface	x

1. Agenda for a comparative European history of diet
   Hans J. Teuteberg — 1

2. British diet since industrialization: a bibliographical study
   Derek J. Oddy and John Burnett — 19

3. Comparative aspects of Irish diet, 1550–1850
   Louis Michael Cullen — 45

4. Modern nutritional problems and historical nutrition research, with special reference to the Netherlands
   Adel P. den Hartog — 56

5. Historical food research in Belgium: development, problems and results in the 19th and 20th centuries
   Peter Scholliers — 71

6. The history of diet as a part of the *vie matérielle* in France
   Eva Barlösius — 90

7. The diet as an object of historical analysis in Germany
   Hans J. Teuteberg — 109

8. Food research from the viewpoint of ethnology, economic and social history in the former German Democratic Republic, 1949–1989
   Rudolf Weinhold — 129

9. Nutrition in Austria in the industrial age
   Roman Sandgruber — 146

10. Food history in Switzerland: a survey of the literature
    Martin R. Schärer — 168

11. Food and foodways as the subject of historical analyses in Hungary
    Eszter Kisbán — 199

12. A methodological approach to the system of food
    consumption in 16th-century Poland
    Andrzej Wyczański — 213

13. Ethnological studies in the traditional food of the Russians,
    Ukrainians and Byelorussians between the 16th and 19th
    centuries: state of research and basic problems
    Michail G. Rabinovich — 224

14. Development and possibilities of historical studies of
    meals and nourishment in Bohemia
    Lydia Petránová — 236

15. Nutritional needs and social esteem: two aspects of diet in
    Sweden during the 18th and 19th centuries
    Mats Essemyr — 256

16. Divergences and convergences in the development of culinary
    cultures
    Stephen Mennell — 278

Index — 289

List of tables

1.1	Social and psychic functions of foodstuff and luxuries	5
4.1	Nutritional advice in the Netherlands, 1847 and 1886	57
4.2	Percentage of household expenditure spent on food by working-class families, 1850–1985	58
4.3	Infant mortality in the Netherlands, 1900–1986	58
4.4	Daily energy and macro-nutrient availability in the Netherlands, 1936/8-1985	58
5.1	Development of per-capita calorie intake in 18th- and 20th-century Belgium (in kcal) a) National average and working-class families b) Middle-class families	83
9.1	Annual Viennese per-capita food consumption, 1784–1910	148
9.2	Weekly income earned and hours worked by an unskilled Viennese industrial worker, 1830–1988	151
9.3	Average expenditure on consumption in Viennese workers' households, 1830–1988	151
9.4	Average annual food consumption in Viennese workers' households	154
9.5	Expenditure on food and luxuries in Viennese workers' households	157
9.6	Annual food consumption per capita in Austria (nutrition balances) 1934–88	160
11.1	Estimated average daily consumption of an adult man, mid-17th-century Hungary	202
11.2	Average annual per-capita food consumption in Hungary, 1881–3	204
11.3	Average annual per-capita food consumption in Hungary, 1934–85	204
12.1	Average daily rations of the royal court in 16th-century Poland	215
12.2	Average daily rations of the gentry in 16th-century Poland	216
12.3	Average daily rations of peasants in 16th-century Poland	217
12.4	Average annual agricultural production in 16th-century Poland	219
14.1	Annual and daily rations of rye bread in Bohemia, 1635–1726	241
14.2	Recommended monthly rations for Bohemian farm domestics, 1701	243
15.1	Daily per-capita energy intake among agricultural workers in Sweden, 16th to 18th centuries	260
15.2	Daily per-capita energy intake among sawmill workers in Sweden	269
15.3	Daily per-capita energy and protein intake in Sweden, 1913–14, 1922 and 1933	269
15.4	Percentage share of energy intake provided by animal products in the diet of Swedish agricultural workers, 16th to 18th centuries	270

List of figures

4.1 Height of army conscripts, 1860–1980 — 59
4.2 Relative frequency of the mention or depiction of the notion of 'tastiness' in food advertisements in Dutch women's magazines, 1900–85 — 64
4.3 Relative frequency of the mention or depiction of health claims in food advertisements in Dutch women's magazines, 1900–85 — 65
4.4 Relative frequency of the mention or depiction of product's ingredients in food advertisements in Dutch women's magazines, 1900–85 — 66
5.1 Meat consumption in the Cities of Ghent and Antwerp and in Belgium in the 19th and 20th centuries — 81
5.2 Belgian food consumption indices, 1896–1940 — 82
15.1 Population growth in Sweden pro mille, 1749–1914 — 258
15.2 Enköping hospital, 1759–81: per-capita energy intake (kcal per day) — 261
15.3 Enköping hospital, 1759–81: per-capita protein intake (g per day) — 262
15.4 Falun hospital, 1659–1750: per-capita energy intake (kcal per day) — 262
15.5 Falun hospital, 1659–1750: per-capita protein intake (g per day) — 263
15.6 Falun hospital, 1756–1837: per-capita energy intake (kcal per day) — 263
15.7 Falun hospital, 1756–1837: per-capita protein intake (g per day) — 264
15.8 Västerås hospital, 1621–1823: per-capita energy intake (kcal per day) — 264
15.9 Västerås hospital, 1621–1823: per-capita protein intake (g per day) — 265
15.10 Weckholm hospital, 1696–1872: per-capita energy intake (kcal per day) — 265
15.11 Weckholm hospital, 1696–1872: per-capita protein intake (g per day) — 267
15.12 Energy intake among forgemen in Forsmarks bruk, 1730–1880 (kcal per day) — 267
15.13 Protein intake among forgemen in Forsmarks bruk, 1730–1880 (g per day) — 268
15.14 Enköping hospital, 1759–1781: percentage share of energy intake provided by animal products — 271
15.15 Falun hospital, 1756–1837: percentage share of energy intake provided by animal products — 271
15.16 Weckholm hospital, 1696–1872: percentage share of energy intake provided by animal products — 272
15.17 Västerås hospital, 1621–1823: percentage share of energy intake provided by animal products — 272
15.18 Forgemen of Forsmarks bruk, 1730–1880: percentage share of energy intake provided by animal products — 273

List of contributors

Dr. Eva Barlösius, formerly: Maison des Sciences de l'Homme, 54, boulevard Raspail, 75270 Paris Cédex 06, France, now: Institut für Agrarpolitik, Marktforschung und Wirtschaftssoziologie, Universität Bonn, Nussallee 21, 5300 Bonn, Germany.

Prof. John Burnett, PhD., Brunel University, Uxbridge, Middlesex UB8 3 PH, United Kingdom.

Prof. Louis Michael Cullen, PhD., University of Dublin, Department of Modern History, Trinity College, Dublin 2, Ireland.

Dr. Mats Essemyr, Uppsala Universitet, Ekonomisk-historika Institutionen, Kyrkogårdsgatan 10, P.O. Box 513, 75120 Uppsala, Sweden.

Dr. Adel den Hartog, Agricultural University, Department of Human Nutrition, P.O. Box 8129, 6700 EV Wageningen, The Netherlands.

Dr. Eszter Kisbán, Magyar Tudomanyos Akademia, Neprajzi Kutato Csoport, Budapest I, Országház u. 30, 1250 Postafiók 29, Hungary.

Prof. Stephen Mennell, PhD., Department of Anthropology and Sociology, Monash University, Clayton, Melbourne, Victoria 3168, Australia.

Prof. Derek J. Oddy, PhD., The Polytechnic of Central London, Faculty of Business, Management and Social Studies, 309 Regent Street, London WIR 8AL, United Kingdom.

Dr. Lydia Petránová, Československá akademie ved ustav pro Etnografia Folkloristiku, CS-120 000 Praha 2, Lazarská 8, Czechoslovakia.

Prof. Michail G. Rabinovich, Institute for Ethnography, Academy of Sciences of the U.S.S.R., ul. Dimitrij Uljanova 19, 117036 Moscow, Russia.

Prof. Dr. Roman Sandgruber, Institut für Sozial- und Wirtschaftsgeschichte, Johannes-Kepler-Universität Linz, Altenbergstr. 69, 4040 Linz, Austria.

Dr. Martin R. Schärer, Alimentarium – Musée de l'Alimentation, Quai Perdonnet-Rue de Léman, B.P. 13, 1800 Vevey, Switzerland.

Dr. Peter Scholliers, Vrije Universiteit Brussel, Centrum Hedendaagse, Social Geschiedenis, Fakulteit der Economische, Sociale en Politieke Wetenschapen, Pleinlaan 2, Lokaal 5 B421, 1050 Brussels, Belgium.

Prof. Dr. Hans J. Teuteberg, Westfälische Wilhelms-Universität Münster, Historisches Seminar, Lehrstuhl für Neuere und Neueste Sozial- und Wirtschaftsgeschichte, Domplatz 20-22, W-4400 Münster, Germany.

Dr. Rudolf Weinhold, Karl-Marx-Str. 52f, O-8080 Dresden, Germany.

Prof. Andrzej Wyczański, Institut Historii Polskiej, Akademie Nauk, Rynek Starego Miasta 29/31, 00-272 Warszaw, Poland.

Preface

This volume contains the proceedings of a conference held by a group of food historians at the University of Münster on 16–19 May 1989. It was the first international symposium which dealt exclusively with the problems and development of food conditions in Europe since modern times and, especially, with their scholarly interpretation. Thus this symposium marked an important step into a new field of historical analysis as well as on the way to international and interdisciplinary cooperation.

The conference, which had been prepared by intensive correspondence and discussions in London and Münster, had three main aims. First, scholars from as many countries as possible, including those of the former Warsaw Pact, were to report extensively on the development and present-day situation of historical food research. At the same time, the essential scholarly literature was to be specified and interpreted in a chronological or other structured form. Within this framework it also seemed desirable to make use of related research methods, especially in the field of quantification, and to obtain information on contemporary sources, which either had been used so far or could possibly be used in the future.

In addition, the participants were free to report on the results of recent individual studies, which concerned the objective, temporal, or local paradigms of the changes in food habits.

Finally, scholars were asked to introduce further topics which seemed especially interesting to research or which could be the subject of a second conference. In preparing the meeting, we agreed to focus on the period since the 16th century. From the beginning, we deliberately excluded the food habits of antiquity and the Middle Ages as well as of all cultures beyond Europe in order to obtain comparable results and to avoid splintering a topic so complicated and so difficult to survey.

In sharply delimiting the themes of the conference in this way, we wished to avoid repeating recent experience of food-history discussions at international conferences on economic history, where papers have tended to be delivered in a vacuum and it has not really been possible to draw conclusions on the general process of food history. It is certainly evident that comparisons between the food conditions of European modern times and earlier eras and other distant regions can be very informative. However, these comprehensive considerations have to be saved for a later phase.

Guided by the motto 'Sometimes a bit less can be a bit more', the number of conference participants, whose names are given after this preface, was deliberately limited to allow more time for each paper and subsequent discussion. It is our conviction that the results of enormous 'mammoth congresses', where orators only have 10 or 15 minutes to read their papers and where there is little time for critical discussion, often bear no relation to the preparatory effort and costs. A considered exchange of ideas in a small group in which everybody has a voice would appear to be much more fruitful.

The contributions are generally presented in the form in which they were delivered in Münster. As usual, they were subsequently reviewed and prepared for printing, and some new material has been added. Some had to be revised with regard to the language, as there were fairly difficult translations from the different mother tongues into the English language. To give this volume a uniform style, we had to adapt the different sources and specifications of literature to the English way of quoting. In addition, all titles which had not been presented in one of the languages of the conference (English, French and German) were translated into English to make this report more readable. The editor hopes that, in this way, the volume will offer a first survey of the development and current situation of historical food research in most countries of Europe, and that it will, at the same time, serve as a *bibliographie raisonnée*, a reference book which has not been published so far.

This first symposium led to the founding of the International Commission for Research into European Food History, with an Executive Committee which was elected to prepare further meetings, and with correspondents for the individual countries. The following conferences of this new association are intended to take place in different European countries every two years; they will deal with specific, closely defined themes.

With its generous financial aid, the private Fritz Thyssen Foundation made the first conference in Münster possible and, in particular, allowed scholars from central and eastern European countries to participate.

Furthermore, we would like to thank Leicester University Press for including this volume in its prestigious programme and Mr Alec MacAulay for the speed with which the volume was published. The publisher and the members of the Commission hope that this book may find interest in many European countries and be the prelude for further publications in the field of food history.

The editor would like to express his warmest gratitude to the representatives of the 16 nations for their eager cooperation during the planning and execution of the conference, for the patience with which they accepted the assignments, and for keeping to the deadlines for the delivery of manuscripts and the manifold corrections to these.

Professors John Burnett and Derek J. Oddy as well as Dr Ludwig Steindorff of the Abteilung für Osteuropäische Geschichte des Historischen Seminars der Westfälischen Wilhelms-Universität Münster have given the editor of this much help in editing individual papers. We are grateful for their contributions to the success of this publication.

Last, but not least, several assistants and students of the Department of Social and Economic History at the University of Münster have made substantial and valuable contributions to the organization of the conference and to the publication of our results. They have eased our work. However, the editor alone bears, as usual, responsibility for any mistakes or omissions which might remain despite all editorial revision.

University of Münster
December 1990   Hans J. Teuteberg

1 Agenda for a comparative European history of diet

Hans J. Teuteberg

For millions of years human history, reduced to the essential chances of survival, had obviously been based on the daily need for food. It was often a desperate fight against crop failures, which continuously recurred, against rising prices, usury and famine. The 18th century, however, saw the onset of the 'diet revolution'; this gathered pace during the 19th century in the course of industrialization and urbanization. In some European countries, as well as in North America, this development led to the breaking of the age-old vicious circle of poverty, low work productivity, and low life expectancy, leading to the creation of our welfare society, with its abundance of food.

More and more nations in the world try to go down this path; yet the gap between the well-fed and the hungry nations, the super-rich and the have-nots, remains very large, and has indeed widened. The less developed countries of the 'Fourth World', with the lowest per-capita income, have the highest population growth rates and the poorest prospects as far as food resources are concerned. Only by decisively intensifying the bilateral and international relief programmes can we solve this global social problem. The recent worrying increase in economic refugees, however, who come from all parts of the world to the few countries with a high standard of living, will most likely intensify this problem within a decade.

In the meantime, the surplus of food has also caused a lot of new problems in the rich industrial states: overweight, which is widespread and leads to many illnesses, is one example; ever increasing forms of alcoholism typical of the affluent society, and unlimited consumption with its damage to the environment, are others. Furthermore, we must not forget in this context that traditional food habits (the family gathering together at the dining table three times a day, for instance) are dying out and that, at the moment, nobody can foresee where this process is leading and what its consequences will be. Food consumption in this context is a reflection of changes in the values of a post-industrial leisure society.

Strangely enough, this fundamental change in our nutrition standards has so far been examined only very unsatisfactorily by scholars. The reasons for this gap in our knowledge are easy to explain. The modern nutrition-related sciences, which developed in the last century, have until now maintained an exclusively scientific focus. In the view of modern scientists, their main task is to examine the nature of the stuff that people use as food and its utilization within the organism. The results of this research are then used for the preservation of human health. In other words, this kind of nutritional research is supposed to examine the processes of digestion within the human body and to gather data for an optimal diet which can be modified according to age, gender and the amount of work humans do. Of special importance is the search for a sound basis for a dietary treatment for diseases of the metabolic, digestive, and excretive processes, and progress towards optimal food conditions, determined by clinical research.

These scientific problems also play a role as far as the question of the agrarian-industrial production of food and its processing and preparation is concerned; the chemical composition of food and the need for nutritive substances, including their effect on metabolism, must be known. Although the interdisciplinary character of the nutritional sciences is underlined here, in general what springs to mind is a cooperation of the individual branches of natural sciences. On the one hand we have physiology, biochemistry, toxicology, and microbiology as basic subjects in our mind, and, on the other hand, we think of food sciences (such as agronomy, food technology, food analysis), and, finally, the different branches of human medicine (pathogenesis, pathophysiology, dietary prophylaxis, epidemiology, therapy, and human genetics).

The humanities, however, are considered by established food scientists only as peripheral, auxiliary means. Of course, scientists concerned with human nutrition know that food is subject to various changes on its way from production to consumption, but all these processes are deliberately excluded from their considerations, as they seem irrelevant from a scientific point of view. Not only political-legal and economic, but also geographical and psycho-social as well as cultural aspects, that is to say, all historical dimensions, are neglected by these scientists.

This obvious neglect of non-scientific aspects has persisted until today and derives from the traditional perceptions of nutrition scientists who, especially in England, France, Germany, and the Netherlands, regard their field of studies exclusively as a branch of biochemistry. Although biased in this way, these nutritional sciences have achieved epoch-making results during the last hundred years. This has been partly because they have confined themselves to a few selected fields of study and deliberately neglected other aspects of research. At the same time, an insight, which had been alive until the end of the 18th century, was lost: the idea that the human as an eating and drinking being is not only a physical object with organs and metabolic processes; he is also a psychic subject with individual signs of life, who can, at least theoretically, arrange his food habits without reference to inborn instincts, although he depends on numerous natural and self-caused behaviour obligations. Scientists failed to see that the substance of human food cannot be derived exclusively from the physical dimension.

Scholars of the humanities, however, add the following considerations. Human existence has a twofold character. On the one hand, nutrition is an absolutely necessary prerequisite for the reproduction of life and is, therefore, strictly subject to natural laws. After his birth, the human being finds himself in a world which he has not created, but which, from then on, becomes his natural environment. All his life, the human being will depend on this natural condition. Thus, the absorption of food is intricately interwoven with the impulse to stay alive and belongs, as much as sleep and breathing, to the important physiological basic needs, the satisfaction of which cannot be delayed. No human can do without the continuous renewal of his life energy by absorbing food. Metaphorically speaking, the human being is an internal-combustion engine which always has to be supplied with fuel in the form of food and drink. The outward appearance is, in that sense, the material product of the foodstuff which the human being daily consumes.

Nevertheless, we know by experience that food, through all times and in all regions, has also been an expression of human desires. This expression was, of course, often limited by the scarcity of economic resources as well as by socio-cultural norms. Although the absorption of food takes place within certain determined limits, there can be no doubt that nutrition is both a process of satisfying the human's basic need for the preservation of his life and, equally, an element of human culture.

The world into which the human being is born is much more determined by the historical process of human development than by natural conditions. In other words, the human's daily meals indicate how man throughout history has changed and differentiated nature according to his needs. In addition, they present a system of social rules and corresponding ways of behaviour. In responding to the given natural and cultural conditions with a creative and reproductive process, the human being creates his own environment. As this world is always a world for other humans as well, this process takes place communicatively with the transmission of information using language, images, symbols and gestures. That is why meals are always welcome occasions for inter-human communication. At this stage, food summarizes and transforms a process which has nothing to do with its original purpose. Eating and drinking are, therefore, indicators for more or less conscious patterns of behaviour, far beyond the mere absorption of food. Eating becomes a behaviour which develops autonomously and persists even after the mere process of absorbing food has been finished. Meals mark and substitute human ways of behaviour which often take place in different spheres of life. On the other hand, conditions of life can also be expressed by the way in which the food is eaten. In this way, every human sphere of life is connected with others by food habits. The typical social norms which are connected with the meals may change, but the intimacy of communication remains. The presentation of food is certainly more commercialized than in earlier times: today, our meals and drinks are more often the products of industry than they are of the domestic kitchen. This, however, has not changed the way in which people like to impress with food. We can even say that the social-communicative character of the meals presents itself the more clearly the faster the physiological need of nutrition is satisfied. For the *beati possidentes,* who have already in early centuries been well fed at the expense of the poor, meals primarily had the function of a 'social protocol' rather than of satisfying physical needs. From this communicative context and from the differences of social classes, ranks, groups and individuals, we can conclude that there is a range of possibilities within the process of adapting to natural conditions and socio-cultural prerequisites which allow the emergence of completely different answers to the same historical situation. The strategies of behaviour differ in regard to the temporal and regional context and to the social and psychic dispositions of the acting humans. We can explain the enormous variety of the courses of action probably best by the term *Ernährungsstil*, which defines the social homogeneity of strategies of action in the context of alternative possibilities. By taking the scholarly discussions on the standard of living and consumption into account, we can understand *Ernährungsstil* as a special form of socio-cultural reproduction on the basis of subjective experiences, judgements and requirements, which exceed the mere materialistic aspect of the absorption of food.

These preliminary considerations show that the human being, like all other creatures, is dependent on the daily supply of food, but they also underline that he does not simply consume without any guiding principle. The taking of meals is determined by the basic scarcity of food, which first has to be produced, and, equally, by socio-cultural patterns of action. As these patterns are connected with ideas on society as a whole, nutrition can always to some extent be explained in cultural and sociological terms. All components which appear in this context constitute a highly complex system of retroaction, which has been subject to very little research. If we combine different efforts to categorize the symbolic content of food, then we obtain the classifications listed in Table 1.1.

According to this summary, meals are connected with representation, prestige and even playful functions, but there is also a link with magical, mythical and religious functions. Eating and drinking play an important role in marking one's own position in society. Since prehistoric man gathered berries, roots and herbs and went hunting and fishing, the composition of meals, the techniques of preparation and preservation and the ways in which the food was consumed have expressed human relations; and they have expressed these relations in a system of intricately interwoven meanings. Once more, we would like to underline that all these relationships contain different categories of meaning. These complex systems have so far been only insufficiently researched. Therefore, food habits are always components of a communicative process that comprises the whole society, as the individual elements adopt the character of coded patterns of behaviour. Thus if we want to analyse food habits, we must decode the commands for a certain behaviour and the motivational impulses which are transmitted by social leaders. In this context, meals and food in general take on the functions of a signal transmitter.

The role of individual foodstuffs within the socio-communicative field becomes even clearer if we point out that there is a difference between eating potatoes in soup during the week and eating them wrapped in aluminium foil with a knob of butter as an accompaniment to a T-bone steak in a fancy restaurant on a Sunday evening.. Sugar is another example: once an expensive luxury good which had to be imported from the colonies, it has become a common sweetener today, offered free of charge in restaurants. Sugar has even been discredited because it causes overweight and

Table 1.1 Social and psychic functions of foodstuff and luxuries

1. Prestige products	are regarded as personal attributes serve as a mark of exhibitionism underline a social elite position
2. Status products	enable socio-cultural identification show social group conformity
3. Fetish and security products	are consumed in situations of stress to gain emotional safety; people think they cannot do without them serve as 'ego-boosters' food for children, the sick and pregnant women
4. Hedonistic products	are consumed to satisfy desire, mostly because of the taste, fragrance and appearance; dependent on the situation as a reward for certain types of behaviour as a demonstration of one's state of mind, of one's pleasure and of communication
5. Functional products	serve exclusively as physiological supply; have no deeper significance and are symbolically neutral

dental decay. Thus it seems evident that the connotation which is connected with certain foods varies as a result of different times and regions and passes different socio-cultural processes, which either revalorize or devaluate the specific foodstuff. None of this could be explained without recognizing the symbolic or communicative character of food.

Anthropology, philosophy and sociology recognized a main attribute of human existence and social action a long time ago: the inseparable combination of compulsive basic needs on the one hand, and the more or less free, individualistic and collective organization of one's environment on the other. In the following, we would like to expand on this idea with regard to food. At the very beginning of mankind, the absorption of food was most likely only a necessity determined by instinct. In the course of his development of over 30 million years, however, the human being gradually lost this instinct; and with his instinct he lost the possibility of regulating his need for food: the human being, in contrast to the animal, is able to overeat. This is not meant pejoratively, for the diminution of his food instinct, the decay of the human's 'inner biological clockwork', made it possible to differentiate food habits in the cultural process more and more and to improve them with regard to taste and aesthetics. This is exactly what the animal cannot do, as it is guided exclusively by instinct. According to the psychologist Maslow, the human being has a primary need for food which is inborn, and a secondary need for food determined by society and culture. The latter necessity mirrors the individual social relations. It is this network of needs and social creativity that constitutes the different cultures. The need for food remains an elemental experience of deficiency and creates an inner state of tension which needs to be overcome. At the same time we can describe this need also as a sociological category with which we can express social identity and social action.

The tension in the individual between the need for food on the one hand and the possibility of meeting that need on the other is also characteristic of the human being. As the needs constantly exceeded the ability to satisfy them, ways had to be found to limit and reduce this demand. This explains the different systems of food distribution by which these needs are limited or by which they are declared as illegitimate. Furthermore, the need for food is always, in addition to the inborn need, subject to a social creative process, which has led to certain patterns of behaviour and distribution. These patterns of behaviour contribute during the process of socialization to the composition of the socio-culturally determined personality of the human being and his system of values.

Therefore, the natural sciences cannot fully explain the major problem of the false nutrition of our modern affluent society. This is a task that can only be carried out by the social and cultural sciences. It is easy to explain why the majority of the people who live in industrial states still eat and drink as if they worked heavily in an agrarian, craft-orientated world: our food patterns do not stem from our high-technology world of today but from the pre-industrial world of yesterday. It was the American sociologist William F. Ogburn who stated many decades ago that the different spheres of our society do not change simultaneously with regard to general temporal changes.

The materialistic culture (that is to say, the sum of scientific discoveries, methods and knowledge) progresses much faster than the immaterialistic culture (the sum of institutions, values and mental norms). According to Ogburn's famous cultural lag theory, there are certain maladjustments which occur regularly when the materialistic and the immaterialistic cultures are out of balance. This theory enables us to explain quite a lot in this context: the patterns of food behaviour, as an element of the immaterialistic culture, obviously lag often behind the faster changes in the materialistic environment. The building and decomposition of food behaviour patterns is a slow process and cannot immediately be changed by simple rational appeals. Here, once more, the limitations of scientific research into food history become evident, as the natural sciences can neither fully explain food habits nor change them.

In analysing the different elements which constitute the meaning of food, we notice that there has long been a trend in the development of nutrition to differentiate and rationalize. The speed and intensity of this trend, however, depend on the different societies and their subsystems, and even slow down or turn into their opposite from time to time. This is primarily connected with the process of the continuous division of labour, the increasing standard of living and the seemingly inexhaustible reservoir of human needs. The trend, we mentioned above, leads in the industrial societies to constant improvements in the production, preparation and preservation of food.

Agriculture increasingly no longer produces simple foodstuffs any more, as it did in earlier times, but regards its main task as enriching the same foodstuffs according to the taste of consumers, tested by market analysis. Within the last hundred years there has been a tendency to shift the activities which belong to the preparation of food (that is to say, sorting, cutting, mixing, colouring and adding spices) from households to industry. Even the realm of the kitchen has been drawn into this process of differentiation and rationalization and has been changed dramatically during the last hundred years. New techniques of preserving food meant that the housewife was no longer dependent on seasonal influences and on the age-old cycle of harvesting and butchering animals.

New kitchen stoves made of cast iron, first supplied with coal and then with gas or electricity, completely new kitchenware, and the 'reform kitchens' influenced by Taylorism and industrial psychology, together with systematic domestic science instruction led to huge improvements in the quality of meals. Moreover, the time needed for the preparation of meals was shortened dramatically. By rationalizing work in the kitchen, people were able to build huge canteens in industrial plants, and eating outside the home grew in popularity. The so-called *Bürgerliche Küche* (middle-class cooking; bourgeois cuisine), which has influenced all social classes since the late 19th century, has led to a lot of industrial innovations, the dimensions of which we have just started to survey. Yet it is remarkable that there have been voices since the late 18th century against the tendency to put cooking into scientific, rationalized, technical and differentiated categories. Since the time of Jean-Jacques Rousseau, these people have demanded a return to 'natural' cooking. The middle-class *Lebensreformbewegung* (health reform movement) which came into being in the late 19th century and which led, among other things, to the temperance movement, to nudism, vegetarianism, health food shops, and dietary nutrition with slimming courses and water cures, accused modern agriculture of ruining 'pure' food by chemical additives and, in this way, of endangering people's health purely for the sake of profit.

However, people failed to see that many basic foodstuffs had been regularly and deliberately tampered with until the period of industrialization and that the hygienic conditions for the daily absorption of food were in general extremely bad. It was the building of the modern food production and distribution system with its mass production that made the introduction of an efficient uniform food quality control possible. Yet, we have also to keep in mind that there is no such thing as 'natural nutrition', except perhaps the mother's milk: the cow's milk is supposed to nourish the calf; the egg is intended to become a chicken and the grain a corn-stalk. What the human being actually did, was to adapt certain plants and animals to his food habits by long evolutionary breeding processes and then declare them to be his food. The improved plants and domesticated animals, however, differ so much from their ancestors that one can hardly determine where nature ends and human art begins. A good example of this is the fattened pig.

Even the oft-reported reproach that 'natural' food has been substituted by industrial products fails to make sense if one takes a closer look at the problem: from the 18th to the 20th centuries, millions of people in Europe, for instance, drank *Ersatzkaffee*, made of chicory rather than real coffee, in order to save money. Moreover, chicory has been known as a salad and healing plant since ancient times; and that is why chicory can actually be regarded as more 'natural' and more 'original'. In the 19th century, financial and fiscal reasons led to the substitution of cane sugar, first by brown syrup and beet sugar, and then, from 1900, by the artificial sweetener saccharin. Furthermore, it is remarkable that this industrial sweetener had, for a very long time, an extremely bad reputation as an artificial and dangerous surrogate, although it is, from a nutritional point of view, quite unobjectionable. These examples show how difficult it has been to separate scientific objectivity from emotion in the field of nutrition. Therefore, we have to interpret the ineradicable and nostalgic longing for 'natural' food as one of the many opposing movements against modern techniques, industry and rationalization.

Even these few examples of the socio-cultural aspects of human nutrition prove that the ambit of a comparative European food history is extremely large. We can paraphrase the main aim of such a comparative history with the following short formula: we wish to clarify not only what and how much was eaten when and where, but above all, for what reasons something was eaten in that specific way. In addition, we wish to take a close look at the changes in food behaviour in different times and regions. Thus, we will need to analyse human activities in the context of natural processes, which constantly repeat themselves, and in connection with individual decisions and the different social and regional patterns of behaviour. In doing so, we will always have to keep in mind that it is nature which offers all the possibilities of food supply, but that it is the human being who finally decides, according to the specific circumstances, how to make use of this supply.

Considering the food problems mentioned above, we can truly say that historical research is confronted with a task that becomes more and more urgent. More than scientists, it is the historians who are able to put the manifold lines of development of human nutrition, which are connected with all other spheres of human life, into a context which also takes different times and regions into account. In contrast to scholars of other disciplines, historians do not examine one development in itself, but look for the interdependence of different causes and effects and try to paint a complete picture. It may sound strange, but it is the comprehensive historical approach which enables us to recognize as well the undoubtedly great achievements of scientists in the field of nutrition and to put these achievements into the right proportion as far as our knowledge of the development of humanity is concerned.

A comprehensive food history must first define terms to describe the multitude of problems which it is confronted with. Leaving food production to one side, it is reasonable to differentiate between the material substance of a food and the different actions necessary to get the food, prepare and consume it. With respect to a logically causal nutrition chain, we then obtain the following complexes of problems:

1. The demand for food within a subsistence economy and on the markets; the different ways of acquiring or buying and storing food; of special interest in this context are the knowledge of goods, the economic margin, the means of transport, the different types of market, the prices, the marketing, and the means of preservation.
2. The preparation and improvement of food especially by cooking, frying, stewing and baking, with the help of special techniques like adding colours, spices, etc.
3. The consumption of food (meals and dining halls; the timing of the meals during the day; the sequence of the different dishes during a meal; the use of leftovers, etc.).
4. The socio-cultural environment of the meals and its individual and collective subjective evaluation (the differentiation of ordinary and festive meals; food as a symbolic, religious and communicative action; the meals as a social division; etc.)
5. The nutritive-physiological contents and the nutritive consequences for health.

Naturally, this is only an initial guideline which has to be differentiated and expanded in various directions. Yet we can conclude from this summary that we will have to take the results of research from different disciplines into account. This is an arduous task, as the scientific methods and specific terms differ greatly, and one has hardly taken notice of any research in other disciplines. Moreover, there has been no coordinated research on the development of food conditions so far.

Nutrition physiologists, biologists and the medical profession, for instance, have several times carried out unprofessional research in the field of food history without considering the results of the history of civilization and without taking notice of its research methods. Books published by these people have borne such promising titles as 'The History of Food' and pretended to present a level of knowledge which, in fact, we have not yet achieved. These books consist of historical notes which are simply gathered together having apparently been obtained in a random manner. In addition, the so-called facts are based on sources which have not been checked, and the notes have not been put into their historical context. The main task of a comparative European food history is to gather the results of different areas of research and to place them in a coherent framework. For the last ten years we have therefore constantly striven to enter this new field of research and to produce a general outline with the help of specialized research presented at national and international conferences. It has, however, become apparent that our knowledge of the development and the present state of the research in the various European countries and of the different historical disciplines is insufficient. This has made it difficult to agree on general explanations on the basis of uniform terms.

To remedy this, we organized the first symposium on European food history, the results of which we will now summarize and evaluate. Some scholars presented, according to the aims of the symposium, an extensive outline of historical food research carried out in their country. They also gave more or less detailed consideration to different methods of research and sources and quoted important authors and their main results. Other scholars based their descriptions of the general change in food conditions rather more on their own research – a method which is of course easier for those who deal with small states. Some preferred to focus their descriptions on specific periods of time; this, as in the case of Poland, depends on the general political history of the country and on the availability of sources. Although we cannot compare the essays of this volume in every respect, a fact that we assumed at the outset because of the cultural and historical diversity of Europe, there are certain similarities, which we would briefly like to mention here.

First, it seems important that in all the countries represented at our symposium there are centres for specific research on food history. The number of scholars and institutes interested in our topic as well as the number of special research programmes, magazines, museums, libraries, and archives exceeded our expectations by far. Equally, there are many more scholars of food history than those who attended our first meeting in Münster. So we hope that future conferences will draw larger audiences and that the research of our newly founded Commission will be given a strong impetus.

As a first common statement we can mention that research is generally hindered by the lack of reliable bibliographies. Even in those countries with advanced research in the field of food history, we mainly found only provisional summaries of earlier and more recent literature which concerned specific problems, times and regions. Most of the scholars had difficulty in gathering information from other collections of literature, for the literature which dealt with food history was often 'hidden' behind titles heralding something different. This meant that a considerable amount of historical knowledge was needed to extract the essential information. The literature on food history is so widely scattered precisely because nutrition is a pervasive social phenomenon connected with nearly all spheres of human life. Apparently, a comprehensive bibliography on cookery books does not exist, although these books present the oldest printed literature in Europe. If we consider the great collections of literature of the different branches of science, then this lack of bibliographies becomes even more visible. Although there have been attempts to collect the material which is relevant to the history of food, reliable collections were never finished because of the abundance of titles, or they simply fell into oblivion. This volume, which is in the first place intended to be an annotated bibliography, fills an important gap, not only for a European but also for a national framework. The titles have been very carefully checked by the authors and they shed light on the question how translations of certain books indicate that a transfer of knowledge has taken place in Europe. It seems that the following causes (in no particular order) were responsible for the genesis of a specific 'food-historical' point of view:

1. The pre-industrial famines in the middle of the last century, with their mass poverty, emigration, and the 'social question' which was especially connected with the workers' wages and the costs of foodstuffs.
2. The development of an autonomous home cooking in connection with an exalted gastronomy and the dispersion of the 'art of cooking' by specific courses in domestic science and by household literature.

Agenda for a comparative European history of diet

3. The general interest in material culture or civilization, with the consumption of specific food and luxury goods as a main factor.
4. The biological and biochemical laboratory experiments on plants and animals which awakened an interest in human nutrition and metabolism, in nutritive values, processes of decay, and improvements in food quality and preservation.

It seems interesting to us that nearly all early general summaries of these topics have been written by nutrition physiologists, physicians, biologists as well as geographers, ethnologists and economists.

It is mentioned in many contributions to this volume that official statistics, which came into being at the beginning of the 19th century, apparently dealt primarily with the consumption of important basic foodstuffs. These statisticians tried to find out the wholesale prices (e.g., for grain and bread) and, in addition, the annual per-capita supply with the help of average harvest incomes, dead weights, and trade and population statistics. At first, their results were fragmentary, but then they developed into long term statistics. Opinions concerning calculations of agricultural output differed widely. They also differed as far as the amount of grain, fodder, organic waste (e.g., bones) and storage loss were concerned. For this reason, the data which have been obtained by macro-economic methods can only mirror relative tendencies in consumption. It has been, however, constantly pointed out that these general per-capita accounts ignore all differences of gender, age, profession, income, social class, education, and, above all, region. Thus, the really interesting aspects of changes in food habits still lie in obscurity. Yet this method of quantification offers the best possibilities for a comprehensive international comparison, as we have a multitude of data and as they can be configured to show consumption trends fairly easily. The per-capita calculations of different towns are more accurate when it comes to the groceries and luxury goods which were subject to taxes. That is why the consumption of meat, sugar, and alcohol has been best researched in Europe so far and can be readily used for initial international comparisons.

In several European countries there exists a more or less great quantity of household budgets, in which the consumption of the family is recorded with regard to prices and quantities and in which this consumption is compared to the family income. These sources present a lucky find for food historians, as the money spent on food constituted by far the major part of household costs until the beginning of the welfare society in the middle of the 20th century. These micro-economic calculations can be used to check the vague per-capita calculations; sometimes they date back to the 18th century and have their roots in account books of great manorial estates, monasteries, hospitals as well as troops and ships' crews. They show up the great differences in the consumption of the various social classes and regions, as well as pointing out gender and age differences. Unfortunately, these household budgets have several grave imperfections: often we cannot be sure that they are truly representative. In addition, the statistical methods differed immensely, so that it has not so far been possible to carry out national or international comparisons. It is also difficult from today's point of view to determine the general minimum of existence at a certain time and place. We know too little about the amount and kind of food people considered to be sufficient. As everyone knows, there is no minimum of existence which is valid for all times and places, but only a subsistence level which is determined anew by every society. These problems can apparently be solved best by gathering as many account books as possible from all countries and preparing them for an initial real comparison by using electronic data processing and new methods of artificial variables (e.g., cluster analysis). It is most likely that until now we have only been able to gather fragments of the account books which have been passed on to us. These calculations became very fashionable in all European countries in the late 19th century, as we can see today, and became an important part of labour statistics, which also bloomed at that time. Edouard Ducpétiaux, Adolphe-Lambert Quetelet, Frédéric Le Play, Ernst Engel and others contributed to the widespread popularity of this method. The statistical offices of the state and the communities, trade unions, public health authorities and other undertakings made an extensive effort to 'measure' nutrition. It became, however, apparent that data on the true consumption of alcoholic beverages, for instance, were often concealed, and that these statistics are therefore mostly wrong. In the 1930s, people became less and less interested in these calculations, so that true long-term statistics are not available; something we can do with the per-capita calculations.

Interestingly enough, there has been additional research on the standard of living of rural and urban labourers in some European states in the 19th century. The people who did this research used in general more precise methods and annotated their work comprehensively. The results are not mere figures like the per-capita statistics and account books but they represent a deeper insight in the nutritional daily life of the lower social classes; often they integrate the people's quotations into their research. Extraordinary examples are the works of Charles Booth and Seebohm Rowntree in England and of the Verein für Socialpolitik in Germany. Historians could use these rich resources (the research consists of several volumes) much more than they have done so far.

After the physiology of nutrition had been institutionalized in the second half of the 19th century, scholars tried for the first time to convert the quantities of food consumed, as determined statistically, into calories and the three most important nutrition units - protein, fat and carbohydrates. Although this method was little used at first, it has become common since the middle of the 20th century. Ernest Labrousse, Robert Philippe, Frank Spooner, John McKenzie, Derek Oddy, Wilhelm Abel, Andrzej Wyczański and the present author have done such nutritional value calculations. As Eva Barlösius, a trained nutritional physiologist, states in this volume, it is astonishing how naively and uncritically some historians have used these physiological calculations in a historical context. These conversions are, like measures of the standard of living, not absolute natural laws which outlive all temporal and regional changes. What they in fact do is mirror certain opinions and interests of their researchers. In addition, we must point out that many results are only apparently exact: the amounts of food, as given by the historical sources, are often not specified. If we then consider how many different kinds of meat, for instance, exist and how different their nutritive and calorie values are, the difficulties immediately become plain. Moreover, nutritional physiologists have been quick to remind us that vitamins, trace elements and even roughage also belong to a balanced diet. And finally, one has to adapt the optimal nutrition requirements to the amount of physical work someone does, that is to say, to one's profession, to one's age, gender, to the climate, etc. If one ignores all these conditions, one can easily produce distorted pictures from fragmentary calculations.

In contrast to nutritional physiology, which operates more or less statically, cultural research into nutrition is principally orientated towards dynamic changes in food habits. Temporal and regional processes set inventions in motion which, if accepted by society, rise to innovations which can truly evoke changes. In addition, these processes lead, through wide diffusion, to a satisfaction of socio-cultural needs and to a new style of nutrition. In this volume, the essays from different European countries show, however, that the scholars of earlier cultural or ethnological food research can explain the genesis of these inventions and their diffusion within the modern consuming society only to a limited extent; for it is the modern consuming society that brings about qualitatively new market mechanisms and new lifestyles but also new ways of communication and diffusion. Since the late 19th century, new impulses for changes in food habits have come into being. These were caused by the development of the modern food industry, by new ways of preserving food, and, at the same time, by growing food trade.

According to these essays, it also seems that the old food habits of pre-industrial towns and rural nobility have been researched far better than the food habits of the industrial age. Apparently, the large quantity of cookery-books, and household, family, and women's magazines with their essays, pictures and advertisements, as well as the catalogues of firms and industrial fairs, the menus of restaurants and the wide range of medical-dietary publications have nowhere been collected and analysed. We have only a fragmentary knowledge of what luxury foods came when and where into the sphere of the kitchen, of how the order of consumption of dishes and meals changed, and consequently of the social esteem connected with them.

So far we can say that historic research has primarily confined itself to the food supply, which has been rashly equated with real consumption. A comprehensive food history, however, must not only deal with food supply, but must also analyse the preparation of meals. In this context, 'meals' are to be defined as one or more foodstuffs made ready to consume. We also have to analyse the technical shifts in the different ways and basic types of preparation and the changes in household appliances, foodstuffs, and recipes. Finally, we must aim to clarify the structural changes within the meals and the actual act of consumption. Here, we will also focus on the changes in the compositions of the courses of meals, the different ways of arranging them, the changes in the decoration of the dining table, the tableware, the table design, etc.

We should not forget, however, that all the innovations in the general field of food have also influenced the different food systems. This fact is mentioned in some essays of this volume. The central question, in this context, is which meals, dishes, and foodstuffs were ousted by others. These processes of substitution are historically extremely relevant, as one also has to keep in mind the different consequences for the overall nutritional balance. They have, furthermore, often caused ardent cultural criticism. This fact explains at least partially the resentment against the introduction of food innovations. This field of study seems so far to have been widely neglected.

As all the contributors to this volume show, innovations in the field of food have also been initiated by the development of modern nutritional physiology. The interactions, however, still remain indistinct. Although there is some brief information on the genesis and development of the different areas of nutritional science in 19th- and 20th-century handbooks on nutritional physiology, one generally does not know how far the inventions of the natural sciences actually changed people's food habits. Most likely, there was a strong interdependence between the propagation of minimum norms of protein, fat and carbohydrates of the daily food supply and the government's attempts to solve the social question in the decades around 1900. In many cases the government, individual communities and charitable and ecclesiastical organizations tried to influence the seemingly unhealthy food habits of urban workers by educational means. The publications of 'cookery-books for the plain household' and cookery courses are only two examples.

Intricately interwoven with this complex of 'food education', which promoted the standards of middle-class cooking, are the attempts to remedy, with the help of uniform national and local laws, the age-old grievances concerning the deliberate adulteration or the careless contamination of foodstuffs. It is astonishing that such an important topic has attracted so little attention, except for a few studies by such scholars as John Burnett. That is why one is often dependent on the inadequate works of doctors, chemists, nutritional physiologists and geographers. Another important field on which research still remains to be done is the genesis of modern governmental food control, which today plays a role in the discussion on improving our natural environment and which sheds light on the history of social hygiene. In this context, it would be interesting to analyse the elements which promoted these laws and those which hindered their progress (the butchers' resistance to the introduction of urban abattoirs with their official meat inspections, for instance). It was with the beginning of the European agricultural market that the standardization of food laws and the examination of 'quality of life' began to play a certain role. The assimilation of the laws will progress further with the development of a uniform European economy and eventual economic union. Thus it seems sensible to trace back the roots of this legislation in the different countries and to compare them comprehensively.

In reading the following contributions, one notices that the description of the different foods varies greatly. While we read a lot about bread and flour, meat and other meat products, alcoholic beverages, tea, coffee and sugar, we hear relatively little of other foodstuffs. This is due to the fact that the taxation of foodstuffs was regularly recorded, so that we have sources which have attracted historians. They were mostly interested in expensive luxury goods, which had always been at the centre of their discussions, rather than in boring everyday food. The proportions of the actual consumption are therefore often blurred: from a quantitative point of view, people consumed mostly meals and drinks of which no historical information has been passed on. Evidently, the nutritional historians' main task must be to 'reconstruct' the neglected elements of daily food consumption. This daily fare has not yet been properly researched and does not yet form part of our historical understanding. Most of the historical descriptions deal with special banquets and 'gala dinners' or expensive luxury goods, and only a small number are concerned with everyday consumption. Significantly enough, there is still no comprehensive cultural history of the simple gruel or the 'small man's' soup, though these two dishes have been an integral part of daily fare for many centuries. We have also to keep in mind that the cheap surrogates (chicory as a substitute for coffee, syrup for sugar, fat and margarine for butter) have been subject to only little research.

We can observe a similar disparity in research concerning the food trade. We know much more about the food supplies of metropolises like London, Paris and Vienna than about the supplies of provincial towns. Although the breakthrough of modern food trade and mass consumption has sometimes been recognized as a problem, historians have not yet studied all sources and aspects. The development from the pre-industrial subsistence economy to households dependent on monetary resources and markets, from the fairs and weekly markets and salesmen to the modern supermarkets with deep-frozen foods, department stores, hypermarkets and mail-order businesses could be an interesting part of transport, trade, and urban history. The growth of modern metropolises would not have been at all possible without a new system of food distribution. The analysis of city directories, of reports from market halls and abattoirs, newspaper advertisements and posters will certainly present substantial results. Scholars from the Netherlands in particular have researched the development and meaning of food advertisements. Target groups for such advertisements were primarily classes with a higher income; it was the aim to promote their consumption of expensive luxury foods (champagne, chocolate, and hot chocolate) or of surrogates which were intended to be put on the market (margarine, meat extracts and canned foods).

In studying historical food research, one is not surprised that the history of food of certain institutions has found special interest in nearly all countries. There are extensive historical sources on the food supply of monasteries, poor- and workhouses, orphanages, hospitals, old people's homes, and prisons, as well as on the food supply of ships, the army, farm-hands, railroad workers and navvies. The cost sheets, for instance, contain an abundance of prices and quantities, which could be converted and made uniform with the help of modern quantitative methods. Social gradation at the table is remarkable everywhere. It underlines once more that meals were used to point out social differences and were also regarded as a means of punishing criminal behaviour. These cost sheets often mirror the lowest nutrition standard and are a good indicator of how nutritional innovations penetrated the lower social classes. Today, we regard monotonous meals with horror; in earlier times, however, they were very much the rule rather than the exception. At the same time, cost sheets present information on regional cooking customs. Swedish research in particular on plain meals dates back to early times and should attract special attention in this volume.

Studies on the development of food conditions in Europe since the beginning of modern times grew to some extent out of the preoccupation with world hunger, the remarkable increase in our population, and the theories of the Neo-Malthusians. Surveys of the literature show that there have been remarkably many studies on regional famines and food crises; yet they are scattered in many journals. These research results should be summarized in a comprehensive and comparative manner. The results include mainly information on agricultural crises, prices and wages, as well as local descriptions of the development of famines; they also point out the correlations between corn prices and birth rates, marriages, fertility and mortality, emigration, and epidemics. These general outlines, like those of W. Abel, W. J. Sheldon, J. D. Post, St. L. Kaplan, F. L. Newman, and I . Komlos, however, are not fully sufficient and do not really satisfy our needs. It is the different European languages which made scholars often ignore famines in other European countries, and that is what often makes the evaluation of the impact of famine imprecise from a temporal and regional point of view. The lack of international comparisons kept alive several 'legends': for instance, the thesis that the Irish famine of 1846–7 was the last great crisis of its kind in Europe: even in the 20th century there were supplies crises during the two world wars and in Eastern Europe. Even the evaluation of the role of the potato has to be rethought. In this context, it also seems necessary to integrate the results of historical climate and environment research. In doing so, completely new interconnections could become apparent.

Summing up, we are convinced that independent historical food research in the different European countries since the beginning of modern times has obtained very similar and astonishing results. Most of the problems, however, need to be rethought, and a lot of historical sources certainly remain in libraries unnoticed. It was the ethnologists who did the most important preliminary work towards a modern history of food. Ethnological food research has a long tradition, more than a hundred years, in Middle and Eastern Europe as well as in Scandinavia and the Balkan states; this tradition is interwoven with the aims of the history of civilization and the history of languages. Early, great works were written in these countries which are still quoted today and which can serve as rich sources.

It was a special characteristic of this ethnological literature that it primarily dealt with the rural food culture of the pre-industrial era. Regional descriptions of certain meals were stressed, as much as kitchen utensils, and in this way an abundance of interesting 'miniature pictures' developed. It seems remarkable that scholars used in many cases linguistic methods to explain the names of certain meals and ways of preparation. Even historic 'doll kitchens' have been used to interpret the past. Ethnologists and anthropologists who were interested in cultures beyond Europe have dealt with the eating habits of the 'natives' since the end of the 19th century. Examples are the field studies of Audrey Richards, Margret Mead, and Mary Douglas. This research has had an immense influence on the psychology and sociology of food habits, first promoted by Kurt Lewin in the 1930s. Yet these studies are more or less static pictures with no overall connection with general history and economic and social changes; they are lacking a more comprehensive attempt at explanation.

It was not until the 1970s that ethnologists became engaged in research on the problems of social and economic history and took over the methods of the social sciences. Since that time, they have also been researching the penetration of food innovations besides the regional and social differences in meals. The subjects of this analysis are the dissolution of the patriarchal table order, the differences in nutrition between towns and villages, the meaning of the seating order at the table as a sign of social hierarchy, the role of food taboos, the changes in meals and manners, etc. Ethnological food research has for the first time used questionnaires and reports to study rural eating and drinking systematically and has established links with anthropogeography and archaeology. In contrast to the research of historians, ethnologists focused on the meals and dishes and their social context rather than on the individual foods. This research threw light for the first time on the changes of the 'meal-patterns'.

Not until the 1960s did historians publish monographs on food history, apart from those scholars of the history of civilization which is strongly connected with ethnology; and in this field, agricultural history and historic demography have assumed the leading role. The problem of world hunger lent a decisive impulse to this preoccupation with food history, as was mentioned earlier. As scholars became increasingly unsatisfied with the mere quantitative analysis of the food supply, they began to study the socio-cultural meaning of meals, the regional differences in foods, and the health implications of nutrition for the different social classes. Today, the trend-setting French food historians study the development of typical regional cuisines and differences in taste rather than mere per-capita consumption. The results of the different scholars, however, vary greatly. Research in the former Soviet Union, Czechoslovakia, and Hungary is dominated by the traditional patterns and methods of the old ethnology of nutrition.

One aim, then, is to combine these unconnected results from the different disciplines and the different countries. And one of the most important tasks is to divide the changes in food conditions into specific periods. Yet these periods will likely be different from the major turning points of political and economic history. The meaning of food in the context of an increasing European population since the beginning of modern times will certainly remain an interesting historical question. It will also be interesting to study the factors and steps which caused the breakaway from the cyclical crises of hunger to the mass prosperity of today. As many of the contributions to this volume show, the character of human nutrition is influenced not only by the improvement of food supplies but also by the enrichment of culinary culture. At the end of his essay, Stephen Mennell points out that what and how people ate is not of overriding importance. Their attitude towards their food is at least as interesting. This concerns the changes in food supplies and the preservation of foodstuffs, the preparation and consumption of meals, using and avoiding specific techniques of cooking, nutrients, and meals. Historical food research gives, in this way, important guidance for social and cultural identification. In the centre of our analysis, therefore, are not only the foodstuffs which are required for meals but also the subjective evaluations and experiences which are connected with the different kinds of food and which, until today, we have imprecisely described as 'taste'.

A European food history is not merely a simple comparative exercise. On the contrary, it is a new and in-depth attempt to gain an understanding of previously unknown facts by researching the sphere of the kitchen. The basis for this new attempt is the old truism that one gets new information at foreign tables. As we all know, peoples have been metaphorically and symbolically characterized by their eating and drinking habits since ancient times. Historical and cultural food research could therefore lead to a better understanding among the European peoples and their cultures.

2 British diet since industrialization: a bibliographical study[*]

Derek J. Oddy and John Burnett

Food supply, consumption and nutritional status

Early in the 1980s, the compiler of a bibliography on the history of food wrote: 'Comparatively few works of scholarly excellence have been written on the history of food. The researcher is obliged to extract bits and pieces here and there from secondary sources whose overall merit may be slight.'[1] While some of us may shrink from accepting the full weight of that judgement, there is a ring of truth about it that we recognize: it remains a matter of surprise that the creation of a bibliography of historical studies of food supply, consumption and nutritional status of the British people is a relatively sparse affair and that the amount of current work in the field is limited.

In the course of writing this survey, only four bibliographical studies of British food history have been found: D. C. Sutton's *The History of Food: A Preliminary Bibliography of Printed Sources*,[2] from which the above quotation was taken, W.H. Chaloner's 'Food and drink in British history. A bibliographical guide',[3] A. Simon's *Bibliotheca gastronomica*;[4] and B. Harrison's 'Drink and sobriety in England 1815–1872: A critical Bibliography'.[5] The neglect of dietary history formed the major theme of T. C. Barker's 'Changing patterns of food consumption in the United Kingdom',[6] and its bibliography should be consulted in conjunction with this paper.

Supply

When I began to examine this topic I was struck immediately by the imbalance in the research which has been undertaken on food supply. Some food commodities have been worked on by researchers throughout the twentieth century. Bread, cheese, and drink are surprisingly popular research subjects; other foods have been

---

[*]The first section of this chapter, on food supply, consumption and nutritional status, was written by Derek J. Oddy; the second, on food distribution, expenditure, cooking and meal patterns, by John Burnett.

almost ignored. One might perhaps expect that bread would attract a good deal of work; its recognition as the staff of life makes it central in the field. But why should one write about cheese? It is not a matter of status, obviously, because meat has always been held in higher esteem. When in the early 19th century William Cobbett rode past agricultural labourers eating their midday meal, he measured their well-being by the size of the piece of bacon or meat that they had, not cheese. Perhaps one explanation for the popularity of cheese as a subject for study is that cheese-making represented a triumph of early food technology. High-status foods were all too frequently also perishable foods: neither fresh meat, white bread, nor fruit kept well or were palatable when preserved, though fresh milk could be converted into cheese (or butter) and retain much of its palatability.

More to the point, flour-milling, baking and cheese-making from the 19th century onwards were carried on in processing plants which were off the farm; so, too, was brewing. Brewing was one of the earliest examples where the demand of the market drew production into large-scale industrial units in Britain. It may be, therefore, that the relatively numerous studies of these branches of food supply reflect the way in which food history has been separated from agricultural history, which has hitherto tended to concentrate on what happened before the product left the farm gate, while studies of food supply have been limited to what went on in markets. In this paper, I restrict my study to production and wholesale trade in food rather than to a discussion of shopping and retail trade in foodstuffs.

Food supply in general terms is an essential part of a number of books: it goes without saying that it is central to much of J. C. Drummond and A. Wilbrahams's *The Englishman's Food*[7] and to W. Crawford and H. Broadley's *The People's Food*.[8] Several other general books on the same theme[9] all touch on the subject to some extent but are often extremely limited in their coverage of the period of industrialization. Anne Wilson's chapter, 'Nineteenth century and after', is less than three pages of text and has not been revised since 1973! Reay Tannahill's chapter, 'The food-supply revolution', is relevant, as is her chapter on 'The scientific revolution', which deals with preservation techniques. Among the general works, only John Burnett's *Plenty and Want*[10] represents the work of an established academic historian working in this field of research and the current edition represents the state-of-the-art knowledge in this field. I do not intend to replicate the bibliography which Professor Burnett provides for this outstanding survey but, instead, will highlight the strengths and deficiencies of recent work on the period of industrialization.

Historians in Britain have provided few monographs on specific topics, periods, or regional studies of food supply. P.E. Dewey's 'Food production and policy in the United Kingdom 1914–1918'[11] has been overshadowed by a larger work by an American, L. M. Barnett.[12] Regionally, Maisie Steven's *The Good Scots Diet* has little quantifiable material on supply and Janet Blackman's 'The food supply of an industrial town: a study of Sheffield's public markets 1780–1900'[13] has not been followed by other writers. Roger Scola, who died last year, published an article on 'Food markets and shops in Manchester 1770–1870',[14] but was prevented by a long illness from completing a work on the food supply of Manchester similar to Janet

Blackman's. One study of Manchester had been published at the turn of the century by W. E. Bear,[15] but we lack similar modern studies for other British towns. At a general level, W. H. Fraser's *The Coming of the Mass Market 1850–1914*[16] has only one chapter on food supply, and we have to turn to J. P. Johnston's *A Hundred Years of Eating*[17] for a more detailed account, or to D. J. Oddy and D. S. Miller's *The Making of the Modern British Diet*[18] in which Part One specifically addresses food supply in terms of a number of commodities. Even so, we can identify several questions which need to be answered in a systematic way before we can be satisfied that we have solved the problem of food supply in Britain during industrialization. We need a comprehensive study which will calculate net food production, allow for the effects of the external trade in food, discuss the mechanism of markets and allow for wastage so that we can have a carefully considered estimation of the food supply reaching consumers.

Commodities

In addition to general studies on food supply, there are also a number of studies on individual commodities. These, again, are somewhat limited. W. Ashley's *The Bread of our Forefathers*[19] is still a useful introduction, but works like R. Sheppard and E. Newton's *The Story of Bread*[20] fall more within the antiquarian's field rather than the academic historian's. E. J. T. Collins's 'Dietary change and cereal consumption in Britain in the nineteenth Century'[21] broadens the concept of bread to include other forms of cereals. Professor Burnett's 'The baking industry in the nineteenth Century'[22] deals with the technical changes which the industry underwent, as does T. A. B. Corley's *A Quaker Enterprise in Biscuits: Huntley and Palmers of Reading*.[23] W. M. Stern's 'The bread crisis in Britain, 1795–96'[24] is one of the few specialist micro-studies on bread.

Surprisingly, the studies of cheese supply are more frequent than those of bread. V. Cheke's *The Story of Cheese-Making in Britain*[25] is a general introduction but as an academic study R. L. Cohen's *The History of Milk Prices*[26] still has to be consulted. Indeed, some of the more detailed studies on cheese supply were written in the interwar period. G. E. Fussell's 'The London cheesemongers of the eighteenth century',[27] and George Fussell and C. Goodman's 'Eighteenth century traffic in milk products'[28] are still valid articles to be read in conjunction with E. H. Whetham's 'The London milk trade 1860–1900'[29] and P. J. Atkins's 'The growth of London's railway milk trade c. 1845–1914',[30] and his subsequent 'The retail milk trade in London c. 1790–1914.'[31] The food supply of large towns such as London was closely linked to transport facilities, as is well illustrated by W.M. Stern's 'Cheese shipped coastwise to London toward the middle of the eighteenth century.'[32]

Perhaps not surprisingly, drink offers the largest set of commodity studies, though the variety in forms of drink, alcoholic and non-alcoholic, may make this a much larger category than other food commodities and may divert the food historian into the social question of temperance instead of food supply. While it is difficult to omit G. B. Wilson's *Alcohol and the Nation*,[33] B. Harrison's 'Drink and sobriety in England 1815–1872: a Critical bibliography'[34] would be an obvious starting point in any survey but one which may divert the reader in this way. N. Longmate's *The Waterdrinkers: A History of Temperance*[35] follows this path. Dr. Harrison's *Drink and the Victorians*[36] reminds us that from the beginning of industrialization drink meant strong liquor. Against this, E. S. Turner's *Taking the Cure*[37] discusses the origins of soft drinks such as mineral and table waters and shows that trade in these commodities, such as Malvern water or Schweppes, dates back to the late 18th century. D. Hartley's *Water in England*[38] is largely antiquarian in character and, being thematic in its coverage of the subject, offers little systematic discussion of the period of industrialization.

Distilling means gin in England, and whisky in Scotland and Ireland (where it is spelt whiskey). It attracts many writers but few historians. D. Daiches's *Scotch Whisky: its Past and Present*[39] is a case in point, but A. Glen's 'An economic history of the distilling industry in Scotland 1750–1914',[40] D. B. Weir's '*The distilling industry of Scotland in the nineteenth and early twentieth Centuries*[41] and M. S. Moss and J. R. Hume's *The Making of Scotch Whisky* treat it in a more academic and analytical vein.[42] D. B. Weir's *History of the Pot Still Malt Whisky Distillers' Association of Scotland: The North of Scotland Malt Distillers' Association 1874–1926*[43] is more concerned with market organization than supply.

The brewing industry has attracted studies which range from the comprehensive to the fragmentary. Fuller works include H. S. Corran's *A History of Brewing;*[44] H. A. Monckton's *A History of English Ale and Beer;*[45] J. Vaizey's *The Brewing Industry 1886–1951: An Economic Study;*[46] I. Donnachie's *A History of the Brewing Industry in Scotland;*[47] and P. Lynch and J. Vaizey's *Guinness Brewery in the Irish Economy, 1759–1876.*[48] E. M. Sigworth's 'Science and the brewing industry, 1850–1900'[49] and P. Mathias's 'Agriculture and the brewing and distilling industries in the eighteenth century'[50] indicate the extent to which one is drawn into technology when studying food supply. O. MacDonagh's 'The origins of porter'[51] is a reminder of just how wide-ranging studies of drink can be.

In this respect, the British have always been categorized as tea-drinkers. D. M. Forrest's *A Hundred Years of Ceylon Tea*[52] and *Tea for the British: a Social and Economic History of a Famous Trade,*[53] together with P. Griffiths's *The History of the Indian Tea Industry*[54] provide narrative accounts of tea as raw material.

Other commodities vary considerably in the extent to which they have been covered. Some have a well-known monograph which has come to be regarded as a standard work and has attracted little revision. R.N. Salaman's *The History and Social Influence of the Potato*[55] occupies such a place, though it must be admitted that the importance of the potato in the Irish diet has produced more recent work by K. H. Connell[56] and L. M. Cullen.[57] The literature on the adoption of the potato is summarized in J. Mokyr, 'Irish history with the potato'.[58] Similarly, the history of the supply of fish has come to be dependent on C. L. Cutting's *Fish Saving: a History of Fish Processing From Ancient to Modern Times,*[59] though there is a short work, to which Dr. Cutting also contributed, which is predominantly a supply-side study.[60]

Meat has lead to several works notably more academic in approach than those on many other commodities. R. Perren's *The Meat Trade in Britain, 1840–1914* is a good illustration of modern work, as are his earlier articles.[61] It is somewhat surprising, therefore, that modern authors still find it necessary to refer back to J. T. Critchell and J. Raymond's *The History of the Frozen Meat Trade*.[62] Some work on meat has been prompted by the interest in the effects of the end of free trade and the introduction of protection in the interwar years. Professor F. Capie's 'Consumer preference: meat in England and Wales, 1920–1939',[63] for example, is really a supply-side analysis of this kind.

Sugar is another commodity in which one book has tended to assume the status of a standard work. N. Deer's *The History of Sugar*[64] is still quoted heavily by other writers. There is also a more recent history by W. R. Aykroyd, *Sweet Malefactor: Sugar, Slavery and Human Society*,[65] and there is also J. Yudkin's *Pure, White and Deadly*,[66] though this is written for a popular audience and is not an academic study of the supply of sugar.

Having discussed cheese in terms of the preservation of milk, it is easy to overlook other dairy foods such as butter and other fats. Surprisingly, margarine, the one completely artificial food created during the period of industrialization, is better documented than butter. J. H. van Stuyvenberg's *Margarine: An Economic, Social and Scientific History, 1869–1969*[67] is not purely concerned with British food supply, but Britain and Germany represented its two chief markets. C. Wilson's *The History of Unilever*[68] is essential reading. There is also A. J. C. Andersen and P. N. Williams's *Margarine*[69] and Andersen's *Margarine*[70] but these are really technical handbooks and have only limited historical introductions.

One commodity group, fruit and vegetables, has been little studied from the point of view of food supply. There is an extensive literature in agricultural and geographical journals which I shall not attempt to cover, except to note that at the turn of the century W. E. Bear wrote several articles in the *Journal of the Royal Agricultural Society of England* which are still cited by modern writers. R. J. Battersby's 'The development of market gardening in England, 1850–1914'[71] is unpublished, but a general account by R. Webber has appeared.[72] Another work by an historical geographer, P. J. Atkins, is 'The production and marketing of fruit and vegetables, 1850–1950'.[73]

Consumption

It is extremely difficult to separate supply from consumption. A number of accounts deal with both aspects but, under closer examination, the consumption figures quoted often turn out to be supply figures expressed per head of the population. However, consumption is more than just the quantities of food consumed, because food quality, tastes, domestic arrangements and social constraints all affect consumption patterns. Professor Burnett's *Plenty and Want*[74] affords the most comprehensive integration of these different aspects of consumption, though few modern scholars examining British food history will not refer also to Drummond and Wilbraham's *The Englishman's Food*.[75] However, even in its revised edition, that work is now very dated. Nevertheless, it offers many ideas which historians have not yet fully explored. In T. C. Barker, J. C. McKenzie and J. Yudkin's *Our Changing Fare*,[76] as in their earlier volume,[77] attempts are made to show changing patterns of consumption of a range of commodities and to assess the factors which affect consumer choice. 'Factors influencing consumption' is also Part II of Oddy and Miller's *The Making of the Modern British Diet*[78] in which studies of the standard of living are set alongside studies of the food-canning and food-manufacturing industries. In the editors' following volume[79] papers on the effects of rationing during and after the Second World War, food technology in the twentieth century, and institutional diets in prisons and schools illustrate how far-reaching modern research has become. In terms of regional development, only Ireland has been studied in any detail. There are two chapters which examine diet in J. M. Goldstrom and L. A. Clarkson's *Irish Population, Economy and Society*,[80] but food is not central to J. Mokyr's *Why Ireland Starved*.[81] The famine in Ireland cannot be omitted: C. Woodham-Smith's *The Great Hunger: Ireland 1845–49*[82] and L. Kennedy's 'Why one million starved: an open verdict',[83] will suffice to indicate the literature on this topic. It should be born in mind that studies of Irish diet in the main describe a pre-industrial society in contrast to the urban-industrial society of mainland Britain. Rural Scotland, therefore, offers a better comparison for the Irish work on diet. A paper reflecting this comparative approach can be seen in R. Mitchison and P. Roebuck's *Economy and Society in Scotland and Ireland*.[84]

Although the 1950s and early 1960s saw a vigorous debate regarding the standard of living during the Industrial Revolution in historical journals, much of this discussion centred on the nature of price data and the construction of an acceptable real-wage index. Little work was done on food consumption. In part, this reflected the availability of sources. Since then, three periods have attracted some detailed attention: the 1860s; the end of the nineteenth century; and the 1930s, when fears of malnutrition arose during the interwar slump. For the 1860s, the Lancashire cotton famine led to two major investigations being carried out for the Medical Officer of the Privy Council by Dr Edward Smith. These have been discussed by D. J. Oddy and J. Yudkin[85] and, more fully, in T. C. Barker, D. J. Oddy and J. Yudkin's *The Dietary Surveys of Dr Edward Smith 1862–3*.[86] The question whether this consumption crisis reached famine proportions has been debated in D. J. Oddy, 'Urban famine in nineteenth-century Britain: the effect of the Lancashire cotton famine on working-class Diet and health'.[87] The interest in late 19th century poverty, national efficiency, and the physical deterioration debate has led to extensive studies of the period extending from 1887, when Charles Booth's surveys were begun in London, to the end of the century, when B. S. Rowntree's survey in York took place. The most comprehensive study of the diet of this period is an unpublished University of London thesis by D. J. Oddy.[88] Other work on the period includes E. M. Schofield, 'Food and cooking of the working class about 1900'[89] which is based on an oral history study. Both are discussed by E. Roberts.[90]

The 1930s have been under scrutiny recently, with the realization that it is half a century since J. B. Orr's *Food, Health and Income*[91] provided the culmination of the 'Hungry England' debate which had been going on since Fenner Brockway's *Hungry England* had appeared in 1932. Fifty years later, C. Webster reactivated the question in 'Healthy or hungry thirties',[92] and it has been further developed by M. Mitchell.[93]

Nutritional status

The assessment of nutritional status depends on quantifiable data surviving for diets during the period of industrialization. Here, therefore, any bibliographical study needs to make some reference to the primary source materials on which dietary analysis can be based.

To date historians in Britain have been daunted by the complexities of the process of nutritional analysis. The published works in which such techniques are demonstrated are few. The earliest example is J. C. McKenzie's 'The composition and nutritional value of diets in Manchester and Dukinfield in 1841',[94] in which the analysis of the diets of nineteen families was computed by hand. This was a limiting factor on the adoption of dietary analysis techniques. Large numbers of diets, or those which were complex with many foodstuffs, or which were expressed only in cooked meals or dishes rather than quantities of food materials, could not be handled except by slow and laborious calculations. The adaption of a computer program to carry out this work was the major breakthrough. The chemical composition of over 660 food items in Britain became available with the publication of work by R. A. McCance and E. M. Widdowson.[95] Values for protein, fat and carbohydrate content, together with minerals, were entered into the University of London computer by the mid-1960s, and various sorting and dietary analysis programs were written at Queen Elizabeth College, (now part of King's College, London). This permitted an expansion in the number of diets which could be analysed and ensured that a standard process of analysis would be used. Simply removing the drudgery of hand calculations also enabled more care to be taken in making allowances for wastage in storage or in cooking losses and in assessing more accurately the edible portions of food materials.

The first diets to be processed by this computer-assisted technique were those collected by Dr Edward Smith in 1862-3. Publications relating to this work have been listed above. The technique has also been used for the analysis of data in F. M. Eden's *The State of the Poor*,[96] D. E. Davies's *The Case of Labourers in Husbandry*,[97] and all major family budget surveys between 1880 and 1938. Preliminary results indicating nutritional status from 1841 to 1913 have been published in D. J. Oddy's 'Food in nineteenth century England: nutrition in the first urban society',[98] and in *Diet of Man: Needs and Wants*,[99] though results for the interwar period are unpublished. Part III of Oddy and Miller's *Making of the Modern British Diet* is concerned with nutritional evaluation, and examines working-class diet in the period 1880-1914.[100]

This represents a major analytical advance in food history work in Britain. However, it is limited by the availability of family budgets and much depends upon interpretation of qualitative evidence in conjunction with quantitative studies. Work on nutritional status is therefore hard to disentangle from studies on health and, particularly, infant or child mortality. Studies of famine especially have lacked the dimension of nutritional status. The literature appears to ask direct questions which require the discussion of nutritional status: in fact many such essays are principally concerned with social disorder, despite the constant reference to hunger: J. Stevenson's 'Food riots in England, 1792–1818',[101] J. Walter and K. Wrightson's 'Dearth and the social order in early modern England',[102] D. E. Williams's 'Were "hunger" rioters really hungry? Some demographic evidence',[103] A. Booth's 'Food riots in the North-West of England, 1790–1801'[104] and W. J. Shelton's *English Hunger and Industrial Disorders*,[105] all tend to fall into this category. J. D. Post's 'Famine, Mortality, and Epidemic Disease in the Process of Modernization'[106] was later developed into *The Last Great Subsistence Crisis in the Western World*.[107] Both contained comparatively little evidence from Britain and were descriptive rather than conceptual in their discussion of famine.

Even more infuriating for the food historian is the explanation offered by T. McKeown's *The Rise of Modern Population*.[108] In choosing to treat food consumption as a residual factor in analysing reasons for the decline in mortality in late 19th-century Britain, Professor McKeown avoided a major issue, when child mortality rates in Britain were so high as to suggest that malnutrition was still widespread. Any Third World country today which showed similar patterns of epidemiological evidence as that of 19th-century Britain would be treated by UN agencies as having problems of low nutritional status. E. M. Crawford's papers, 'Dearth, diet and disease in Ireland, 1850: a case study of nutritional deficiency'[109] and 'Scurvy in Ireland during the Great Famine',[110] M. W. Beaver's 'Population, infant mortality and milk'[111] and I. Buchanan's 'Infant feeding, sanitation and diarrhoea in colliery communities 1880–1911'[112] are examples of the type of work which is essential for the application of studies of nutritional status to the explanation of population change. Another excellent example of the application of dietary studies to a particular aspect of history is J. Watt, E. J. Freeman and W. F. Bynum's book, *Starving Sailors: The Influence of Nutrition on Naval and Maritime History*,[113] which arose from a symposium at the National Maritime Museum, Greenwich, in 1890.

The consideration of physical stature is a further area which may engulf the food historian: D. J. Oddy's 'The health of the people'[114] tries to link dietary evidence with physical development, while longer trends have been examined by R. C. Floud and K. W. Wachter.[115] Professor R. W. Fogel has been engaged in similar studies of long-term changes in nutrition, labour welfare, and labour productivity in the United States and his collaboration with Professor Floud has led to some comparative work on British and American heights. How far food history may become marginalized in such studies is illustrated by M. Mitchell's 'The effects of unemployment on the social conditions of women and children in the 1930s',[116] when feeding becomes only a minor part of a debate on the human environment.

Conclusion

Over the last twenty-five years or so there has been a surprising variety of work on the history of food supply, consumption, and nutritional status in Britain. Any survey of it reveals a wide variety both in the topics undertaken and in the standards of the work. The bulk of what has been written is by general authors who have been dealing at a level not included in this bibliographical essay, that of the popular cookery writer. Academic writing, by contrast, has been diffused, and some of it, under closer examination, reveals itself as being marginal to food history. As a subject, food can be a case study to illustrate the work of urban historians, urban geographers, labour historians, transport historians and even medical historians. All of them make use of it but none of them see it as central to their particular discipline.

In consequence, much food history research in Britain is widely diffused, both in location and topic. Those associated with the meeting of food historians, nutritionists and food technologists which began at Queen Elizabeth College, Kensington (now part of King's College, London), in the 1960s tend to regard it as the longest-running and most productive source of work on food and dietary history. Its early conferences produced *Changing Food Habits* and *Our Changing Fare;*[117] its later, more regular seminar meetings provided the basis for the publications on *The Dietary Surveys of Dr. Edward Smith, Fish in Britain, The Making of the Modern British Diet*, and *Diet and Health in Modern Britain*.[118] A recent series of meetings of the seminar has produced papers with the theme 'First World past : Third World present', which are to be published shortly. For the last six years, the Economic and Social Research Council has been providing limited support for this seminar, while some royalties from books published have also contributed a tiny amount towards its expenses. The Historians and Nutritionists Group at King's College, London, may therefore regard themselves with some justification as the leading centre of food history research in Britain. However, there is no formal institutional framework for this research: the Social Nutrition Research Unit on which the early work was based was wound up in the early 1970s, and since then the seminar and its publications have resulted from the efforts and interests of individual scholars.

There is other work as well. Dr Zeldin runs a seminar at the University of Oxford which has provided stimulus for a number of scholars, including Dr Mennell and Dr. Harvey Levenstein, whose *Revolution at the Table*[119] deals with the transformation of the American diet. Dr Zeldin is also associated with the journal *Food and Foodways*, though during its first three years there have only been three somewhat peripheral articles on food and drink in Britain. There have also been a number of ethnological studies carried out by Alexander Fenton in Edinburgh. Some regional work, mainly that on Irish diet, also exists. At the University of Belfast, Professor Leslie Clarkson and Dr Margaret Crawford have been working on a new set of studies of Irish diet based more firmly on a framework of nutritional analysis than earlier work in Ireland.

The Past and Present Society attempted to revive its earlier interest in diet recently, and one meeting of a Past and Present Seminar took place in Oxford two or three years ago. The unfortunate demise of Mr T. S. Aston, the Society's honorary secretary, seems to have brought this initiative to an end.

There are a number of research units and institutes which might be involved in some aspects of food history, though their major concern is with questions of contemporary policy and present-day research. These include the London Food Commission; the University of Glasgow, which has a medical sociology unit and also houses the Strathclyde Health archives; the Rowett Research Institute in Aberdeen, where a considerable amount of John Boyd Orr's original material has been preserved and is available for consultation; and the University of Bradford, where Dr Wheelock's Food Research Unit has attempted to obtain funding for a food supply study of the British diet. There has been little, if any, contact between these different groups and, to date, there has been no attempt in Britain to coordinate the work of these separate centres of research.

Food distribution, expenditure, cooking and meal patterns

Professor Oddy has examined the literature on the history of food products and supplies in Britain since industrialization, on changes in consumption levels and nutritional status of the population. This part of our paper follows food from the quantitative level to its destination as household meals.

Food distribution

Although the histories of many of the major food commodities have been studied, historians have given less attention to the processes by which foods reached domestic larders, that is, to the distribution as opposed to the production process. The outstanding change brought about by industrialization and urbanization was the growth of a commercial market for food as the opportunities for self-sufficiency declined, and as traditional skills such as home baking and brewing disappeared in many parts of Britain. During the eighteenth century a network of local corn markets covered the country,[120] soon supplemented by longer-distance trade in meat and potatoes. It is not clear to what extent the expansion of the canal network after 1760 facilitated the movement of food, but given their slow speed they can hardly have been important for the transport of perishable foods such as fruit, vegetables or dairy products. Only from the 1840s onwards did the new railways begin to transform internal trade and to create more of a national market for food products.

The problems of food supply to London, which already contained more than 2.5 million people in 1851, early attracted attention,[121] while Henry Mayhew also wrote much about the London markets and the street traders in all kinds of food.[122] Dr Blackman has examined the changing provision of food supply to a provincial city, Sheffield, between 1780 and 1900,[123] and to northern industrial towns more generally in a subsequent paper.[124]

Markets served not only the wholesale but also the retail trade, especially for vegetables, fruit and meat, where the working-class practice of buying the Sunday joint from market stalls on Saturday evening continued throughout the nineteenth century. The hawking of some foods such as tea was also common, especially in rapidly growing suburban areas not well supplied with shops. But the fixed shop, which had been usual in towns for the sale of groceries well before the 18th century, generally came to dominate most food retailing in the 19th. Its history has been surveyed by James Jeffreys,[125] David Alexander,[126] and Roger Scola[127] who shows the remarkable growth in the number of shops in Manchester between 1770 and 1870. The importance of the small 'corner shop' (often known by contemporaries as the chandler's shop), supplying a range of basic foods in working-class neighbourhoods, has also been studied,[128] as have the trading practices of an 18th century shopkeeper in a small Lancashire town.[129]

Shopkeeping on what would now be described as a multiple basis began with the co-operative movement in 1844. Trading on the principles of purity of food and a dividend on purchases, co-operative stores became important in the later 19th century, especially in northern industrial towns: their history has been extensively studied by Redfern,[130] Cole,[131] Pollard[132] and others. The transition from the individual, commercial shop to multiple chains of stores, often described as 'the retailing revolution', is documented by Professor Mathias,[133] while the histories of individual firms include those of Lipton,[134] Sainsbury[135] and Tesco.[136] The rise of other modern chains of supermarkets, and the effects of self-service on consumer behaviour, await their historians.

Food expenditure and budgeting

Examinations of shopping inevitably involve questions of the allocation of household resources to food. Over the last 200 years food has remained the largest item of domestic expenditure, though with rising incomes and relative reductions in the prices of many foods, the proportion has declined substantially. From budgets collected in the 1790s[137] it has been estimated that 69% of the income of rural labourers' families went on food and drink, and almost half on bread and flour alone.[138] William Neild's study of the budgets of Lancashire textile factory workers in 1841 showed a not dissimilar pattern for this considerably better-paid group: the family with the highest income, where several members were earning, spent 44% of its income on seven items of food (bread, meat, bacon, potatoes, butter, tea and sugar), while the lowest-income family, earning 16*s* (80p) a week, devoted 72% to these items:[139] it is worth noting that 16*s* was twice the weekly wage of many agricultural labourers. Dr Edward Smith's investigation into the effects of the cotton famine on Lancashire textile workers in 1862 is important in this context.[140] Smith found that when workers suffered a reduction of income as a result of unemployment or short-time working, they did not simply cut out meat and other expensive foods in favour of bread, but reduced their consumption of all foods, though by different amounts.

Most historians agree that the standard of living of the working classes improved notably from the 1870s as Britain became a mass importer of cheap wheat and, later, meat, but this had no dramatic effect on the proportion of income spent on food. Levi calculated in 1885 that the working classes spent 71% of their incomes on food and drink compared with 44% by the middle and upper classes,[141] but although food still took such a large share, the working-class diet now included a wider variety of foods such as tea, sugar, butter, milk, eggs and fruit previously consumed only in small quantities. In a study of 1881 the British Association for the Advancement of Science estimated that the working classes now spent more on meat than on bread, and more on milk and eggs than on potatoes, the most generally consumed vegetable.[142] By the beginning of the twentieth century some reduction in the proportion of the food budget was noticeable, a government enquiry of 1903 suggesting that 61% of income was now the average working-class expenditure on food and non-alcoholic drink.[143]

Around the turn of the century the plight of the poor in an affluent society received the attention of social investigators who included budgetary details in their surveys in their efforts to determine a 'poverty line': Charles Booth did so in his study of the East End of London,[144] Benjamin Seebohm Rowntree in his investigation of York[145] and, with a collaborator, in a study of the condition of agricultural labourers.[146] These demonstrated the persistence of a problem of absolute poverty, among perhaps one-third of the population, defined by Rowntree as an income insufficient to purchase sufficient food for 'mere physical efficiency'. In south London Mrs Pember Reeves found families who had less than 2*d* (1p) per person per day to spend on food, where bread was still the mainstay of the diet, supplemented by whatever tiny quantities of 'condiments' could be afforded.[147]

Also towards the end of the century, middle-class budgets came under scrutiny at a time when some items of expenditure such as domestic servants and public school education were becoming more costly. Two independent estimates assigned 39%[148] and 37%[149] to food in households with incomes of between £700 and £800 a year: such expenditure naturally allowed a luxurious diet, with large quantities of meat, in sharp contrast to that described by Mrs Reeves for families who lived on *Round About a Pound a Week*.[150]

The appearance of depression and mass unemployment between the two world wars prompted a number of social investigations which included analyses of the cost and content of working-class diet. In addition to employing more advanced statistical techniques, some surveys incorporated the new knowledge of nutrition to make more refined measurements of the intake of nutrients, vitamins and minerals. The most important included *Has Poverty Diminished?*,[151] *The New Survey of London Life and Labour*,[152] *A Social Survey of Merseyside*,[153] *Work and Wealth in a Modern Port*,[154] *Food, Health and Income*,[155] and *The People's Food*.[156] The last showed that the wealthiest socio-economic group, with incomes over £1,000 a year, now spent only 11.8% on food, while the poorest with less than £125 a year, spent 46.6% – still significantly less than before 1914. Boyd Orr's work was particularly significant in drawing attention to the 'nutritional gap' between rich and poor, especially in the 'health protective' foods, and his claim that less than half the population were able to secure the optimum diet for health caused much controversy. Other studies of the diets of low-income groups in the 1930s included *Poverty and Public Health*,[157] *Men Without Work*[158] and *Poverty and Progress*,[159] Rowntree's second social study of York based on data collected in 1935.

During the Second World War the food of the nation, in terms of quantity, cost and nutritional value, came to be monitored by the Ministry of Food, and this has been subsequently continued in the annual reports of the National Food Survey Committee (now a division of the Ministry of Agriculture, Fisheries and Food). We therefore have a valuable continuous series from 1940 to the present, measuring the food entering domestic larders (but not food consumed outside the home) of the different socio-economic groups and household sizes. In 1985 people in the United Kingdom devoted, on average, only 20.2% of total household expenditure to food, the poorest group 29.4% and the wealthiest 15.5%,[160] indicating the long-term reduction in the share of food in the family budget consequent upon generally rising standards of living. Recent public anxiety has tended to focus on problems of overeating rather than undernutrition, though with the reappearance of large-scale unemployment in the last few years there has been some revival of concern about its effects on nutritional status, represented by the findings of some pressure groups and researchers[161] rather than by official enquiries.

Cooking

Historians have paid little attention to the stages between the purchase of food and the meal on the table. There was much criticism of the working classes in the nineteenth century for abandoning home-baked bread and home-brewed beer in favour of 'shop bread' and tea: though still expensive, tea had crept into use by agricultural labourers in the South of England as early as the 1790s[162] and was roundly condemned by traditionalists such as William Cobbett as wasteful extravagance.[163] He was only one of several authors who tried to re-educate the poor into sound practices of domestic economy which they believed were threatened by new, inappropriate social habits: their writings took the form of manuals containing household hints and recipes for supposedly cheap dishes which often showed a lack of understanding of the domestic difficulties of the poor.[164] The kind of cooking which they recommended required equipment, time and, often, a variety of ingredients not easily available. In many rural cottages and in the tenemented houses where many poorer town-dwellers lived there was only an open fireplace, and not always enough fuel for that. In these circumstances the stewpot, the frying-pan and the kettle were the main cooking utensils, especially when housewives also worked on the land, in factories or at domestic industries: 'convenience foods' such as bought bread, tea and cheese were not so much luxuries as necessities, and meat, when it could be afforded, was usually bacon which could be quickly fried, rather than butcher's meat which required stewing or roasting. Small cast-iron ranges, with an oven and a water-boiler on each side of an enclosed fire, began to be fitted in new 'model' cottages in the countryside and in back-to-back houses in towns from the 1840s,[165] but for many working-class housewives the most important innovation was the gas cooker, which began to spread from the 1890s when cookers could be rented and the gas paid for on the penny-in-the-slot system.[166] Even so, outside London and other large towns gas installation often came only between the two world wars; its progress, and that of cooking by electricity which also grew between the wars, merits further attention by historians.

We should not assume, therefore, that in poorer households before 1914 cooking was done on a daily basis, and in her social study of a Wiltshire village in 1909, Maude Davies discovered that wives cooked only once or twice a week in winter.[167] Oral history has been usefully employed in a study of cooking practices at the turn of the century;[168] much depended on the cheapness and availability of coal, and in this respect industrial towns in the North were more fortunate than remote villages in the South, a fact which helps to explain the survival of traditions of home-baked bread, pies and cakes in Yorkshire and Lancashire. The history of domestic heating and cooking has been written by Lawrence Wright,[169] while Giedion has included useful sections on the development of kitchen design and equipment in his history of technology:[170] recent accounts are *The British Kitchen* and *Five Hundred Years of Technology in the Home*,[171] both profusely illustrated.

In middle-class, servant-keeping households cooking was a very different matter. Here, where meat rather than bread was the most important item in the diet, roasting on spits in front of the large open fire was the preferred method and continued for much of the 19th century, only slowly being replaced by the closed range or 'kitchener': the origins of this have been traced to Leamington in the 1820s,[172] but it was still regarded as experimental in Webster's *Encyclopaedia of Domestic Economy*.[173] Some versions ran to 18 feet in length and contained numerous ovens, roasters, water-boilers and hotplates, and required much coal and attention. Details of the equipment of a middle-class kitchen may be gathered from numerous cookery books and manuals, of which Isabella Beeton's[174] was the most widely read. When domestic service became more expensive in the late 19th century, and middle-class wives increasingly had to undertake their own cooking, books such as *The Servantless House*[175] offered them advice. With the great expansion of lower-middle-class suburban housing between the wars, typically represented by the three-bedroom semi-detached house, there was an explosion of such advice literature in books and women's magazines, typified by the writings of Mrs C. S. Peel[176] and by 'Ideal Home' exhibitions: the social context of women's lifestyles in these new environments has recently been researched.[177]

Meals and mealtimes

Over the last two hundred years the trend has been for regional and, to a rather lesser extent, social class differences in food to diminish, and for common food and meal patterns to develop under the influence of commercial marketing and advertising: formerly, there were wide differences between England and Scotland, between northern and southern England, and between rich and poor within any one region. The supposed 'preference' of a labourer in southern England for a diet of white bread, tea and, if possible, bacon in contrast to the barley bread, hasty pudding, milk and potatoes of the North was noticed by Eden:[178] further north, in Scotland, the common foods were oatmeal porridge, potatoes, milk, cheese and kale. These differences probably reflected the different availability of foods such as dairy products rather than a true preference based on choice.[179] In all regions, as incomes rose the dependence on bread and potatoes declined and the consumption of meat increased,[180] so that among the wealthy vegetables and bread became mere accompaniments to the preferred food. Over the long term, rising standards of living gave more choice to the working class, and socio-economic differences in diet tended to narrow, but regional differences, especially between England and Scotland, were still strong in the interwar years and even since 1945.[181] Regional variations in the consumption of different foods are still sufficiently important to be recorded in the annual reports of the Food Survey Committee reflecting the survival of local tastes and cooking traditions even in a national market. Changes in tastes and fashions in food in Britain between 1940 and 1980 have been examined by Christopher Driver,[182] and on a world-wide scale from prehistoric times to the present by Reay Tannahill,[183] while Stephen Mennell has contributed an illuminating comparative study of the sociology of taste in England and France.[184]

In leisured society in the 18th century the pattern was essentially for only two meals a day: a large, late breakfast, which included meat and fish as well as bread and preserves, and dinner eaten at around 3 or 4 p.m. in the country and up to 6 p.m. in town; there might be a small snack of a sandwich or biscuits at midday (Dr Johnson's 'nunchin') and a little cold supper at 9 or 10 p.m.[185] Dinner was the principal meal of the day, solid and lengthy, with a profusion of meats, game, fish and puddings placed together on the table from which guests helped themselves. This was 'English service', which came to be divided in the later 18th century into two large courses, each containing numerous dishes and little apparent logic. French cuisine, which was becoming fashionable in England before the Revolution, was delayed by the subsequent hostilities but triumphed after 1815 in wealthy urban society. French dishes, preferably cooked by French chefs, implied *service à la français*, in which dishes followed a progression from soup to dessert, the main courses being divided by entrées and entremets.[186]

With a lengthening day due to longer Parliamentary and court sittings and more extended business hours, the gap between an earlier breakfast and a later dinner – now at around 8 p.m. in fashionable Victorian society – came to be filled by a more substantial and formal luncheon at around 12.30 – 1.00 p.m.: it might almost be said that the early Victorians 'invented' luncheon as the third meal of the day, though not all approved of the innovation and some declined to observe it. Dinner was transformed again in the 1870s and 1880s when *service à la Russe* was introduced, each of ten or more dishes being brought round and served to each guest by waiters.[187] This established the meal pattern which still survives in modified form for formal occasions: the middle class simplified it for domestic use into the four-course pattern of soup, fish, roast and pudding or dessert.

Working-class meal patterns had much less formality, dictated by available income, work patterns and cooking resources. 'Respectable' families followed the three-meals-a-day pattern of the middle classes, though for them 'dinner', the main meal, was eaten at midday, followed by a family tea shared with the children, and a slightly later supper for adults.[188] Lower down the scale there was less regularity. Agricultural labourers and other heavy manual workers often had as many as five meal occasions during the day: breakfast, a 10 a.m. snack, midday lunch (usually cold), a 4 p.m. snack, and evening supper at home, often the only cooked meal of the day. In such households Sunday dinner was the only occasion when all the family ate together. Among the better-off working classes, and in the middle classes, 'high tea' on Sundays was also something of a ritual occasion, with cold meats or fish and salads as well as bread, cakes and pastries; by the end of the century the newly imported canned tropical fruits also made an appearance at such festivities.

No systematic studies have been made of working-class meal patterns before 1914. For the interwar years *The People's Food*[189] surveys the content and timing of meals across the range of socio-economic classes, followed up twenty years later by Warren.[190] Despite the war and rationing which finally ended only in 1954, it was surprising how little had changed either in the time or content of meals. Thirty years further on, it is regrettable that there was no third Crawford survey in 1988, which would have provided a unique longitudinal analysis over half a century. Recent changes in meal patterns are principally available only through private market research agencies, among which Taylor Nelson Ltd has conducted a Family Food Panel on a continuous basis since 1974. These most recent findings suggest a fragmentation of meal occasions in contemporary Britain, a polarization of meals towards the beginning and end of the day and a growth of 'snacking' replacing formal meals, particularly the midday meal and tea. There are some interesting parallels here with the pattern in 18th-century leisured society of only two main meals a day.[191]

References

1 Sutton (1982).
2 Sutton (1982).
3 Chaloner (1960).
4 Simon (1953).
5 Harrison (1967).
6 Barker (1978).
7 Drummond and Wilbraham (1957).
8 Crawford and Broadley (1938).
9 Hartley (1954); Tannahill (1973); Wilson (1973).
10 Burnett (1989b).

11 Dewey (1980).
12 Stevens (1985).
13 Blackman (1962–3).
14 Scola (1975).
15 Bear (1899).
16 Fraser (1981).
17 Johnston (1977).
18 *The Making* (1976).
19 Ashley (1928).
20 Sheppard and Newton (1957).
21 Collins (1975).
22 Burnett (1962–3).
23 Corley (1972).
24 Stern (1964).
25 Cheke (1959).
26 Cohen (1936).
27 Fussell (1928).
28 Fussell and Goodman (1934–7).
29 Whetham (1964–5).
30 Atkins (1978).
31 Atkins (1980).
32 Stern (1973).
33 Wilson (1940).
34 Harrison (1967).
35 Longmate (1968).
36 Harrison (1971).
37 Turner (1967).
38 Hartley (1964).
39 Daiches (1969).
40 Glen (1969).
41 Weir (1974).
42 Moss and Hume (1981).
43 Weir (1970).
44 Corran (1975).
45 Monckton (1966).
46 Vaizey (1960).
47 Donnachie (1979).
48 Lynch and Vaizey (1960).
49 Sigsworth (1964–5).
50 Mathias (1952–3).
51 MacDonagh (1963–4).
52 Forrest (1967).
53 Forrest (1973).
54 Griffith (1967).
55 Salaman (1949).
56 Connell (1962).
57 Cullen (1968).
58 Mokyr (1981).

59 Cutting (1955).
60 Barker and Yudkin (1971).
61 Perren (1978); Perren (1971); Perren (1975).
62 Critchell and Raymond (1912).
63 Capie (1976).
64 Deerr (1949–50).
65 Aykroyd (1967).
66 Yudkin (1986).
67 Stuyvenberg (1969).
68 Wilson (1954, 1968).
69 Andersen (1954); Andersen and Williams (1956).
70 Andersen (1954).
71 Battersby (1960).
72 Webber (1975).
73 Atkins (1985).
74 Burnett (1989).
75 Drummond and Wilbraham (1939, 1957).
76 *Our Changing Fare* (1966).
77 *Changing Food Habits* (1964).
78 *The Making* (1976).
79 *Diet and Health* (1985).
80 Goldstrom amd Clarkson (1981).
81 Mokyr (1983).
82 Woodham-Smith (1975).
83 Kennedy (1984).
84 *Economy and Society in Scotland* (1988).
85 Oddy and Yudkin (1970)
86 *The dietary surveys* (1970).
87 Oddy (1983).
88 Oddy (1971); part of it appeared as Oddy (1970).
89 Schofield (1971).
90 Roberts (1977).
91 Orr (1936).
92 Webster (1982).
93 Mitchell (1988).
94 McKenzie (1962).
95 McCance and Widdowson (1960).
96 Eden (1797).
97 Davies (1795).
98 Oddy (1970a).
99 *Diet of Man* (1978).
100 *The Making* (1976).
101 Stevenson (1974).
102 Walter and Wrightson (1976).
103 Williams (1976).
104 Booth (1977).
105 Shelton (1973).
106 Post (1976).

107 Post (1977).
108 McKeown (1976).
109 Crawford (1984).
110 Crawford (1988).
111 Beaver (1973).
112 Buchanan (1985).
113 Watt, Freeman and Bynum (1981).
114 Oddy (1982).
115 Floud and Wachter (1982).
116 Mitchell (1985).
117 *Changing Food Habits* (1964); *Our Changing Fare* (1966).
118 *The Dietary Surveys* (1970); *Fish in Britain* (1971); *The Making* (1976); *Diet and Health* (1985).
119 Levenstein (1988).
120 Fay (1923–5).
121 Dodd (1856).
122 Mayhew (1851).
123 Blackman (1962–3).
124 Blackman (1966).
125 Jeffreys (1970).
126 Alexander (1970).
127 Scola (1975).
128 Blackman (1976).
129 Willan (1970).
130 Redfern (1913); Redfern (1938).
131 Cole (1945).
132 Pollard (1971).
133 Mathias (1967).
134 Waugh (1951).
135 Boswell (1969).
136 Corina (1971).
137 Davies (1795).
138 Richardson (1976).
139 Neild (1841).
140 *The dietaries* (1970).
141 Levi (1885).
142 British Association (1881).
143 Board of Trade (1903).
144 Booth (1889).
145 Rowntree (1901).
146 Rowntree and Kendall (1913).
147 Reeves (1913).
148 Layard (1888).
149 Colmore (1901).
150 Burnett (1989b).
151 Bowley and Hogg (1925).
152 Smith (1930).
153 Jones (1934).

154 Ford (1934).
155 Orr (1936).
156 Crawford and Broadley (1938).
157 McGonigle and Kirby (1936).
158 Pilgrim Trust (1938).
159 Rowntree (1941).
160 Social Trends (1987).
161 Lang et al. (1984).
162 Eden (1797).
163 Cobbett (1823).
164 *The Family Economist* (1848-9); Copley (1849); Francatelli (1977); Soyer (1855); Thompson (1884).
165 Burnett (1986).
166 Daunton (1983).
167 Davies (1909).
168 Schofield (1972).
169 Wright (1964).
170 Giedion (1970).
171 Yarwood (1981); Yarwood (1983).
172 Ravetz (1968).
173 Webster (1884).
174 Beeton (1861).
175 Panton (1884)
176 Peel (1914); Peel (1919).
177 North (1989).
178 Eden (1797).
179 Campbell (1966).
180 Engels (1958).
181 Stevens (1985).
182 Driver (1983).
183 Tannahill (1973).
184 Mennell (1985).
185 Palmer (1952).
186 Dolby (1830).
187 Burnett (1989a).
188 Rowntree (1901).
189 Crawford and Broadley (1938).
190 Warren (1958).
191 Burnett (1989).

Literature

Alexander, David, *Retailing in England During the Industrial Revolution* (London, 1970).
Andersen, Age Jorgen Christian, *Margarine* (Oxford, 1954).
Andersen, Age Jorgen Christian and Percy Noel Williams, *Margarine* (1954; 2nd rev. edn Oxford, 1956).
Ashley, Sir William, *The Bread of Our Forefathers* (Oxford, 1928).

Atkins, Peter J., 'The growth of London's railway milk trade, 1845–1914', *Journal of Transport History*, 4 (1978), pp. 208–26.
Atkins, Peter J., 'The retail milk trade in London, 1790–1914', *Economic History Review*, 2nd series, 33(1980), pp. 522–37.
Atkins, Peter J., 'The Production and marketing of fruit and vegetables, 1850–1950', in Derek John Oddy and Derek Stanborough Miller (eds), *Diet and Health in Modern Britain* (London, 1985).
Aykroyd, Wallace Rudell, *Sweet Malefactor: Sugar, Slavery and Human Society* (London, 1967).
Barker, Theodore Cardwell and John Yudkin, *Fish in Britain* (London, 1971).
Barker, Theodore Cardwell, 'Changing patterns of food consumption in the United Kingdom', in John Yudkin (ed.), *Diet of Man: Needs and Wants* (London, 1978), pp. 163–86.
Barnett, Louise Margaret, *British Food Policy during the First World War* (London, 1985).
Battersby, Roy John, *The Development of Market Gardening in England, 1850–1914* doctoral thesis (London, 1960).
Bear, William E. (ed.), *Journal of the Royal Agricultural Statistical Society*, 3rd series, 10 (1899).
Beaver, M. W., 'Population, infant mortality and milk', *Population Studies*, 27 (1973), pp. 243–54.
Beeton, Isabella, *The Book of Household Management* (London, 1861).
Blackman, Janet M., 'The food supply of an industrial town. A study of Sheffield's public markets 1780–1900', *Business History*, 5 (1962–3), pp. 83–97.
Blackman, Janet M., 'Changing marketing methods and food consumption' in Theodore Cardwell Barker, John Crawford McKenzie and John Yudkin (eds), *Our Changing Fare. Two Hundred Years of British Food Habits* (London, 1966), pp. 30–46.
Blackman, Janet M. 'The corner shop: the development of the grocery and general provision trade' in Derek John Oddy and Derek S. Miller (eds), *The Making of the Modern British Diet* (London, Totowa, New York, 1976), pp.148–60.
Board of Trade, *Memoranda, Statistical Tables and Charts*, Cd. 1761 (London, 1903).
Booth, Alan, 'Food riots in the North-West of England, 1790–1801', *Past and Present*, 77 (1977), pp.84–107.
Booth, Charles, *Life and Labour of the People in London* (London, 1891).
Boswell, James, *JS 100. The Story of Sainsbury's* (London, 1969).
Bowley, Arthur Lion and Margaret A. Hogg, *Has Poverty Diminished?* (London, 1925).
British Association for the Advancement of Science, *Report of the Committee on the Present Appropriation of Wages* (51st meeting, 1881).
Brockway, Archibald and Baron Brockway Fenner, *Hungry England* (London, 1932).
Buchanan, Ian, 'Infant feeding, sanitation and diarrhoea in colliery communities 1880–1911', in Derek John Oddy and Derek Stanborough Miller (eds), *Diet and Health in Modern Britain* (London, 1985), pp. 148–77.
Burnett, John, 'The baking industry in the nineteenth century', *Business History*, 5 (1962–3), pp. 98–103.
Burnett, John, *A Social History of Housing 1815–1985* (London, 1986).
Burnett, John, *Changing Meal Patterns in the Twentieth Century* (Manchester, 1989a).
Burnett, John, *Plenty and Want. A Social History of Food in England from 1815 to the Present* (3rd rev. edn, London, 1989b).
Campbell, Roy H., 'Diets in Scotland – an example of regional variation', in Theodore Cardwell Barker, John Crawford McKenzie and John Yudkin (eds), *Our Changing Fare. Two Hundred Years of British Food Habits* (London, 1966), pp. 47–60.
Capie, Forrest, 'Consumer preference: meat in England and Wales, 1920–1939', *Bulletin of*

Economic Research, 28(1976), pp. 85–94.
Chaloner, William Henry, 'Food and drink in British history. A bibliographical guide', *Amateur Historian,* 4(1960), pp. 315–19.
Changing Food Habits, ed. John Yudkin and Johan Crawford McKenzie (London, 1964).
Cheke, Valerie, *The Story of Cheese Making in Britain* (London, 1959).
Cobbett, William, *Cottage Economy* (London, 1823).
Cohen, Ruth Louisa, *The History of Milk Prices* (Oxford, 1936).
Cole, George Douglas Howard, *A Century of Co-operation* (London, 1945).
Collins, Edward John T., 'Dietary change and cereal consumption in Britain in the nineteenth century', *Agricultural History Review,* 23(1975), pp. 97–115.
Colmore, G., '£800 a Year', *Cornhill Magazine,* new series, 60(1901), June, pp. 790–800.
Connell, K. H., 'The potato in Ireland', *Past and Present,* 23(1962), pp. 57–71.
Copley, Esther, *Cottage Cookery* (London, 1849).
Corina, Maurice, *Pile it High, Sell it Cheap. The Authorised Biography of Sir John Cohen, Founder of Tesco* (London, 1971).
Corley, Thomas Anthony Buchanan, *Quaker Enterprise in Biscuits: Huntley and Palmers of Reading* (London, 1972).
Corran, Harry Stanley, *A History of Brewing* (Newton Abbot, 1975).
Crawford, E. Margaret, 'Dearth, diet and disease in Ireland 1850: a case study of nutritional deficiency', *Medical History,* 28 (1984), no 2, pp. 151–61.
Crawford, E. Margaret, 'Scurvy in Ireland during the Great Famine', *Social History of Medicine,*1 (1988), no. 3, pp. 281–300.
Crawford, Sir William and H. Broadley, *The People's Food* (London, 1938).
Critchell, James Troubridge and Joseph Raymond, *The History of the Frozen Meat Trade* (London, 1912).
Cullen, Louis Michael, 'Irish history without the potato', *Past and Present,* 40(1968), pp. 72–83.
Cutting, Charles Latham, *Fish Saving: A History of Fish Processing from Ancient to Modern Times* (London, 1955).
Daiches, David, *Scotch Whisky. Its Past and Present* (London, 1969).
Daunton, Martin J., *House and Home in the Victorian City* (London, 1983).
Davies, David, *The Case of Labourers in Husbandry* (London, 1795).
Davies, Maude Frances, *Life in an English Village* (London, 1909).
Deerr, Noel, *The History of Sugar,* 2 vols, (London, 1949, 1950).
Dewey, Peter E., 'Food production and policy in the United Kingdom 1914–1918', *Transactions of the Royal Historical Society,* 30(1980), pp. 71–89.
Diet of Man: Needs and Wants, ed. John Yudkin (London, 1978).
Diet and Health in Modern Britain, ed. Derek John Oddy and Derek Stanborough Miller (London, 1985).
The Dietary Surveys of Dr Edward Smith 1862–3, ed. by Theodore Cardwell Barker, Derek J. Oddy and John Yudkin, London, 1970.
Dodd, George, *The Food of London* (London, 1856).
Dolby, Richard, *The Cook's Dictionary and Housekeeper's Directory* (London, 1830).
Donnachie, Ian, *A History of the Brewing Industry in Scotland* (Edinburgh, 1979).
Driver, Christopher, *The British at Table 1940–1980* (London, 1983).
Drummond, Sir Jack Cecil and Anne Wilbraham, *The Englishman's Food* (London, 1939;. rev. by M. Hollingsworth, London,1957).
Economy and Society in Scotland and Ireland, 1500–1939, ed. Rosalind Mitchison and Peter Roebuck (Edinburgh,1988).

Eden, Sir Frederic Morton, *The State of the Poor*, 3 vols (London, 1797).
Engels, Friedrich, *The Conditions of the Working-Class in England in 1844*, trans. and ed. by W.O. Henderson and W.H. Chaloner (Oxford, 1948).
The Family Economist, London 1848–9.
Fay, Charles Ryle, 'The miller and the baker: a note on commercial transition 1770–1837', *Cambridge Historical Journal*, 1(1923–5), pp. 85–91.
Fish in Britain, ed. Theodore Cardwell Barker and John Yudkin (London, 1971).
Floud, Roderick C. and Kenneth W. Wachter, 'Poverty and physical stature: evidence on the standard of living of London boys 1770–1870', *Social Science History*, 6(1982), pp. 422ff.
Ford, Percy, *Work and Wealth in a Modern Port* (London, 1934).
Forrest, Dennis Mostyn, *A Hundred Years of Ceylon Tea, 1867–1967*, (London, 1967).
Forrest, Dennis Mostyn, *Tea for the British: A Social and Economic History of a Famous Trade* (London, 1973).
Francatelli, Charles Elmé, *A Plain Cookery Book for The Working Classes* (London, 1852; repr. 1977).
Fraser, W. H., *The Coming of the Mass Market 1850–1914* (London, 1981).
Fussell, George Edwin, 'The London cheesemongers of the eighteenth century', *Economic Journal (Economic History)*, 1 (1928), pp. 394–8.
Fussell, George Edwin and C. Goodman, 'Eighteenth–century traffic in milk products', *Economic History*, 3 (1934–7), pp. 380–7.
Giedion, Siegfried, *Mechanization Takes Command* (Oxford, 1970).
Glen, Isabel A., *An Economic History of the Distilling Industry in Scotland 1750–1914* (doctoral thesis, Strathclyde, 1969).
Goldstrom, Joachim Max and Leslie Albert Clarkson (eds), *Irish Population, Economy and Society* (Oxford, 1981).
Griffiths, Sir Percival Joseph, *The History of the Indian Tea Industry* (London, 1967).
Harrison, Brian, 'Drink and sobriety in England 1815–1872: a critical bibliography', *International Review of Social History*, 12 (1967), pp. 204–76.
Harrison, Brian, *Drink and the Victorians* (London, 1971).
Hartley, Dorothy, *Food in England* (London, 1954).
Hartley, Dorothy, *Water in England* (London, 1964).
Jeffreys, James Bavington, *Retail Trading in Britain, 1850–1950* (Cambridge, 1954).
Johnston, James P., *A Hundred Years of Eating* (Dublin, 1977).
Jones, David Caradog, *A Social Survey of Merseyside* (London, 1934).
Kennedy, Liam, 'Why one million starved: an open verdict', *Irish Economic and Social History*, 11 (1984), pp. 101–6.
Kitchiner, William, *The Cook's Oracle* (London, 1817).
Lang, Tim et al., *Jam Tommorow. Report of a Pilot Study on the Food Circumstances of 1,000 People on Low Incomes in the North of England* (Manchester, 1984).
Layard, George James, 'How to Live on £700 a Year', *Nineteenth Century*, (1888), February, pp. 329–44.
Levenstein, Harvey A., *Revolution at the Table* (London, 1988).
Levi, Leone, *Wages and Earnings of the Working Classes* (London, 1885).
Longmate, Norman, *The Waterdrinkers: A History of Temperance* (London, 1968).
Lynch, Patrick, and John Ernest Vaizey, *Guinness's Brewery in the Irish Economy, 1759–1876* (Cambridge, 1960).
MacDonagh, Oliver Gerard Michael, 'The origins of porter', *Economic History Review*, 2nd series, (1963–4), pp. 530–5.

The Making of the Modern British Diet, ed. Derek John Oddy and Derek Stanborough Miller (London, Totowa, New York, 1976).
Mathias, Peter, *Retailing Revolution. A History of Multiple Retailing in the Food Trades Based upon the Allied Suppliers Group of Companies* (London, 1967).
Mathias, Peter, 'Agriculture and the brewing and distilling industries in the eighteenth century', *Economic History Review*, 2nd series, 5 (1952–3), pp. 249–57.
Mayhew, Henry, *London Labour and the London Poor*, 3 vols (London, 1851).
McCance, Robert Alexander and Elsie May Widdowson, *The Composition of Foods* (3rd rev. edn, London, 1960).
McGonigle, George Cuthbert Mura and J. Kirby, *Poverty and Public Health* (London, 1936).
McKenzie, John Crawford, 'The composition and nutritional value of diets in Manchester and Dukinfield in 1841', *Transactions of the Lancashire and Cheshire Antiquarian Society*, 72 (1962), pp. 123–40.
McKeown, Thomas, *The Rise of Modern Population* (London, 1976).
Mennell, Stephen, *All Manners of Food. Eating and Taste in England and France from the Middle Ages to the Present* (Oxford, 1985).
Mitchell, Margaret, 'The effects of unemployment on the social conditions of women and children in the 1930's', *History Workshop Journal*, 19(1985), pp. 105–27.
Mitchell, Margaret, 'The 1930's nutrition controversy', *Journal of Contemporary History*, 23 (1988), pp. 445–64.
Mokyr, Joel, 'Irish history with the potato', *Irish Economic and Social History*, 8 (1981), pp. 8-29.
Mokyr, Joel, *Why Ireland Starved: A Quantitative and Analytical History of the Irish Economy, 1800–1850* (London, 1983).
Monckton, Herbert Anthony, *A History of English Ale and Beer* (London, 1966).
Moss, Michael Stanley and John R. Hume, *The Making of Scotch Whisky* (Edinburgh,1981).
Neild, William, 'Comparative statement of the income and expenditure of certain families of the working classes in Manchester and Dukinfield in the years 1836 and 1841', *Journal of the Statistical Society of London*, 4(1841), pp. 320–34.
North, David L., 'Middle class suburban lifestyles and culture in England 1919–1939', (doctoral thesis, Oxford, 1989).
Oddy, Derek John and J. Yudkin, 'The English diets of the 1860's', *Proceedings of the Nutrition Society*, 28, p.13A.
Oddy, Derek John, 'Food in nineteenth–century England: nutrition in the first urban society', *Proceedings of the Nutrition Society*, 29(1970a), pp. 150–7.
Oddy, Derek John, 'Working–class diets in late nineteenth–century Britain', *Economic History Review*, 2nd series, 23 (1970b), pp.314–23.
Oddy, Derek John, 'The working–class diet, 1886–1914' (doctoral thesis, London, 1971).
Oddy, Derek John, 'The health of the people', in Theodore Cardwell Barker and Michael Drake (eds), *Population and Society in Britain 1850–1980* (London, 1982), pp. 121–41.
Oddy, Derek John, 'Urban Famine in nineteenth–century Britain: the effect of the Lancashire cotton famine on working–class diet and health', *Economic History Review*, 2nd series, 36(1983), pp. 68–86.
Our Changing Fare, ed. Theodore Cardwell Barker, John Crawford McKenzie and John Yudkin (London, 1966).
Orr, John Boyd, *Food, Health and Income* (London, 1936).
Palmer, Arnold, *Movable Feasts* (Oxford, 1952).
Panton, J. E., *From Kitchen to Garret. Hints for Young Householders* (London, 1884).

Peel, Constance S., *How To Keep House* (London, 1902).
Peel, Constance S., *The Labour–Saving House* (London, 1914).
Peel, Constance S., *The 'Daily Mail' Cookery Book* (London, 1919).
Perren, Richard, 'The North American beef and cattle trade with Great Britain, 1870–1914', *Economic History Review*, 2nd series, 24 (1971), pp. 430–44.
Perren, Richard, 'The meat and livestock trade in Britain 1850–70', *Economic History Review*, 2nd series, 28(1975), pp. 385–400.
Perren, Richard, *The Meat Trade in Britain 1840–1914* (London, 1978).
Pilgrim Trust (Report to), *Men without Work* (Cambridge, 1938).
Pollard, Sidney, 'Nineteenth–century co–operation: from community building to shopkeeping', in Asa Briggs and John Saville (eds) *Essays in Labour History 1866–1923* (London, 1971), pp. 74–112.
Post, John Dexter, 'Famine, mortality and epidemic disease in the process of modernization', *Economic History Review*, 2nd series, 29 (1976), pp.14–37.
Post, John Dexter, *The Last Great Subsistence Crisis in the Western World* (Baltimore, Maryland, 1976).
Ravetz, Alison, 'The Victorian coal kitchen and its reformers', *Victorian Studies*, 11(1968), pp. 435–60.
Redfern, Percy, *The Story of the C.W.S: The Jubilee History of the Co–operative Wholesale Society Ltd. 1863–1913* (Manchester, 1913).
Redfern, Percy, *The New History of the C.W.S.* (London, 1938).
Reeves, Magdalen, Stuart Pember, *Round About A Pound a Week* (London, 1913).
Richardson, Thomas L. 'The agricultural labourer's standard of living in Kent, 1790–1840', in Derek John Oddy and Derek S. Miller (eds), *The Making of the Modern British Diet* (London, Totowa, New York, 1976), pp. 103–16.
Roberts, E., 'Working Class Standards of Living in Barrow and Lancaster, 1890–1914', *Economic History Review*, 2nd series, 30 (1977), pp. 306–321.
Rowntree, Benjamin Seebohm, *Poverty: A Study of Town Life* (London, 1901).
Rowntree, Benjamin Seebohm and May Kendall, *How the Labourer Lives: A Study of the Rural Labour Problem* (London, 1913).
Rowntree, Benjamin Seebohm, *Poverty and Progress* (London, 1941).
Salaman, Redcliffe Nathan, *The History and Social Influence of the Potato* (Cambridge, 1949).
Schofield, E.M. 'Food and cooking of the working–class about 1900', *Transactions of the Historical Society of Lancashire and Cheshire*, 123(1971), pp. 151–68.
Scola, Roger, 'Food markets and shops in Manchester 1770–1870', *Journal of Historical Geography*, 1(1975), pp. 153–67.
Shelton, Walter James, *English Hunger and Industrial Disorders. A Study of Social Conflict During the First Decade of George II's Reign* (London, 1973).
Sheppard, Ronald and Edward Newton, *The Story of Bread* (London, 1957).
Sigsworth, Eric Milton, 'Science and the brewing industry 1850–1900', *Economic History Review*, 2nd series, 17 (1964–5), pp. 536–50.
Simon, André, *Bibliotheca gastronomica* (London, 1953).
Smith, Edward, *Practical Dietary for Families, Schools and the Labouring Classes* (London, 1864).
Smith, H. Llewelyn, *The New Survey of London Life and Labour* (London, 1930).
Social Trends, Central Statistical Office 17, Her Majesty's Stationery Office (London, 1987).
Soyer, Alexis, *A Shilling Cookery for the People* (London, 1855).
Stern, Walter Marcell, 'The Bread Crisis in Britain 1795–96', *Economica*, 31 (1964), pp. 168–87.

Stern, Walter Marcell, 'Cheese shipped coastwise to London towards the middle of the eighteenth century', *Guildhall Miscellany*, 4(1973), pp. 207–21.
Stevens, Maisie, *The Good Scots Diet* (Aberdeen, 1985).
Stevenson, John, 'Food riots in England. 1792–1818', in Roland Edwin Quinault and John Stevenson (eds), *Popular Protest and Public Order* (London, 1974), pp. 33–74.
Stuyvenberg, J. H. van (ed.), *Margarine: An Economic, Social and Scientific History, 1869–1969* (Liverpool, 1969).
Sutton, David C. *The History of Food: a Preliminary Bibliography of Printed Sources* (Coventry, 1982).
Tannahill, Reay, *Food in History* (London, 1973).
Thompson, Sir Henry, *Food and Feeding* (3rd edn. London 1884).
Turner, Ernest Sackville, *Taking the Cure* (London, 1967).
Vaizey, John Ernest, *The Brewing Industry 1886–1951: An Economic Study* (London, 1960).
Walter, J. and Keith Wrightson, 'Dearth and the social order in early modern England', *Past and Present*, 71 (1976), pp. 22–42, 84–107.
Warren, Geoffrey C., *The Foods We Eat* (London, 1958).
Watt, Sir James, E. J. Freeman and W. F. Bynum (eds), *Starving Sailors: the Influence of Nutrition on Naval and Maritime History* (London, 1981).
Waugh, Alec, *The Lipton Story* (London, 1951).
Webber, Ronald, *Market Gardening: The History of Commercial Flower, Fruit and Vegetable Growing* (Newton Abbot, 1975).
Webster, Charles, 'Healthy or hungry thirties', *History Workshop Journal* 13(1982), pp. 110–29.
Webster, Thomas, *An Encyclopaedia of Domestic Economy* (London, 1884).
Weir, Donald B., *History of the Pot Still Malt Whisky Distillers' Association of Scotland: The North of Scotland Malt Distillers' Association, 1874–1926* (Elgin, 1970).
Weir, Donald B., *The distilling industry of Scotland in the nineteenth and early twentieth centuries*, doctoral thesis (Edinburgh, 1974).
Whetham, Edith Holt, 'The London milk trade 1860–1900', *Economic History Review*, 2nd series, 17 (1964–5), pp. 369–80.
Willan, J.S., *An Eighteenth-Century Shopkeeper: Abraham Dent of Kirkby Stephen* (Manchester, 1970).
Williams, Dale Edward, 'Were "Hunger" Rioters Really Hungry? Some Demographic Evidence', *Past and Present* 71 (1976), pp. 70–5.
Wilson, Charles Henry, *The History of Unilever*, 3 vols (London, 1954, 1968).
Wilson, Constance Anne, *Food and Drink in Britain* (London, 1973).
Wilson, George Bailey, *Alcohol and the Nation* (London, 1940).
Woodham-Smith, Cecil, *The Great Hunger: Ireland 1845–49* (new edn, London, 1975).
Wright, Lawrence, *Home Fires Burning* (London, 1964).
Yarwood, Doreen, *The British Kitchen* (London, 1981).
Yarwood, Doreen, *Five Hundred Years of Technology in the Home* (London, 1983).
Yudkin, John, *Pure, White and Deadly* (rev. edn, London, 1986).

3 Comparative aspects of Irish diet, 1550–1850

Louis Michael Cullen

Irish dietary history is highly unusual. It is also marked by more controversy than that of other countries, a fact which underlines the problems of generalization that lie in it. Three features bring out this unusual character. First, it is the country which earliest and most extensively adopted the potato. Second, it is the last western European country to have experienced a famine. Professor Devine's recent book on the highland famine in Scotland in 1846–7, in stressing how slight was the rise in highland mortality, gives a new emphasis to the uniqueness of the Irish situation.[1] Third, it has often been claimed that dietary changes associated with the advent or spread of the potato accounted for the accelerated growth of Irish population between 1750 and 1845. A fourth factor might be adduced: the base of Irish diet was probably less stable than elsewhere – its marked butter content declined in the seventeenth century, and it shifted in post-famine times towards a more modern structure.

Within this framework, continuities and discontinuities have to be allowed for: regional ones and, because Ireland was a country in a colonial setting, cultural ones, quite apart from class differences. All this means that the study of Irish diet is not easy. It has also been complicated by assumptions, sometimes nationalist, sometimes Marxist, which tended to exaggerate Irish poverty, itself quite real, and I believe, the deepest in north-west Europe. Of these the extreme statement is Hobsbawm's assertion of 'eight and a half million Irishmen pauperized beyond belief'.[2]

The potato has been a subject of controversy from the time of Salaman's book on the subject up to the recent writing of Ó Gráda and Mokyr.[3] Indeed, the standard historical investigation of Irish diet by Lucas is simply entitled 'Irish food before the potato': it speaks of the 'dark reign of the potato' and 'a quite abnormal truncation of many aspects of Irish diet in the eighteenth and nineteenth centuries'.[4]

However, the topic becomes even more complicated if it is borne in mind that the introduction of the potato in the first instance was not associated with poverty. Indeed, the first evidence of the potato comes from the fields or storehouses of English settlers, not of natives,[5] and settlers of English origin who migrated to America brought the potato with them. A Quaker born in 1685 into an English family in Ireland who had emigrated to America advised a coreligionist to bring potatoes with him rather than any other item, regretting that on his own voyage he had not done so – as a result 'I longed so much for them that I dreamed night after night that I had left the ship and got home and there I was sacking them in barrell sacks'.[6] The potato was widely imported from Ireland, and consignments were extensively advertised in 18th-century colonial newspapers.[7] Very striking, too, is the fondness for potatoes evident among the Irish brandy merchants, Catholic and Protestant, who settled in Cognac, one of whom may have been the first man to plant the potato in the Charente region.[8] It is hardly surprising in these circumstances that potato and meat consumption are frequently mentioned in the same context both at popular and higher social levels. Diet in the population at large was varied before mid-century, and for many rural families including all middling families even after mid-century it was in no sense confined to a single item. Moreover, when the potato diet became much more widespread from the 1760s onwards, the phenomenon was not necessarily poverty-related. The spread of the potato has often been related to the famine of 1740–1, but the real situation is far more complex. Indeed, security in food supply and in income seems to have improved on balance in the 1750s and 1760s.[9] Increased potato consumption may simply and paradoxically reflect the fact that cereal cultivation intensified in the 1750s and 1760s. This entailed growing reliance on the potato as a root crop in rotations. In joint supply with grain, not storable beyond at best a single season and too bulky for distant markets, it made good sense at the time to consume more of it and release grain for other purposes. Significantly, spirit production greatly increased in Ireland at this stage. While spirits had long been known in Ireland, more imported than domestic spirits were consumed and only at the end of the 1770s did domestic production pull ahead of imports. Cheap potatoes, too, enabled the production of more pigs and bacon. In the 17th century pork had been a food of 'people of condition',[10] but pork now became the most widely consumed meat among the lower classes.

The lack of a clear association at this stage between the dietary pattern and poverty may seem to suggest an approach consistent with recent anti-Malthusian writing, and which claims that the potato was an adequate diet and the basis of a healthier and better-fed population than in the past. If the potato let the people down, it was not because of inadequate diet, it is argued, but because of the novel fact of potato blight.[11] This case is not convincing. There is much evidence of undernourishment and seasonal shortage. Besides, the thesis makes no allowances for the growing shortage of milk at the end of the 18th century for the lower classes, and for the effects of this on their health and condition. It is true that in the currently fashionable exercise of measuring heights Irishmen emerge as tall.[12] As for the usefulness of heights in the study of physical condition, many other factors may enter: Morincau has noted that though Breton conscripts were not as tall as other Frenchmen, they also experienced a lower rejection rate for army service.[13] D'Avaux, the French ambassador in Ireland in the military campaigns of 1689, hence long before the great advances of the potato, was already struck by the height of Irishmen.[14]

Irish diets before the potato were retarded ones, and as almost medieval diets they were a reflection of backwardness more immediately than of poverty in the modern sense. The latter point is a particularly important one, as modern comments on earlier Irish diet rarely make enough allowance for the fact that quite a lot of meat was consumed. Significantly, d'Avaux noted in 1689 that skill as butchers was the only skill among the Irish soldiers: 'c'est le seul métier de tous les irlandais, et il n'y a un soldat qui ne le soit'.[14] Moreover, fowl were numerous, their prevalence around cabins drawing the comments of visitors like Arthur Young, and the boiled egg was a basis of an impromptu meal.

Indeed, in the less intensively farmed regions with waste land at hand there was often more variety in diet than among the labourers in the rich eastern counties. In Coquebert de Montbret's account of County Mayo, for instance, there is an absence of reference to the poverty and malnutrition which he witnessed even on the rich plains of Kildare.[15] Sometimes staying in the cabins of the poor, he was prompted on one occasion to observe that 'this was not the first time when expecting nothing he was better served than elsewhere'.[16]

The simplicity of the dietary base and the absence of a highly stratified pattern may have admitted of the comparatively rapid adoption of the potato as a food. This, combined with the fact that farmers provided for the potato in their crop rotations by the economical expedient of renting potato plots for a year to their labourers, explains why labourer diets shifted progressively towards heavy potato consumption. In the early 19th century, despite few comparative advantages for wheat, now the main focus of expansion in the cereal acreage, exports of grain and flour doubled to 2 million quarters in the 1820s and rose to above 3 million quarters by 1838. This achievement, and at high yields per acre, was made possible not only by heavy labour investment (much of the land was cultivated by spade, but also by a massive increase in potatoes as the basic cleansing crop in crop rotations. In this situation the potato surplus was not only consumed by the poor but increasingly began to invade the diets of the better-off. Whereas the potato had been consumed in the first half of the harvest year with other foods widely used in the second half, better keeping qualitites were now sought out and it was consumed in the second half of the year as well. The potato had also usually been the food of one meal only of the two or three daily meals; it now became a food of two or more meals. This development, it should be repeated, was not confined to the poor but affected the better-off as well. It seemed superficially attractive as it maximized income. It went hand in hand with increased purchases of whiskey, clothing, and, for the better-off, tea. The French consul in Dublin in 1834 contrasted the abundance of food at local level in France with the sale of so much in Ireland.[17] Rising food disposals on the market are not in themselves unusual. But in the Irish context they seem to have been carried to extremes simply because of the accident of the original pastoral character of so much of the country and of the abrupt rise in cereal cultivation from the 1760s.

Ultimately Irish diet, even before the rise in population, seems to have been a poor one by European standards. This is borne out both in the dependence on dairy products and in the widespread reliance on oats, the cereal of light soils and shady or slow ripening summers. Oats were the basis, even in the capital, Dublin, of the staple alcoholic beverage, ale, a product castigated in the 17th century by both English and French visitors. The shift to increased grain cultivation in the next century, combined with growing reliance on the potato as a foodstuff, left a surplus of cereals which made possible the production of beverages that were far more palatable than their oaten predecessors, and hence the growth of a huge domestic alcoholic beverage industry. Increased barley production was the basis of the invigorated whiskey industry of the mid-18th century. Somewhat more slowly, the urban beer industry recovered, with a barley-based product rather than an oat-based one, replacing the huge imports of mid-century. Domestic cider production, once vigorous in the southern half of the country, also faded away. This switch, with its reliance on cereals with a heavier demand on soil, further entrenched the dependence on potatoes as a root crop.

The commercialization of the food economy was reflected in growing sales of butter and pork by smallholders. By the end of the 18th century, even farmers were disposing of much of their butter, which had now lost its overwhelming place in their own diet. For the poor, as commercialization gave every acre an enhanced cash value, land to graze a cow was no longer available as a supplement to their potato plot, and by 1800 a scarcity of milk in their diets was in evidence. In Brittany in 1800 most peasants still had a cow; in Ireland this had already ceased to be the case. Cottiers and labourers were frequently milk buyers when they could afford it, and also, often of necessity, food buyers in the spring. In such conditions commercialization often made more headway through necessity among the poor than among the better-off who were slower to change their ways. Weavers were quicker to take to tea-drinking than farmers. If the family potato supply failed, the income that bought whiskey, cloth, tea or tobacco could be switched to purchase food. Indeed, the very poor, those who relied on casual labour and who in the absence of regular employment were not always able to rent a plot, were invariably food purchasers. Humphrey O'Sullivan's diaries are an account of the food market in the poor rural town of Callan in the late 1820s and early 1830s. Written from the perspective of a comfortable but sympathetic townsman, they do not provide any basis for optimism about the condition of the poor or marginal population on the fringes of a small Irish country town in one of the richest tillage districts in Ireland.[18]

The extensive changes in both diet and food marketing suggest low incomes and a readiness to change dietary standards in the interest of making some desirable cash purchases. Irish incomes were probably about half English incomes, and they were also lower than French incomes. Even more important in this context is the fact that the unequal distribution of income in Ireland was probably more marked than in other countries. Certainly the landed classes had large incomes, much larger than in *ancien régime* France, for instance. Leaving higher incomes aside, what is striking is the contrast in incomes between skilled and unskilled workers and the wide range within unskilled incomes. The wages of skilled workers were as high as in England or Scotland, and skilled wages in the country towns were often close to city rates. On the other hand, unskilled workers in the more favoured locations earned only half the rates of skilled workers, and in other districts the disparity could widen to a quarter. The wage disparity between skilled and unskilled and among the unskilled themselves is a hallmark of a less developed country. It is the disparities within the country which make generalization difficult and even admit of conflicting trends. Thus, while the potato diet increased in the early 19th century, food diversification was in some respects increasing. Tighe, who commented on the decline in vegetables in popular diet, at the same time noted that in County Kilkenny 'the cultivation of vegetables by market gardeners had increased three or four-fold, within these twenty years'.[19] In fact, given the new wealth of many, and the greatly enhanced commercial channels which meant that cash could be turned into food, the circumstances of many rural dwellers had actually greatly improved. The famine did not put the community at large at risk. For many – a majority in the richer areas, a minority in the poorer areas – the situation was simply one of economic crisis, often of entirely manageable proportions, not one of survival. It entailed some reduction in cash income because they ate some of the grain they would have sold if the potato had not failed and because the cottiers to whom they had rented plots defaulted on their rent payments.

Estimates of the poor in the 1830s suggested that about 3 million out of Ireland's 8.25 million population lived in dire poverty. This figure corresponds rather neatly to the figure actually receiving relief a decade later at the height of the Irish famine in the summer of 1847. The underlying depth of Irish poverty serves to remind us that the blight of itself is not the basic factor in the Irish famine of 1845–8. Long before the Great Famine, Malthus had taken sharp issue with the potato optimist, Arthur Young, because, pessimistically and correctly as events proved, he saw the problems of replacing a sole foodstuff in the event of failure. It was not the potato but reliance on it as a sole foodstuff and especially such reliance in the more marginal lands in the West and South-West which was the problem. The potato failure posed less of a problem to the often more poorly dieted labourer in a market economy in rich eastern districts than it did on the western fringe of the island. Almost paradoxically some of the most disastrous consequences of the potato failure were witnessed in some of the comparatively rich coastal districts of south-west Cork, where moderately good land combined with massive use of seaweed as fertilizer had made extraordinarily heavy food cropping possible and precipitated dependence on a potato diet.

Evidence of diets helps to make international and class comparisons clearer. Dietary budgets, of course, have limitations: we cannot be sure that they are representative, and they are rarely full enough to admit of conversion into satisfactory comparative measures such as calorie content. But they are invaluable for all that. Thus on the eve of the famine on a middle-sized county Dublin farm, the hired labourers dieted by the family were each given a pound of bacon at dinner on three days a week and on the other three days a quarter pound of butter and four duck eggs.[20] What the proportions were at other meals we do not know, but the diet also included wholemeal bread, porridge and potatoes. The records of religious houses afford much evidence of food purchases, though rarely in a form which admits of quantification. Those of the Franciscan community in the city of Cork in the 1760s and 1770s do, however, admit of some quantification. Their per-capita income would have amounted to half the wages of an artisan in regular employment. Their meat consumption averaged about 38 lb per head, butter consumption 10–20 lb, and, in addition (if we dare generalize from details of fish in four months in a single year), roughly 24 lb of fish per annum, in addition to bread and potatoes.[21]

A number of other statistical estimates of diet can be put together. For instance, the masons employed on Christ Church Cathedral in 1565, who were dieted by the clerk of works, were fed up to 2 lb of salted beef per day, 2 lb of wheaten bread and 8 pints of largely oaten ale.[22] The invalids in the Royal Hospital in 1692 were fed a pint of water gruel for breakfast; for the six non-fish days they were fed for four days 1 lb. of beef or mutton, and for two days 8 oz of cheese or 3 pints of pease porridge and butter, in addition to a daily ration of 1 lb bread and 3 pints of beer.[23] In 1577 the diet of the English army in Dublin was 1.5 lb of white bread, 2 quarts of beer and 2 lb of salt or fresh beef (on the fish day 8 oz butter or 1 lb of cheese or eight herrings).[24] The diet of seamen on merchant vessels in 1695 at Kinsale was 2 lb of beef or pork, 1 lb of bread and 1 gallon of beer per day, plus 1 lb of butter or cheese per week.[25] The victualling of seamen at Charlesfort in Kinsale in 1686 was not dissimilar.[26] The French hospital regime in Ireland in 1690 allowed for each officer's servant 1.5 lb meat, 1.5 lb bread and 2 quarts of beer plus wine.[27] These figures seem to represent an upper limit for working-class diets, and have something of an international quality or concordance about them. If they are treated as the diets of skilled workers, and the Christ Church Cathedral diet is, of course, explicitly that, they are by definition unrepresentative of Irish conditions at large. D'Avaux, the French ambassador in Ireland in 1689–90, who in his correspondence often gave as much attention to the French soldiers' rations as to their munitions, was in fact astonished at the rudimentary dieting of the soldiery of his Irish allies:

> on leur donna à chacun un peu de farine d'avoine dont ils font une paste dure et des gâteaux force minces qu'ils font sècher devant le feu, ils n'ont que cela et de l'eau assez mauvaise pour toute nourriture.[28]

Family diets even of a skilled worker with dependents must have fallen short of these per-capita levels. Unskilled diets in an urban context could not have rivalled them, and unskilled diets outside the towns may frequently have been even poorer. These figures admit of some international comparisons within categories; they do not admit of international comparisons in a wider context.

Of course, we can make qualified comparisons on many bases other than attempted food balance sheets. Evidence of what was on sale is quite common, and gives us a good idea not only of what could enter into diets but also of changes over time. Among the most interesting documents are actual recipe books which reveal the repertoire of a family, even if they do not tell us much about what they ate on a daily basis. The drawbacks of recipe books are that they are almost invariably the recipes of the well-to-do, and that they give us some idea of the festive fare rather than the daily repertoire of the family. But within these limits they are quite good, and afford some idea of the range and variety of the diet. Kilkenny is perhaps the richest location in Ireland in such material.[29] By coincidence, the diaries of the schoolteacher and shopkeeper Humphrey O'Sullivan in the same region afford an idea of festive fare at a more modest level on a number of occasions where he was host or guest. Another diary, *The Retrospections of Dorothea Herbert 1770–1806*, gives a rather good idea of what festive fare was in a very comfortable family (a rich rector with perhaps £2000 per annum) on the fringe of the same region.[30] Such accounts also help us form an idea of the degree of sophistication of the food traditions of the house. There is a contrast between the mere abundance denoted by several joints of meat, with or without the addition of fish or rare vegetables like asparagus, and more elaborately prepared meals, including the eye-catching as well as elaborately prepared desserts. Indeed, in the context of domestic festive fare, a question is the extent of the diffusion of culinary skills in the community. In the Irish context such skills were not widely available in the community (though the question of the role of domestic service in better-off houses in diffusing knowledge of cooking techniques and of making new products, notably tea, more widely known, is itself an interesting one). However, they did exist, and the food writer, Maura Laverty, in a novel drawing on memories of her own youth in County Kildare, provides an interesting and sympathetic account of a rural virtuoso of the kitchen.[31] Evidence of fare at inns is another dimension which in some respects reflects the culinary capacity of the country accurately enough. It understates the high points in cuisine, of course, but, then as now, it nevertheless gives a telling idea both of the repertoire and even of the expectations of the customers.

A striking feature of the difficulty of generalizing is that of bread. The basic food of rural Ireland originally was porridge rather than bread. However, oaten cakes, baked on a griddle, were widely known and, indeed, even at a very low social level were essential because they were the food both of the traveller and of the worker absent for the day in the fields. Indeed, there was a wide range of breads in use in the countryside. Humphrey O'Sullivan in the rich South-East made a distinction between three types of bread (unleavened, leavened, and with currants).[32] In many areas barm was not readily available, and the decline in rural brewing must have aggravated the shortage: the traveller Coquebert de Montbret, covering the long journey from Galway to Westport, noted that even the wheaten bread was baked as the traditional flat cakes on the griddle due to the lack of barm.[33] Even in a prosperous northern region, County Down, although there was a variety of griddle cakes, there was no leavened bread.[34] Where barm was present, the wall bread oven was quite common in comfortable houses in the 18th century, and reflected a wide range of baking alternatives.

In post-famine times, incomes rose perhaps three-fold between 1845 and 1911. There were dramatic changes in food patterns as well. The per-capita consumption of flour perhaps doubled between 1860 and 1900. This implied both an increased reliance on shop bread and even in domestic baking a growing replacement of traditional cereals by white flour. In County Limerick even as early as 1858, at the comfortable farm house of the O'Briens at Lough Gur, one of the regular callers was a woman who 'went her round twice a week carrying on her back a large hamper of baker's bread from a neighbouring village'.[35] This bread did not wholly displace domestic baking in comfortable homes, and in fact the Irish baking repertoire is actually a richer and more varied one than in much of western Europe. However, a diet based on shop bread, butter, tea and sugar became increasingly the diet of the urban poor and of the labourers in the countryside. It has been suggested that in vitamin content this was a poorer diet than the largely potato diet it replaced.[36]

The analytical study of Irish diet is in its infancy. The composition of diet and its evolution have both received little attention. In broad terms, it is true to say that Irish diet has been studied either as part of a descriptive account of traditional rural practices without serious effort to get to grips with the mechanisms of dietary patterns or change, or as a subsidiary dimension to controversies among historians about the potato, the land system or the Great Famine. In the case of ethnological study, the sources have lain both in early and more modern literary texts and in data gathered into the archives of the Irish Folklore Commission, more extensively for the western seaboard than elsewhere, as part of its collecting work, some of it conducted by questionnaire. In the folkloral study of food Dr Anthony T. Lucas has been the great exponent,[36] and more recently Dr Patricia Lysaght of the Department of Folklore (University College, Dublin) has continued with the same thorough approach, though diversifying to take innovation into account.[38] Dr T. P. O'Neills's work also stands out as one of the best ethnological surveys of Irish food.[39]

In the case of historians, diet has received little attention. It has cropped up incidentally in the study of agriculture and attains controversial dimensions in discussion of the reasons for the spread of the potato in the diet, and in examination of the Great Famine. In general, in Irish history, diet has tended to be simplified to that of the poor (just as in ethnological study interest has lain in traditional foods rather than in the continuing experimentation with diet). In Irish rural history writing, there is often an absence of clear-cut distinction between social classes within regions or between regions with widely differing standards of living. There is only one broad historical survey of diet: it also explores the relationship between hospitality and diet.[40] There is also a short survey of dairy foods.[41] Dr Margaret Crawford's unpublished dissertation on 19th-century workhouse diets, however, represents the first stage in a more detailed study of diet: in association with Professor L.A. Clarkson of Queen's University, she has now extended her research into a wider survey of Irish food. She has already published an initial account of the spread of maize in 19th-century Irish diets.[42] This is an interesting topic not only because of the importance maize assumed in the Irish diet during the Famine but also because maize was already making its appearance and was to remain, in contrast to rural diets elsewhere in northern Europe, perhaps unique in its persistence for the remainder of the century. Indeed, if Irish diet in earlier centuries was both dairy-based and fitted in the potato precociously, it remained slow, even in comfortable districts, in post-Famine times, to shed both the potato and maize. The mechanics of all this are far from simple, and it would be rash to seek to explain them in a narrow context.

There are two questions or problems in diet which are of interest. The first is that it is dangerous to assume that diet changed during or because of the famine. There are indications that, while maize and domestically produced cereals made post-Famine diets more varied, the potato still loomed large quite late in the 19th century, and that food patterns may still have continued to be influenced by the urge to maximize cash income. Indeed, there are some indications even of comfortable rural families both using the low-grade maize and retaining a surprisingly high potato content in their diet for several decades. Hence the question of changing expectations and use of income in the late 19th century is quite important. The second is the extent to which the First World War may have changed things. Certainly conscription and long periods at the front are said to have brought novel foods from the French countryside to the attention of young Irish men, and to have promoted novelty in diets on their return home.[43] As the Irish rural population did not serve in great numbers, it is not clear to what extent diets changed in rural Ireland in the period. There was certainly a dramatic rise in farm incomes during the First World War. Farm incomes fell back in the postwar years, though the savings made during the war and postwar inflation were reflected in an enhanced liquidity of the farm population. However, the fact that in the 1920s the old pattern of exporting the good bacon and importing cheap American bacon re-established itself almost without change suggests that there may have been few dietary changes at large in Ireland in the 1920s and that the main changes may in fact be post-1945. This may also put a greater emphasis than is perhaps appreciated, and at the expense of assumptions made about widespread changes in earlier or later times, on developments within the twenty years preceding 1914.

References

1 Devine (1988).
2 Hobsbawm (1968), p. 73.
3 For surveys of the literature on this subject, see Cullen (1968); Mokyr (1981); Ó Gráda (1988), pp.8–12.
4 Lucas (1960–2), pp.8, 30.
5 Cullen (1983), p. 159.
6 Goodbody (1975), p. 111.
7 Truxes (1988).
8 Cullen (forthcoming).
9 Cullen (1986), pp. 160–3.
10 National Library of Ireland, MS 392, p. 269.
11 Mokyr (1985); Ó Gráda (1984); Ó Gráda (1988), pp. 9–12, 34–5.
12 Ó Gráda (1988), pp. 16ff.
13 Morineau (1984), p. 380.
14 *Négociations* (1934), pp. 29, 573.
15 Ní Chinnéide (1976), p. 58.
16 Ní Chinnéide (1971), p. 66.
17 Archives Nationales, Paris, AE 13 iii 436: Quelques notes sur l'Irlande, 29 June 1834.

18 *The Diary* (1936/37). See also Cullen (1983), pp. 179–82.
19 Tighe (1802), p. 498.
20 *The Material for Victory* (1958), pp. 5ff.
21 O'Connell (1942).
22 Mr Michael Ashworth's Transcript of the Christ Church Cathedral Building Accounts 1564–1565. I am indebted to Prof. J. F. M. Lydon for making them available to me.
23 Public Record Office of Ireland, Royal Hospital records.
24 Gerrard papers in *Analecta Hibernica*, vol. 2, p. 159.
25 Caulfield (1879), p. lxiv.
26 Ibid., p. lvii.
27 *Négociations* (1934), p. 727.
28 Ibid., p. 100.
29 *Cookery and Cures* (1983).
30 *The Retrospections* (1988).
31 Laverty (1942).
32 *The Diary* (1936–7), Vol. II, p. 361.
33 Ní Chinnéide (1976), p. 58.
34 Dubourdieu (1802), pp. 80, 87ff.
35 Carbery (1942), p. 65.
36 Clarkson and Crawford (1988), p. 190.
37 See Ó Danachair (1976), pp. 9–14, for a list of the published work of Dr Lucas.
38 Lysaght (1987).
39 O'Neill (1977).
40 'Diet in a changing society' and 'Hospitality and menu' in Cullen (1981, 1983), pp. 140–92.
41 *A History of the Irish Dairy Industry* (1982). This has also quite a useful short bibliography.
42 Crawford (1981).
43 Bonnain-Moerdijk (1975).

Literature

Bonnain-Moerdijk, Rolande, 'L'Alimentation paysanne en France entre 1850 et 1936', *Études rurales*, no. 58 (April–June 1975), pp. 29–49.
Carbery, Mary, *The Farm by Lough Gur* (London, 1942).
Caulfield, Richard, *Council Book of the Corporation of Kinsale* (Guildford, 1879).
Clarkson, Leslie A. and Margaret Crawford, 'Dietary directions: a topographical survey of Irish diet, 1836' in Peter Roebuck and Rosalind Mitchison (eds), *Economy and Society in Scotland and Ireland 1500–1939* (Edinburgh, 1988), pp. 171–92.
Cookery and Cures of Old Kilkenny (Kilkenny, 1983).
Crawford, Margaret, 'Indian meal and pellagra in 19th-century Ireland', in J. M. Goldstrom and Leslie A. Clarkson (eds), *Irish Population, Economy and Society: Essays in Honour of the Late K. H. Connell* (Oxford, 1981), pp. 113–33.
Cullen, Louis Michael, 'Irish history without the Potato', *Past and present*, 40 (1968), pp. 72–83.
Cullen, Louis Michael, *The Emergence of Modern Ireland 1600–1900* (London, 1981; Dublin, 1983).
Cullen, Louis Michael, 'Economic development 1750–1800', in *A New History of Ireland*, vol.

4, *Eighteenth-century Ireland, 1691–1800* (Oxford, 1986), pp. 150–65.
Cullen, Louis Michael, forthcoming volume on the seventeenth- and eighteenth-century brandy trade.
Devine, T. M., *The Great Highland Famine* (Edinburgh, 1988).
The Diary of Humphrey O'Sullivan, 4 vols, ed. M. McGrath (Dublin, 1936–7).
Dubourdieu, James, *Statistical Account of the County of Down* (Dublin, 1802).
Gerrard papers in *Analecta Hibernica*, vol. 2, Irish Manuscripts Commission (Dublin, 1931), p. 159.
Goodbody, Olive, 'Two letters of Benjamin Chandler', *Quaker History*, 64 (1975), pp. 110–15.
A History of the Irish Dairy Industry, National Dairy Council (Dublin, 1982).
Hobsbawm, Eric, *Industry and Empire* (London, 1968).
Laverty, Maura, *Never No More* (Springfield, Illinois, 1942).
Lucas, Antony T., 'Irish food before the Potato', *Gwerin*, 3(1960), pp.8–43.
Lysaght, Patricia, '"When I makes tea, I makes tea" ... Innovation in food: the case of tea in Ireland', *Ulster Folklife*, 33(1987), pp. 44–71.
The Material for Victory being the Memoirs of Andrew Kettle, ed. L.J. Kettle (Dublin, 1958).
Mokyr, Joel, 'Irish history with the potato', *Irish Economic and Social History*, 8(1981), pp. 8–29.
Mokyr, Joel, *Why Ireland Starved. A Quantitative and Analytical History of the Irish Economy 1800–1845* (London, 1985).
Morineau, Michel, 'Richesse et pauvreté des regions: Une nouvelle approche', in *Congreso de historia rural siglos XV al XIX*, Madrid 1984, pp. 373–92.
Négociations de M. le Comte d'Avaux en Irlande 1689–1690, ed. J. Hogan (Dublin, 1934).
Ní Chinnéide, Síle, 'A journey from Cork to Limerick in December 1790', *North Muster Antiquarian Society Journal*, 14(1971), pp. 65–74.
Ní Chinnéide, Síle, 'A Frenchman's tour of Connacht in 1791, part I', *Journal of the Galway Archaeological and Historical Society*, 35 (1976), pp. 30–42.
O'Connell, W.D., *Cork Franciscan Records 1764–1831* (Cork, 1942).
O Danachair, Caoimhin, *Essays in Honour of A. T. Lucas* (Dublin, 1976).
Ó Gráda, Cormac, 'Malthus and the pre-famine economy', in A. E. Murphy (ed.), *Economists and the Irish Economy* (Dublin, 1984), pp. 75–95.
Ó Gráda, Cormac, *Ireland before and after the Famine* (Manchester, 1988).
O'Neill, T. P., *Life and Tradition in Rural Ireland* (London, 1977).
The Retrospections of Dorothea Herbert 1770–1806 (new edn, Dublin, 1988).
Tighe, William, *Statistical Observations Relative to the County of Kilkenny* (Dublin, 1802).
Truxes, Thomax M., *Irish-American Trade 1660–1783* (Cambridge, 1988).

4 Modern nutritional problems and historical nutrition research, with special reference to the Netherlands

Adel P. den Hartog

Introduction

In western Europe and other industrialized regions an excessive diet and related nutritional problems for most of the population are a point of concern for public health and society as a whole. It is necessary to study not only the nature and extent of present nutritional problems but also the socio-economic and cultural changes in society which have led to this situation. The aim of this paper is to indicate how social sciences may contribute to a better understanding of present nutritional problems by making use of historical research methods and social history.

The modern diet of western Europe and North America is largely the result of the Industrial Revolution and subsequent developments. In view of this, socio-historical approaches to a better understanding of present nutritional problems will largely be focused on the 19th and 20th centuries.

The study of the social relationship between man and his food may be done from two different angles. First, it may be approached from a sociological and a historical point of view, as a contribution to our knowledge and theory of society and culture. Second, cases of nutritional problems, overnutrition or malnutrition, may be studied in order to find an answer to questions such as why there is a nutritional problem in a particular society or section of the population and what can be done to solve this problem. It is of importance to stress that approaches from the social sciences directed at nutrition have an applied character and should look for theoretical and methodological guidance from their disciplines of origin.

Development of nutritional-scientific thinking

Before discussing the role of social history and social sciences in relation to nutritional problems, it is necessary to give a brief analysis of the development of nutrition as a science and of changes in scientific thinking. Human nutrition may be defined as an anthropo-biological science, studying the relationship between man and the food he eats and, in particular, what it means for his health.

The science of nutrition, as Magnus Pyke points out, is the fruit of a century of revolutionary intellectual activity. In the 19th century, during the Industrial Revolution, the idea of combining scientific principles with technology was developed which resulted in the biochemical and physiological understanding of what food means for man.[1] In the development of the nutritional sciences two major approaches can be distinguished: the first is a physiologically and biochemically oriented approach, based on experimental work in the laboratory, often carried out on animals;[2] the second is an epidemiologically oriented approach concerned with public health. Needless to say, these two approaches are very much interrelated. The work of nutritionists in the field of public health and epidemiology is of great importance to social scientists with an interest in the sociological, anthropological or socio-historical aspects of food. The early scientific interest in nutrition is closely associated with the problem of mass poverty in Europe at the beginning of the 19th century. It was the Dutch physician and later professor of chemistry at the University of Utrecht, Gerrit Jan Mulder (1803–80), who in 1847 published the first scientific study on nutrition with a strong public health component.[3] In his booklet he pointed out that people do not consume those kinds of foods that are essential for mental and physical vigour (see Table 4.1). Mulder rejected the prejudices of the well-to-do on the so-called

Table 4.1 Nutritional advice in the Netherlands, 1847 and 1986

1847	1986
G. J. Mulder	Nutrition Council
• For the poor: more beans, less potatoes	• Introduce variety into diet
• Special care for poor children: protein-rich food	• Restrict consumption of fat (less saturated fat and enough unsaturated fat)
• For the well-to-do: less meat, less fat	• Restrict consumption of cholesterol
• A varied diet to prevent desire for excessive drinking	• Eat plenty of starch and fibre, less sugar
	• Restrict consumption of alcohol
	• Restrict use of salt

Source: den Hartog (1987), p. 35.

laziness of the labourers. The lack of vigour is, according to Mulder, due to a diet solely based on potatoes which lacks sufficient albumen or egg-white. Since egg-white is so important he introduced the term 'protein' at the suggestion of the Swedish chemist Berzelius. At the end of the 19th century the nutritional way of thinking was determined by the following concepts: first, that food may be a threat to health when infested by microorganism or as a result of poisoning; and second, that when a sufficient quantity of food is available in terms of energy, proteins, fats and carbohydrates there will be no threat to health.

In this period the medical sciences were strongly influenced by the newly acquired knowledge on infectious diseases caused by microorganisms. Under these

Table 4.2 Percentage of household expenditure spent on food by working-class families, 1850–1985

1850	1900	1950	1985
70	50	39	20.5

Source: den Hartog (1980); CBS (1988), p. 327.

Table 4.3. Infant mortality in the Netherlands, 1900–86 (per thousand births)*

1900	1910	1920	1930	1940	1950	1960	1970	1980	1986
155.5	107.9	82.5	51.3	39.4	26.7	17.0	12.7	8.6	7.8

* Infant mortality in the years 1860–1874 may be estimated at 204 per thousand
Source: den Hartog (1980), p. 354; CBS (1988), p. 85.

Table 4.4 Daily energy and macro-nutrient availability in the Netherlands, 1936/8–85

	1936–8	1950	1960	1970	1985
Energy, kcal	2830	2813	2931	2959	3102
Protein %	11.9	11.0	10.5	11.0	11.5
Fats %	33.7	32.5	37.0	38.5	39.0
Carbohydrate %	54.4	54.0	51.0	48.0	45.0
Alcohol %	—	1.0	1.5	3.0	4.5

Source: Hautvast and Hermus (1982), p. 194; LEI (1987), p. 15.
(The figures of 1950 and 1970 are rounded off).

circumstances it was very difficult to conceive of the idea of contracting a disease from a diet due to the lack of a certain substance in the food rather than from an infection or an intoxication.[4]

In the discovery of the vitamins, as these unknown substances in food were called, Dutch investigators played an important role.[5] Although in various European countries some investigators surmised the existence of small organic compounds in food to be essential to human life, their ideas did not gain a firm hold because of the prevailing concept of infectious diseases. In 1905 A.C. Pekelharing, a professor of hygiene at the University of Utrecht, was the first to demonstrate the existence of unidentified nutrients essential to human life. Outside the Netherlands his work received little attention as he published his findings in Dutch. However, the Englishman F.G. Hopkins independently did the same type of research, and was awarded the Nobel Prize for this breakthrough in nutritional science.

From about 1900 the nutritional situation of large sections of the Dutch population improved. Although the food pattern of the working class still lacked variety, the obvious forms of malnutrition disappeared.[6] So far nutritional work was concentrated on the problems of shortages during the economic crisis of the 1930s

Modern nutritional problems and historical nutrition research 59

Figure 4.1 Height of army conscripts, 1860–1980

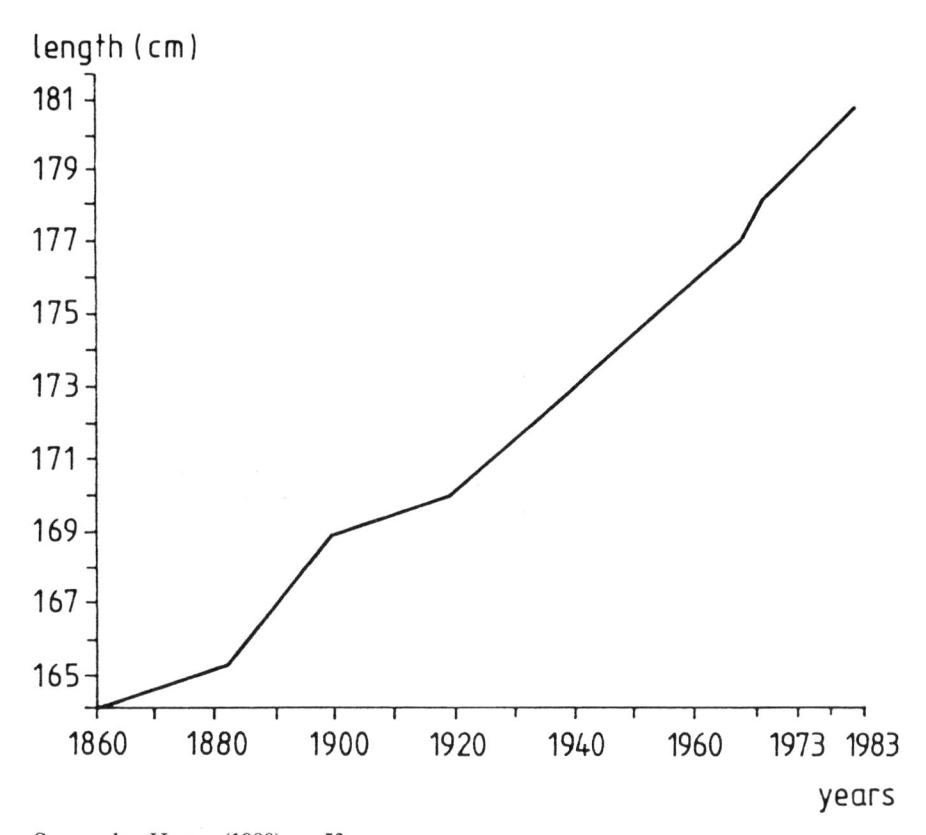

length (cm)

[Line graph showing height increasing from ~165 cm in 1860 to ~181 cm in 1983, with x-axis years: 1860, 1880, 1900, 1920, 1940, 1960, 1973, 1983]

years

Source: den Hartog (1988), p. 52.

and the Second World War. In November 1949 the last remnants of the food rationing system of the war disappeared: the last rationed foods – meat, bacon and cheese – became freely available to the consumer. The rapid economic growth led to an unprecedented situation where practically the entire population no longer had to cope with a marginal food supply (see Tables 4.2–4.4 and Figure 4.1).

The problem now was how to make the best possible choice from a large range of different foods. However, it took quite some time before nutritionists realized that in the industrialized countries nutritional problems were developing into problems related to overconsumption. Nutritional research gradually shifted towards overconsumption and problems such as heart disease, hypertension, diabetes and cancer. The concept of a prudent diet was introduced, a diet which would both promote good health and contribute to the prevention of nutrition-related diseases[7] (see Table 4.1). The concern with health became so predominant that it overlooked somewhat the fact that man also eats for pleasure.

Since the 1970s nutrition as a science and profession has increasingly been challenged by the so-called alternative food systems and by critical consumers. The abundant food supply, with its industrially processed foods, resulting in a widening gap between consumers and producers, has led certain consumers to take a sceptical stance with respect to the ideas of modern science. At first some nutritionists were rather disturbed by such often unscientific interference from outsiders in their work. Gradually, however, it was realized that supporters of alternative food systems were justified in looking carefully at the ethical and environmental aspects of food production and food consumption.

Since the 1980s the nutritional sciences in the Netherlands, as well as in other western European countries, have been confronted not only with nutritional problems related to affluence, but also with the beginning of a new poverty resulting from economic recession and unemployment. What does unemployment mean as far as nutrition is concerned? Are those who are now dependent on a minimum social benefit gradually drifting towards a situation of nutritional deficiency? There are indications that this is not yet the case, although the diet may become marginal. On the other hand it should be realized that poverty is a relative concept. When economic problems cause a diet to become frugal, it loses its most important social function – the joy of eating.

Sociological and socio-historical studies on food and nutrition

Approaches to food and food habits from the social sciences find their origin in anthropology, in southern Africa and the United States. It was Audrey Richards who published two anthropological food studies in the 1930s on Northern Rhodesia, now Zambia.[8] In this period there was a considerable interest in nutrition in England and an urgent need to raise the economic standard of the various populations of the British Empire.[9] The work of Richards has stimulated others to study the social relationship between man and his food.

As for the industrialized countries, during the Second World War American authorities became concerned about the food situation in the United States and Europe. In 1940, the National Academy of Sciences created a Committee on Food Habits, consisting of social scientists and health specialists, among them Margaret Mead and Kurt Lewin.[10] This led to the development of further studies on food habits. When, in the 1950s, the food situation in western Europe was back to normal and the first signs of a new prosperity became visible, interest in the study of food habits in relation to health and well-being diminished somewhat. However, some important studies with a strong theoretical base by such authors as Claude Lévi-Strauss, Mary Douglas and Frederick Simoons appeared, but these were mainly concerned with non-western societies. In particular the work of Simoons, with its historical-geographical approach, should be mentioned.[11]

In the early 1970s, interest in the study of food habits revived again. Society is increasingly confronted with problems of overnutrition. Consumer concern for the quality of diet and growing interest in culinary matters have further stimulated food studies since the 1980s. It is known that the *Annales School* has carried out a number of important studies on food and drink from a historical perspective.[12] Pioneering work towards a better understanding of the development of the modern diet due to the process of industrialization in western Europe has been done in the UK by Burnett and Oddy and in Germany by Teuteberg and Wiegelmann.[13]

In the Netherlands, until the 1970s, there were hardly any professional contacts between the nutritional and social sciences. Likewise, food as an object for historical research hardly received any attention.[14] An exception should be made for the physician, Lambertus Burema, who published a study on nutrition in the Netherlands from the Middle Ages to the 20th century. Although the book lacks a certain vision and is not very systematic, it nevertheless can be considered as a brave effort in a period when food studies were not *en vogue* as they are now. It is still a good source of information.[15]

Based on an analysis of publications partly or wholly devoted to food habits, carried out in the Netherlands, in the period 1975-88, the following approaches can be distinguished: studies on food marketing, studies on food habits from a nutritional point of view, sociological, ethnological, and socio-historical studies.[16] These studies were carried out by researchers from different disciplinary backgrounds. It is of interest to note the relatively large share of sociological and ethnographical studies taking into account the dimension of time and socio-historical work. This accounts for 53 out of 204 titles.

Methodological issues

In 1975 Maurice Aymard published in the *Annales* a stimulating paper on methodological aspects of the history of nutrition.[17] Aymard considers three major approaches of importance to research: the social and cultural meaning of food and diet to man; trends in food availability and food consumption patterns; changes in the nutritional value of the diet and its health implications. One aspect received less attention from Aymard: the necessity to include work on the social or socio-economic mechanisms which brought these changes about.

In the Netherlands Lucassen and Trienekens[18] underlined the need for socio-historical nutrition research for two reasons: first, nutrition is a basic need and has a central place in people's standard of living; second, nutrition and food habits are an essential part of society and culture, and hence of the history of the mentalité of the people.

As far as nutrition as part of the standard of living is concerned, there are several important research sources: food production figures; so-called food balance sheets; budget surveys; demographic data; health reports, and anthropometrical data (in particular height) on army recruits, which have been collected since 1860 on a regular basis (see Figure 4.1). Food consumption surveys, the first of which took place in 1907 among a small group of labourers in the city of Utrecht,[19] should also be added.

Trienekens published his extensive study on food policy, food production and the food distribution system in the Netherlands during the Second World War.[20]

Young children belong to the so-called vulnerable groups; infant and child mortality figures are good indicators of the health and nutritional situation of a society. Historical demographic research of the 19th and early 20th centuries has clearly demonstrated the relation between high infant mortality, the quality of drinking water, and breast feeding practices.[21] In the Netherlands the first childcare centre was established in 1901, inspired by the French system of 'consultations de nourisson et gouttes de lait'. However, infant mortality was already decreasing before a network of childcare centres was set up, because of the introduction of a safe water supply. Some work has been done to indicate the improvements in the nutrition of the Dutch population from 1900 to 1914. Mention should also be made of a study on economic development and the standard of living in the Netherlands during the first part of the 19th century, with extensive data on food and nutrition.[22]

Increasing attention has been given by ethnologists and sociologists to the central question of changes in food habits and the meaning of food to man, including taste and culinary aspects. Various research methods have been used, among them use of informants and oral history, content analysis of cookery books and food advertisements, and study of marketing archives. Some aspects of these methods will be discussed in more detail below.

Informants and oral history in the study of modern diet

It is known that oral history as a research method was developed by anthropologists for use in non-western societies where written records are scarce or almost non-existent. For contemporary history, of which the study of the modern diet is a part, oral history has also proved to be a useful research tool. One should realize that many aspects of our food and food habits are so normal and even prosaic in contemporary eyes that they have been ignored and not recorded.

Ethnographic research by the P. J. Meertens Institute in Amsterdam has included a number of studies on foodstuffs such as bread, fat, coffee and tea, and the preserving of meat.[23] This work is based on information received from a vast network of correspondents in rural areas. Questionnaires are sent to correspondents selected on their knowledge of local ethnography. By means of this method it is possible to go back to the situation of 1900–20. The validity of this method may be challenged because of possible misinterpretation of the questionnaire, personal bias and recollection problems. On the other hand written sources, however scarce they may sometimes be, are helpful not only as a secondary material but also to check the data collected. Maps are often used to present the data because they allow regional differences to be seen.

The *huishoudschool* and changing food habits

As to the question of why food habits change, it is very likely that, leaving aside factors such as rising incomes and the separation between home and place of work, education and advertisements have influenced our food habits. Home economics as an object for studying changes in food habits was initiated by our department in 1982 and further developed by Jobse-van Putten and van Otterloo; the latter did extensive work in this field, inspired by the civilization process theory of Norbert Elias.[24] The development of the special school for home economics, or *huishoudschool*, for girls at the end of the 19th century can be seen as a part of the wish of the more enlightened bourgeoisie to 'raise' the level of the working classes.

Training in home economics for girls is a good source of information on the ideas on nutrition, food preparation, and eating habits developed by the upper classes and spread among the population. Formal training in home economics started about 1885 and was first directed towards girls from well-to-do families. Gradually, it included girls from the working class and from the families of small farmers. In the 20th century up to the end of the Second World War it was one of few opportunities for working-class girls to receive an additional education of two years after primary school. The elementary courses in home economics were intended as a training for the future housewife. Analysis of the educational material reveals the following major elements:

1. Primary responsibility of women for the food and nutrition of the household.
2. Practical lessons in food preparation and cooking.
3. Some basic knowledge of nutrition and hygiene.
4. Emphasis on a varied diet, bearing in mind limited household resources. New was the attention given to vegetables and fruit as healthy and tasty food. A varied diet in a well-managed household was seen as a way to diminish the desire of the husband for alcoholic beverages, in particular *genever* (Dutch schnapps) and as a means of making a 'home' for him.
5. Good table manners, which meant eating with knife and fork, waiting at table until every member of the household had finished, and a cosy, sociable atmosphere during mealtimes. It also included eating from individual plates. Of great interest is that much attention was given to the meal as the occasion when all members of the household could be together.

Apart from studying the content of the curriculum and textbooks, much use is made of informants, such as retired teachers and former pupils. After the 1960s the *huishoudschool* is of less importance as a source for studying changes in food habits. This is due to the process of emancipation in which educational aspirations of girls went beyond the traditional confinements of food, nutrition and household tasks in general. As a result the contribution of home economics in the education of girls declined drastically.

Another angle for study is the analysis of the cookery pages of those women's

Figure 4.2 Relative frequency of the mention or depiction of the notion of 'tastiness' in food advertisements in Dutch women's magazines, 1900–85

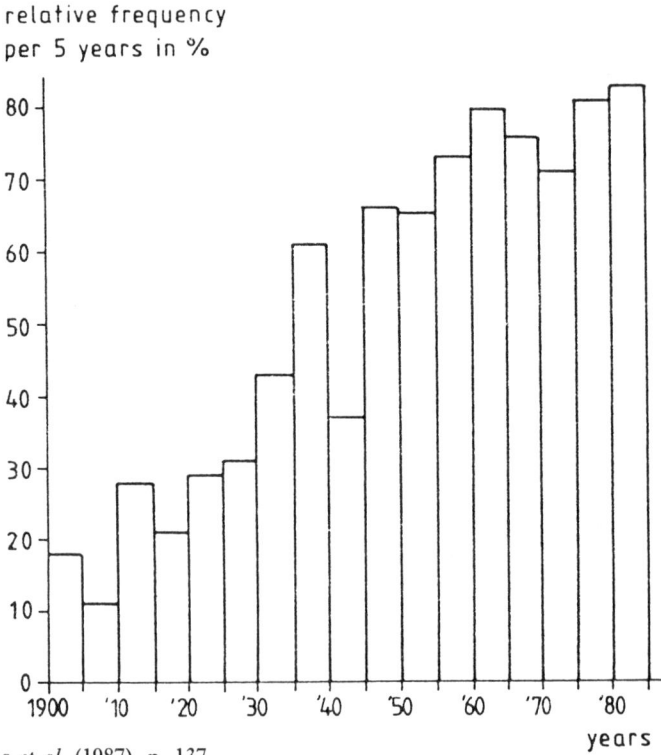

Source: Bos et al. (1987), p. 137.

magazines with a wide circulation and directed to a general readership. The American-born historian, Catherine Salzman, studied Dutch culinary history between 1945–1975 using the recipes published in a women's magazine and a popular cookery book as primary sources.[25] Particular attention was paid to the extent to which dishes from abroad, especially from Indonesia and North America, were adopted. The study indicates that during the period covered there was greater change in the ingredients used than in the meal pattern as a whole. The main daily dietary pattern remained the same: two cold meals based on bread and one hot meal.

Content analysis of food advertisements

The food industry is criticized from time to time for creating unhealthy food habits. The possible effects of food advertisements on food habits and nutritional knowledge are difficult to measure. However, it is possible and useful to analyse what kind of information on nutrition has been directed towards the general public.

A content analysis was carried out on nutrition information as presented in food

Figure 4.3 Relative frequency of the mention or depiction of health claims in food advertisements in Dutch women's magazines, 1900–1985

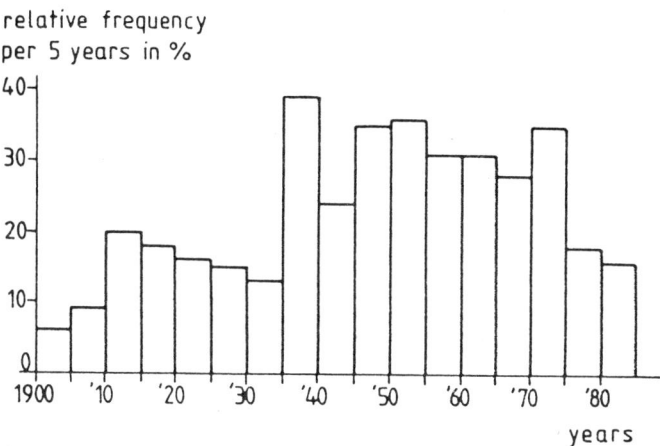

Source: den Hartog et al. (1989), p. 226.

advertisements in four Dutch family and women's magazines between 1900 and 1985.[26] The food advertisements were analysed on the basis of 47 characteristics which may be divided into three groups: general characteristics; information on food, nutrition and health; and social aspects such as target groups, industrial development, distribution and economy. Four issues per year of each magazine were analysed. In total, 4,203 food advertisements were recorded and analysed by computer, using the SPSS statistical package. It is of interest to note that in the period 1900–85 food advertisements as a percentage of total advertisements increased from 20 in 1900 to 35 in 1985. Mention of the concept of 'tastiness' associated with a product increased gradually from 11% of all food advertisements at the beginning of this century to 83% in 1985 (Figure 4.2).

It is striking that the increase in food advertisements and the greater emphasis on the hedonistic aspects of food coincide to a certain extent with the growth of the standard of living. Food advertisements have always been directed towards women. In the 1950s and 1960s more than 30% of all food advertisements clearly depicted women in the role of the housewife or mother.

Health claims have always played a major role, both directly and indirectly. They appear in about 30% of all food advertisements after the Second World War. Nutritional information appears at best in no more than 10% of food advertisements. The speed with which newly obtained scientific data on nutrition are presented in food advertisements has increased during recent years. In 1912 the word 'vitamin' was introduced by Funk and only in the period from 1935 to 1939 the term vitamin appeared in the advertisements. In this respect the manufacturers of margarine were quick to introduce to the general public terms such as 'cholesterol'. A relative new element in the early 1980s was to mention what a product does not contain, such as additives and sugar (see Figure 4.4).

Figure 4.4 Relative frequency of the mention or depiction of a product's ingredients in food advertisements in Dutch women's magazines, 1900–1985

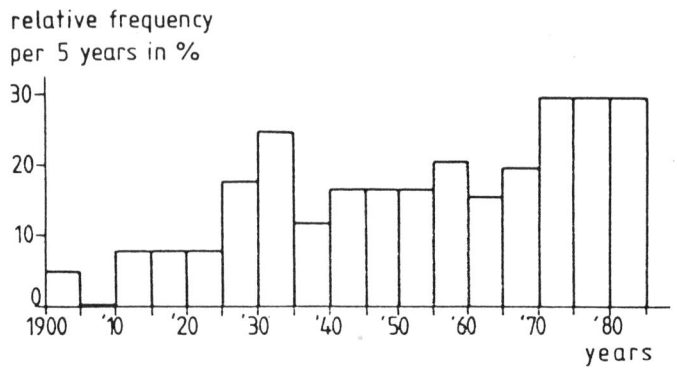

Source: den Hartog *et al.* (1989), p. 227.

Discussion

The dimension of time plays a major role in present-day nutrition. At the individual level during the life cycle of man, the effects on health of early inappropriate food will only be visible at a much later age. This aspect is even more apparent in view of the increased age of the population of Europe. Healthy food habits need to be acquired at a young age for a better chance of a long and healthy life. At the group or society level, the present dietary pattern is the result of a lengthy process of socio-economic and cultural change. Sociological approaches making use of historical research methods and social history are of importance for a better understanding of the genesis of the modern diet and its nutritional problems.

Not all researchers will favour this because their primary objective is not to work out nutritional problems, but to contribute to theories on the place of food in society and culture. Needless to say, for a better understanding of present nutritional problems theoretical guidance from the historical and social sciences is indispensable.

Several methodological issues have been discussed in this paper. However, one question still needs to be mentioned. To what extent should we try to study nutrition as a social phenomenon in its entirety, which is, as we know, very complex? On the other hand, is it more practical to study only one aspect for the sake of clarity, such as a particular foodstuff, a particular dish or particular social groups?

As far as further research is concerned, it may be useful to give more attention to problems of food innovation and the role of food technology and marketing activities. Archives of food manufacturers and marketing firms are interesting sources for the study of changing food habits. The problem, of course, is that these archives are not easily accessible, even for the study of the period before the Second World War. Another problem is that old-established and well-known firms may have cleared their shelves so that most of the material is lost.

As a result of European expansion and later colonial imperialism, European food habits spread to many other parts of the world. A great variety of foods, such as bread, biscuits and other wheat products, all sorts of sweets, tinned meat and fish, condensed milk and milk powder, ice-cream, beer and soft drinks, which originated in Western Europe and North America, have become increasingly accepted in tropical Africa and Asia.[27] This suggests that the study of the dietary history of Europe should not be confined to Europe itself.

References

1. Pyke (1968).
2. Widdowson (1985).
3. Mulder (1847).
4. A useful source for the development of the nutritional sciences is the study of McCollum (1957). One may also consult Darby (1985) and Todhunter (1976).
5. See van den Briel-van Ingen (1983), pp. 168ff.
6. Den Hartog (1980), pp. 352–5.
7. Marks (1985); see also *Richtlijnen goede voeding* (1986), with a summary in English.
8. Richards (1932); Richards (1939); Richards (1977).
9. Richards (1977), p. lx.
10. Guthe and Mead (1945).
11. Simoons (1962) made a study on taboos and avoidance of meat as food based on geographical and historical material.
12. See *Food and Drink* (1979).
13. Burnett (1979), the first edition of which appeared in 1966; *The Making* (1976); Teuteberg and Wiegelmann (1972).
14. A notable exception is the work of Baudet (1904), pp. 164ff., on meal and kitchen in the Middle Ages.
15. Burema (1953).
16. Den Hartog and Kroes-Lie (1988).
17. See Aymard (1979), pp. 3–5.
18. Lucassen and Trienekens (1983), pp.183–7.
19. Moquette (1907).
20. Trienekens (1985).
21. See, for example, Hofstee (1983), Vandenbroeke, van Poppel and van der Woude (1983).
22. Meere (1982), pp. 80–113.
23. See, for example, the study of Jobse-van Putten (1976) on fat utilization in 1920–5 and Jobse-van Putten (1989) on rural food conservation.
24. Den Hartog (1982), p. 83, and an unpublished study on schools for home economics prepared by M. Baggerman in 1983; Jobse-van Putten (1987).
25. Salzman (1985).
26. Bos *et al.* (1987).
27. Den Hartog (1986).

Literature

Aymard, Maurice, 'Towards the history of nutrition: some methodological remarks', in Robert Forster and Orest Ranum (eds), *Food and Drink in History. Selections from the Annales* (Baltimore, 1979), pp. 1–16.

Baudet, F. E. J. M., *De maaltijd en de keuken in de middeleeuwen [Meal and kitchen in the Middle Ages]* (Leiden, 1904).

Bos, Gerda *et al.*, '85 jaar voedingsmiddelen advertenties in Nederlandse tijdschriften [85 years of food advertisements in Dutch weekly magazines]' in Annemarie de Knecht-van Eekelen and Marian Stasse-Wolthuis (eds), *Voeding in onze samenleving, een cultuurhistorisch perspectief* (Alphen a.d. Rijn, Brussels, 1987), pp. 135–59.

Briel-van Ingen, Tina van den, 'Beknopte geschiedenis van de voedings wetenschap in Nederland [A concise history of the nutrition sciences in the Netherlands]', *Voeding*, 44(1983), pp. 160–9.

Burema, Lambertus, *De voeding in Nederland van de middeleeuwen tot de twintigste eeuw [Nutrition in the Netherlands from the Middle Ages to the twentieth century]* (Assen, 1953).

Burnett, John, *Plenty and Want. A Social History of Diet in England from 1815 to the Present Day* (2nd rev. edn, London, 1979).

CBS, Centraal Bureau voor de Statistiek, *Statistisch Zakboek 1988 [Statistical Yearbook 1988]* (The Hague, 1988).

Darby, William D., 'Some personal reflections on a half century of nutrition science, 1930s–1980s', *Annual Review of Nutrition*, 5 (1985), pp. 1–24.

'Dietary goals for the Netherlands', *Voeding*, 47 (1986), pp. 153–81.

Food and Drink in History. Selections from the Annales, ed. Robert Forster and Orest Ranum (Baltimore, 1979).

Guthe, Carl E. and Margaret Mead, *Manual for the Study of Food Habits* (Washington, D.C., 1945).

Guthe, Carl E. and Margaret Mead, *The Problem of Changing Food Habits. Report of the Committee on Food Habits 1941–1943* (Washington, D.C., 1943).

Hartog, Adel P. den, 'De beginfase van het moderne voedselpatroon in Nederland, voedsel en voeding in de jaren 1850–1914 [The early phase of the modern food patterns in the Netherlands, food and nutrition in the years 1850–1914]', *Voeding*, 41 (1980), pp. 334–42; 348–57.

Hartog, Adel P. den, 'De ontwikkeling van het moderne voedselpatroon in Nederland [Development of the modern food pattern in the Netherlands]', in Adel P. den Hartog (ed.), *Voeding als maatschappelijk verschijnsel* (Utrecht, 1982), pp. 56–115.

Hartog, Adel P. den, *Diffusion of Milk as a New Food to Tropical Regions: the Example of Indonesia 1880–1942* (Wageningen, 1986).

Hartog, Adel P. den, 'Voedingsgewoonten en een veranderende samenleving [Food habits and a changing society]', in Annemarie de Knecht-van Eekelen, and Marian Stasse-Wolthuis, (eds), *Voeding in onze samenleving, in cultuurhistorisch perspectief* (Alphen a. d. Rijn/ Brussels, 1987), pp. 15–37.

Hartog, Adel P. den and Sioe Kie Kroes-Lie, *Bibliografie van onderzoek naar voedingsgewonten in Nederland 1975–1988 [Bibliography of Food Habits Research in the Netherlands]* (Wageningen, 1988).

Hartog, Adel P. den *et al.*, 'Voedingsinformatie in reclame, een analyse van 85 jaar voedingsmiddelen reclame [Nutrition information in advertisements, an analysis of 85 years of food advertising]', *Voeding* 50 (1989), pp. 224–9.

Hartog, Cornelis den, Jo G. A. J. Hautvast, Adel P. den Hartog, Paul Deurenberg, *Moderne Voedingsleer [Modern Nutrional Sciences]* (Utrecht, 1988).
Hautvast, Jo G. A. J. and Hermus Ruud J. J., 'Suggesties voor een voedsel en voedingsbeleid [Suggestions for a food and nutrition policy in the Netherlands]' in Adel P. den Hartog (ed.), *Voeding als maatschappelijk verschijnsel* (Utrecht, 1982), pp. 188–217.
Hofstee, Evert W., 'Geboorten, zuigelingenvoeding en zuigelingensterfte in hun regionale verscheidenheid in de 19e eeuw [Births, infant feeding and infant mortality in their regional diversity in the 19th century]', *Bevolking en Gezin suppl.*, 2 (1983), pp. 7–60.
Jobse-van Putten, Jozien, 'Een boterham met tevredenheid? [Just a crust?]', *Mededelingen van het Instituut voor Dialectologie, Volkskunde en Naamkunde*, no 28 (1976), pp. 15–24.
Jobse-van Putten, Jozien, '"Met nieuwen tijd, komt nieuw (w)eten". Invloed van het voedingsonderricht op de Nederlandse voedingsgewoonten, ca. 1800–1940 [Influence of nutrition training on Dutch food habits]', *Volkskundig Bulletin*, 13 (1987), pp. 1–29.
Jobse-van Putten, Jozien, *Van pekelvat tot diepvrieskist [From salting to the deep freezer]* (Amsterdam, 1989).
Knecht-van Eekelen, Annemarie de, 'Opvattingen over zuigelingenvoeding in de negentiende eeuw [Ideas on infant feeding in the 19th century]', *Voeding*, 47(1986), pp. 16–23, 190–5.
LEI, Landbouw Economisch Instituut, *Consumptie van voedingsmiddelen in Nederland [Consumption of Foodstuffs in the Netherlands]* (The Hague, 1987).
Lucassen, Jan and Gerard Trienekens, 'Ten geleide. Sociaal-historisch voedingsonderzoek [Introduction. Social-historical nutrition research]', *Tijdschrift voor Sociale Geschiedenis*, 9 (1983), pp. 183–7.
The Making of the Modern British Diet, ed. Derek J. Oddy and Derek S. Miller (London, Ottawa, New York, 1976).
Marks, Linda, 'Policies for a prudent diet', *Food Policy*, 10 (1985), pp. 166–74.
McCollum, Elmer V., *A History of Nutrition, the Sequence of Ideas in Nutrition Investigations* (Boston, Mass., 1957).
Meere, J. M. M. de, *Economische ontwikkeling en levensstandaard in Nederland gedurende de eerste helft van de negentiende eeuw [Economic Development and Standard of Living during the First Half of the Nineteenth Century]* (The Hague, 1982).
Moquette, J. R. R., 'Onderzoekingen over volksvoeding in de gemeente Utrecht [Studies on nutrition of the people of the municipality of Utrecht]' (doctoral thesis, Utrecht, 1907).
Mulder, Gerrit J., *De voeding van Nederland in verband tot de volksgeest [Nutrition in the Netherlands and the Spirit of the People]* (Rotterdam, 1847).
Otterloo, Anneke H. van, 'Voedzaam, smakelijk en gezond. Kookleraressen en pogingen tot verbetering van eetgewoonten tussen 1880 en 1940 [Cookery teachers and efforts to improve dietary habits between 1880 and 1940]', *Sociologisch Tijdschrift*, 12 (1985), pp. 495–542.
Pyke, Magnus, *Food and Society* (London, 1968).
Richards, Audrey, *Hunger and Work in a Savage Tribe* (London, 1932).
Richards, Audrey, *Land, Labour and Diet in Northern Rhodesia* (London, 1939).
Richards, Audrey, 'Preface', in T. Fitzgerald (ed.), *Nutrition and Anthropology in Action* (Assen, Amsterdam, 1977), p. IX.
Richtlijnen goede voeding, ed. Nutrition Council (1986).
Salzman, Catherine, 'Margriet's advies aan de Nederlandse huisvrouw [Advice of the woman's weekly magazine *Margriet* to the Dutch housewife]', *Volkskundig Bulletin*, 11(1985), pp. 1–17.
Simoons, Frederic J., *Eat Not This Flesh. Food Avoidances in the Old World* (Madison, Wisconsin,1962).

Teuteberg, Hans-Jürgen and Günter Wiegelmann, *Der Wandel der Nahrungsgewohnheiten unter dem Einfluss der Industrialisierung* (Göttingen, 1972).

Todhunter, Neige, 'Chronology of some events in the development and application of the science of nutrition', *Nutrition Reviews*, 34 (1976), pp. 353–65.

Trienekens, Gerard, *Tussen ons volk en de honger: de voedselvoorziening 1940–1945 [Between Our People and Starvation: Food Distribution 1940–1945]* (Utrecht, 1985).

Vandenbroeke, Christiaan, Frans van Poppel and Ad M. van der Woude, 'De zuigelingen- en kindersterfte in België en Nederland in seculair perspectief [Infant and child mortality in Belgium and the Netherlands in secular perspective]', *Bevolking en Gezin*, suppl. 2(1983), pp. 85–115.

Voeding in onze samenleving in cultuurhistorisch perspectief, ed. Annemarie de Knecht-van Eekelen and Marion Stasse-Wolthuis, (Alphen a.d. Rijn, Brussels, 1987).

Widdowson, Elsie Marion., 'Animals in the service of human nutrition', in T. G. Taylor and N. K. Jenkins (eds), *Proceedings of the 13th International Congress of Nutrition* (London, 1985), pp. 52–7.

5 Historical food research in Belgium: development, problems and results in the 19th and 20th centuries*

Peter Scholliers

Food and drink habits can be considered to be quite reliable witnesses of the stages of society's development. This is the case not only from a purely economic point of view, but also from the point of view of class relations, state policy, social distinction and cultural aspiration. One can regard food history as a synthesis of these very complex, interrelated phenomena (including varied topics such as trade policy, ceremonial dinners, taxes, labour conditions, incomes, industrialization, outdoor eating, price formation, agricultural output, dinner parties, etc). So to study the food of the past is to look at numerous developments on various levels.

This paper considers the way in which this theme has been dealt with by historical research in Belgium. It aims to give a survey of historical food research in Belgium with regard to the 19th and 20th centuries.

Time and place are of much interest. Belgium was one of the nations which saw early industrialization, adhering to the practice and ideology of *laisser faire, laisser passer*. It therefore had an open economy, sensitive to innovations of all kinds (be it steam machines, co-operative stores, Fordist modes of production, canned tomatoes or even *nouvelle cuisine*). Belgium was not a trendsetter, but neither was it a laggard. Thus, to look at Belgian food habits is to reach beyond the boundaries of this small country and to examine the development of industrial capitalism in general.

The first step towards the analysis and interpretation of Belgium's food industry under industrial capitalism is to examine the methods, the source material, the aims, the approaches, the questions, the results and the controversies of Belgian historical food research. Most topics will no doubt be familiar to all food history researchers.

Early efforts

Food is at the core of people's minds and activities; this is true above all when it is in short supply. In the middle of the 1840s, the poor availability of rye and potatoes led to increasing prices while at the same time the incomes of thousands declined due to the collapse of the textile cottage industry. The consequence was starvation, leading to a higher mortality, huge migration, social unrest and severe repression. Contemporaries were eager to contribute to the solution of the *crise des Flandres* by suggesting new agricultural techniques, the extending of the arable land or the abolition of consumption taxes. They made severe moral judgements on workers' 'inadequate management' of their pay (too much gin drinking). But, most important to us, they made some hasty comparisons with the food conditions of the first quarter of the century.[1] Thus, although brief, they made the very first contributions to the history of food in Belgium.

Food conditions improved because of successful harvests in the late 1850s and early 1860s. Attention now turned to the monotonous diet of the working class. Although this diet generally provided sufficient calories, researchers found that it lacked animal products, while the quality of the food was very bad because of the widespread adulteration.[2] Labourers were eating too many potatoes and too little meat. Some researchers believed that, due to this deficient nutrition, the labour productivity of the Belgian working class was less than in neighbouring countries.

The so-called 'agricultural invasion' in the 1870s attracted much more attention from researchers interested in the history of prices than from those involved with the history of food consumption. The German statistician, Ernst Engel, used Belgian data of working-class family budgets of 1853 (Ducpétiaux) and 1891 (official inquiry) to calculate not only the average expenditure by income category, but also the average food consumption of adult male workers. His work led to the formulation of the famous 'consumer law'.[3]

Obviously, historical food research in Belgium during the 19th century was not a major area of investigation. It was restricted to some very general impressions and resulted in only vague knowledge, primarily dealing with working-class food consumption in mid-century. Interest in historical research was directed by contemporary questions and was influenced by ideology.

Although the young Belgian state developed a flourishing statistical activity in the 1840s and 1850s (Adolphe Quetelet and Edouard Ducpétiaux were among the prominent statisticians of their time), it did not provide food consumption figures (nor did it provide statistics of agricultural output). Its main interest was clearly not in the food consumption of the masses. But the state surely was no exception at that time; generally speaking, and with the exception of some inquiries into working-class budgets, very few people were then interested in living conditions and in the (food) consumption of the working class.

The first quantitative contributions

The First World War led to an enormous amount of publications dealing with how to cope with food shortages and giving recipes for cheap cooking. The shifts in the consumption of food brought about by war were studied by A. Henry (of the Ministry of Agriculture), who was the first to attempt to calculate annual per-capita food consumption figures, based on estimates of agricultural output.[4]

Also, the state showed some interest in food consumption statistics. The central bank, the Banque Nationale de Belgique, introduced a retail sales (bakery and grocery) index from 1928 onwards.[5] These figures are for current prices but give no direct information on quantities consumed.

In the middle of the economic crisis of the 1930s, L.H. Dupriez, an economist from the University of Leuven, needed information on the quantity of food consumed for his study of economic cycles. Macro-economic data on wages, prices, industrial output, savings, profits and so on were studied with a view to forecasting economic development. Dupriez's main interest was to provide an index of national average consumption. There were few official consumption statistics at his disposal, contrary to the situation in Germany or the Netherlands, for example. He calculated annual indices for the total consumption of wheat, groceries (sugar, coffee, rice), fruit, drinks, and tobacco for the years 1897-33, and presented indices of total meat consumption for the years 1920-1933.[6] He did not compute per-capita figures.

The choice of goods was dictated by the available source material. Dupriez used national tax statistics for drinks, tobacco and margarine, which were taken directly from official publications. Next, he used data on agricultural output in combination with trade statistics, but he regarded the results as not very satisfactory. Finally, official statistics of abattoirs were used from 1920 onwards. Dupriez constructed a weighted index of total food consumption, which he cautiously considered as representative of Belgiums's food consumption (see Figure 5.2 below).

Dupriez's contribution fits perfectly well with the aims of the economic cycle studies which became popular in those days: one is able to follow the general year-to-year development of food consumption and to relate this to the course of other macro-economic indicators dealing with wages, prices, unemployment, etc. But the specific approach does not allow consideration of per capita intake of foodstuffs, nor does it allow calculation of average calorie intake or of the composition of the average food basket. Moreover, social or regional differences are pushed aside, which is, of course, the case with all averages. Therefore, Dupriez's contribution has restricted significance with regard to historical food research.

A completely different approach was adopted by sociologists working during the 1930s, who wanted to measure the progress of working-class nutritional standards and the standard of living in general from the end of the 19th century onwards. These authors were astonished by what they considered to be a sensational improvement in workers' living conditions.[7] Their writings had ideological aims, stressing the fact that the capitalist system was, in the long run, capable of ensuring a decent living standard for all people. This research was published at the lowest point of the economic crisis and the optimistic findings stood in stark contrast with the everyday reality of unemployment, declining real wages and falling purchasing power. However, the investigations did not consider the 1930s. Use was made of inquiries into working-class budgets, containing data on food quantities consumed. The results of an inquiry carried out in 1929 were published in 1931.

The data of this large-scale official inquiry were compared with those of previous budget inquiries of the 'extensive' type (where the large number of budgets prevailed over the in-depth analysis of but a few budgets, the latter being the Le Play approach). Quite a lot of such inquiries had been carried out in Belgium. The inquiries aimed at establishing the living conditions of the working class in order to shape an adequate policy dealing with *la question sociale* (outbreaks of labour unrest) and after the First World War to provide the weighting coefficients for the calculation of the official price index.

The very first data were collected as early as 1841. E. Ducpétiaux studied numerous working-class budgets in 1853, and the Ministry of Labour repeated this exercise in 1891 and 1921. In 1910, the Institut de Sociologie Solvay of the University of Brussels studied the food habits of the Belgian working class. The work of Ernst Engel, using Belgian data of 1853 and 1891, strongly influenced Belgian historical diet research. He calculated the monthly food consumption of an adult male worker, and this standard was also used by the Belgian sociologists. The consumption of ten basic foodstuffs of an adult worker (3.5 'quets') was calculated for the years 1891, 1910, 1921 and 1929 (see the average calorie intake in Table 5.1 below). Budget inquiries proved to provide many possibilities for research into the diet of the past.

However, one must be very careful in using the results of these data, since they are concerned with a specific sample of people at a specific historical moment. This should be kept in mind when various budget inquiries are compared. The first thing to do is to look at the composition of the sample (industrial activity, income, family structure, age) in order to investigate whether the data are representative, reliable and, above all, comparable. For instance, a closer look at the data of the Belgian budget inquiries shows that the investigations of 1891 and 1910 considered primarily well-paid workers in the Walloon part of Belgium and the big cities, whereas the investigations of 1921 and 1929 provided data covering the whole of the country, including unemployed workers.

A brief prewar *status quaestionis* with regard to historical food research was given in 1944 by M. Neirynck, a sociologist from Leuven University.[8] He investigated the development of the purchasing power of Belgian workers and considered real wages alone as an inadequate indicator of the development of the standard of living. Therefore, he looked at working-class consumption patterns. He used the studies of E. Engel, M. Gottschalk, A. Julin, H. Denis and others, relying on the results of the above-mentioned budget inquiries. He used new information which was made available by research in 1932 dealing with the spending patterns of unemployed workers. He was struck by the improvement in the diet of the working class from the middle of the 19th century, an improvement confirmed by his investigations into real wages. He stated that the labour movement was not able substantially to influence real wages and consumption, which were primarily directed by the performance of industry. This was a neo-corporatist statement of someone who was to become the head of the Scientific Department of the Belgian Christian Union.

How did these first quantitative studies contribute to historical diet research? Attention was paid mainly to working-class food habits, thus excluding other classes. This was due to the use of budget inquiries which exclusively considered the working class. All of this research concentrated on working-class diet, without worrying much about general social and economic development (meaning that, for instance, diet development was not compared with profit rates or with GNP). On the other hand, Dupriez concentrated on macro-economic changes, using weighted indices. Average per-capita consumption remained unknown, together with regional differences of food and drink habits. However, very important work was done: source material was tested, methodological problems were tackled, and the first fruits of historical food study were presented.

The influence of the *Annales*

Of the two approaches mentioned above, only the macro-economic one enjoyed any success after the Second World War. The Service de Conjoncture of the University of Leuven continued to research long-run consumption data.[9] The Banque Nationale published index numbers of retail sales. The Department d'Économie Appliquée of the Université de Bruxelles began the study of food consumption, but using family expenditure statistics, without considering quantities consumed.[10] The analysis of budget inquiries was abandoned. Only when the results of a new inquiry were made available was a brief historical consideration made.

The French *Annales* School was a major influence on historical food research in Belgium from the late 1950s onwards. *Annales* historians showed an interest in the history of economic and social structures, the history of attitudes, regional development, the history of the daily life of the common people and the history of the so-called *vie matérielle*. Food consumption was one of the numerous topics tackled.[11]

At first, most studies by Belgian historians were devoted to pre-industrial times.[12] Very soon, some researchers turned to the early 19th century. The leading historian in this field was Christiaan Vandenbroeke of the University of Ghent. His interest was in the social, demographic and economic development of the 18th and early 19th centuries, and particularly in the diet history of that period. He well understood that food history had to be integrated into the history of agriculture, population, prices, trade, wages and social policy. He became a specialist in most of these fields. His impressive list of publications dealing with diet history started in the late 1960s.[13] Important findings were published in his doctoral dissertation. Based on new calculations, he presented agricultural, price and trade statistics with regard to cereals, potatoes, meat, and drinks as well as a table of per-capita food consumption in Flanders at the end of the 18th century.[14] Any investigation into the diet history of Belgium should start with this table, which provides reliable diet data during the very beginning of industrial capitalism. An average of 2,580 kcal per day and per head was achieved, 16% of which came from animal products, including meat, eggs, butter, milk and some fish and cheese. Bread accounted for 48% and potatoes for 21% of the daily calorie intake.

Some quite new findings were presented with regard to the food consumption of the city of Ghent during the first half of the 19th century. The originality of this research lay in the use of statistics concerning taxes on imported food (the *octroi*), which existed for some Belgian cities from the beginning of the 19th century until their abolition in 1859.[15] On very few occasions, this type of source material had already been used by contemporaries. C. Vandenbroeke studied the year-to-year per-capita consumption of the most important foodstuffs and was able to describe accurately the development of the diet in Ghent (see the example of meat consumption in Figure 5.1 below).

The *octroi* was also used by Catharina Lis and Hugo Soly, in an article dealing with the food consumption in the city of Antwerp.[16] The authors set their research in the context of the British standard-of-living debate between the 'optimistic' and 'pessimistic' views on the social consequences of the industrial revolution. This was a refreshing contribution at a time when the debate was above all concerned with real wages and price statistics. Lis and Soly looked at the consumption of various foodstuffs, and concluded that there was a marked impoverishment and polarization in Antwerp during the first half of the 19th century. These results were confirmed by data from charity institutions dealing with average calorie intake of the people receiving relief. This latter source material was also used by Patricia van den Eeckhout in a study on the poor of Brussels.[17] She calculated the daily calorie intake of the beggars, living in the Dépôt de la Cambre between 1811 and 1850.

It is obvious that the 1960s and 1970s were a time when the study of food habits in the recent past flourished. Usually directly inspired by the *Annales*, the authors mentioned here integrated their research into a broader historical framework, and considered food history as the predominant part in studying the development of the standard of living. Their contribution was decisive for the further research of food habits: new approaches were proposed, new source material was used, and above all new questions were put.

'Political economy' of food consumption

The first generation of Belgian historians working in the 1970s paid but little attention to the development of nutritional standards in the second half of the 19th century and the early 20th century (a period which had already been studied by economists and sociologists in the 1930s). Historical research in the strict sense was started by Patricia van den Eeckhout when studying the poor of the city of Brussels. She used the results of budget inquiries of 1841 and 1891 and calculated the average daily calorie intake of Brussels working-class families (see Table 5.1).[18] Thus, use was again made of the results of budget inquiries. This work led to new insights with regard to the progress of workers' standard of living during the second half of the 19th century. Progress only seemed sensational because the starting point (which was the middle of the 19th century) was so extremely low. Moreover, not all workers benefited equally from the improvement and many had to choose whether they were going to eat sufficient vegetable foodstuffs or whether they were going to increase their consumption of animal foodstuffs. A combination of the two was impossible for many working-class families.

I also had the opportunity to reconsider the data from budget inquiries concerning the years 1890-1930, which were used previously.[19] These were tested for their reliability, and the results were confronted with new series of real wages. This research was done in order to obtain information on the development of the standard of living, but also in order to contribute to the history of the labour movement and to the history of the relations between labour and capital. If it is relatively easy to explain the development of nutritional standards during the first three quarters of the 19th century, things get more complicated from the 1880s onwards, when food habits and consumption in general of the working class were to become part of the economic cycle, meaning that food consumption and workers' total consumption meant much more than the mere procreation and reproduction of the labour force: producers proved to be consumers, too.

I used new source material to refine the picture of food consumption at the turn of the century (accounts of institutions and sales figures of co-operative stores).[20] This approach clearly differed from previous ones (except for the calculations of the Banque Nationale), since no use was made of quantities of food consumed. Use was made of the average amount of money spent by the customers of co-operative stores. Year-to-year indices of per-capita spending on bread, groceries and meat were calculated in current and fixed prices (an example is shown in Figure 5.2).

A survey of historical diet research in Belgium was written for the International Economic History Conference in Budapest in 1982.[21] Food history was seen as forming part of a broad history of living conditions and attention was paid to food consumption as well as to consumption of other goods and services and to leisure preferences. An attempt was made to link the research dealing with the first half of the 19th century with the research on the second half of the 19th century and the early 20th century. The weaknesses of Belgian historical food research clearly were made apparent on that occasion. There was, for instance, no information whatsoever on the development of average calorie intake: there were data dealing with average food consumption of cities on the one hand, and with food consumption of male adult workers on the other hand, and both sets of data were hard to combine; there were no annual per-capita statistics of food consumption, though such figures did exist in such countries as France, Germany, Sweden, the Netherlands and Great Britain.

Therefore an attempt was made to calculate the annual per-capita consumption of certain foodstuffs from the 1830s to the 1930s.[22] Such calculations became possible because of the recent availability of statistics of agricultural output.[23] The work was of a purely descriptive nature, dealing with methodological problems and presenting the results of the calculations. The problems known to be involved with this type of computation (such as reliable output and trade statistics, deductions for losses, fodder and seed for sowing) had to be solved. For some foodstuffs (such as coffee, rice, fruit, drinks, tobacco and margarine) there were no problems at all. As for wheat, rye and potatoes, calculations were more complicated. Average year-to-year figures of consumption of meat and of dairy products were not calculated because of the enormous difficulties involved. This work resulted in many graphs and tables and in conclusions on the level of per-capita calorie intake in the 1850s, the 1900s and the 1930s. It goes without saying that all differences of age, activity, income, culture, etc., are blended together in one average. One can ask what the exact meaning is of this kind of informat∑ion. Perhaps the main importance offered by national average consumption figures is to provide a framework that can be used in international comparisons. However, it remains a very general indicator!

Criticism of these food statistics was formulated by Jan Blomme, who wrote a dissertation on the agricultural history of Belgium in the 19th and 20th centuries. He used the results of the budget inquiries, converted the data into national per-capita averages and concluded that the bread consumption figures were too high in the years 1910 and 1921. But according to the authors of the annual statistics, his estimates were too low.[24] This debate continues.

The research by J. Blomme was part of a much broader study of the reconstruction of the Belgian national accounts, conducted at the University of Leuven and directed by Herman van der Wee. Parts of his research deal with the diet history of industrial Belgium. There is, for instance, the work done by Martine Goossens on the annual meat consumption in Brussels between 1819 and 1846.[25]

Research of a somewhat different kind considered the influence of the First World War on diet patterns and on living conditions. This relatively brief but quite radical outburst was studied in relation to the food supply of a country confronted with a very sudden and radical change in agriculture, trade, employment and retailing.[26] The consequences of food shortages on demographic development (mortality, migration, nuptiality) were studied. Use was made of reports, data on bread rations, calorie intake figures for people receiving public and private charity, numbers of those attending public soup distributions, etc. In short, an exceptional period required the use of very specific source material.

A very brief survey of diet history in Belgium was presented at the Conference on Economic History in Berne in 1986.[27] Again, this occasion served to make weak areas of Belgium's diet history all too apparent. Although new information was collected, data were still lacking with regard to calorie intake, while levels of protein and vitamin consumption remained totally unknown. An attempt was made to consider food history as part of Belgium's industrial development and to link per-capita food consumption to the needs of industry ('crude' work in textile mills and coalmines required particular energy intake levels; Fordist work methods had different needs; white-collar work, which was spreading, required fewer calories; the mass consumption period required 'industrialized' and commercialized food habits).

The historical food research of the late 1970s and 1980s benefited from historical work in general, because of the huge amount of social and economic historical data made available during that period (e.g., output, trade, wages and price statistics). Attention was paid to the late 19th and early 20th centuries. At the same time, the history of diet was linked to problems dealing with the development of social policy, demography and industry, but especially to the development of the standard of living and to the economic performance.

Social inequality, food consumption and culture

During the same period interest grew in the food consumption of different social classes. Until then information on diet in the past only considered the working class or the population as a whole. Of course, capitalist development influenced the food and drink habits of the various social groups and classes in very different ways.

Daniel Bauters of the University of Ghent was the first to study the diet habits of Belgium's better-off classes. Inevitably, this involved a micro-economic approach. He used the accounts of a school community in Melle, a village near the city of Ghent, catering for the children of wealthy people.[28] He showed the possibilities of this type of source material together with the extreme differences which existed between the diet habits of the bourgeoisie and those of the labouring classes. This supposes that food consumption within the school did not differ a great deal from the diet patterns of the rich at home. It did not differ very much, but both the quantity and the quality of food consumed were probably underestimated, since any information with regard to ceremonial dinners, banquets, suppers and so on (which were very important to the 19th-century bourgeoisie) is completely lacking.

I tried to look at social differences with regard to food consumption, but I was not very successful due to a complete lack of data.[29] The main finding was a very large inequality in food consumption, thus confirming the results of Bauter's research. Consumption of meat and of dairy products formed the dividing line between the poor, the working classes, the petty bourgeoisie and the rich.[30] Accounts of rich families can be used to improve the knowledge of food habits of the wealthy (quantities consumed, the frequency of parties and cost) and also to know the cultural values of these classes. Attention should be paid to *étiquette*, *haute cuisine*, dinners and suppers – in short, to food used as a means of distinction between social classes and groups, as a means of showing pretension to a higher social group, or as a means of communication.

'Culture', of course, does not only refer to rich people. The food consumed by the working class, particularly on 'social occasions', also has a clear cultural significance. Moreover, food and drink consumption on special occasions (marriages, funerals, fairs) informs us of people's preferences, which can be of use with regard to working-class standards and values in general.

A recent book by the sociologist, Léon Moulin, deals with the cultural history of food of better-off people in Europe, primarily during the pre-industrial period.[31] It is an expensive, abundantly illustrated work, but with only few references to present-day historical food research, apart from some articles from the *Annales*. Though it was not the explicit aim of the author, the cultural and social meaning of food and drink of the elite clearly emerges.

A *status quaestionis* of Belgian food history

It must be stressed that 'modern' historical food research in Belgium started quite late, but that a lot of work has been done since then, using the experience of neighbouring countries. How did Belgian research contribute to the knowledge of the past in general? What are the weaknesses, and what remains to be done?

Sources and methods

Several types of source material have been used. Budget inquiries and tax statistics were used from the beginning of the investigations into the history of diet. Annual national per-capita food consumption figures were calculated based on statistics of output, trade and taxes. Annual local per-capita statistics were calculated based on the *octroi*. Both national and local series are important contributions from Belgian historians to the general knowledge of the diet in the past. Also historical data on food intake were sought in accounts of charity institutions, in sale figures of co-operative stores, in reports by contemporaries and in accounts of rich families. It goes without saying that the quality of the data provided by this source material varies greatly. One must keep in mind that these data were rarely collected with a view to the construction of food consumption statistics!

As for the methodology, quantitative techniques, even if not very sophisticated, were used from the beginning of the investigations. The more narrative style - qualitative source material and a 'literary' approach - is rather neglected. At the very beginning, historical food research was carried out by doctors. They were followed by economists and sociologists from the moment quantitative techniques came into use after the First World War. More recently, historians have become the predominant researchers in this field, while other representatives of the social and human sciences remain absent. Nowadays, historical food research in Belgium is, alas, not an interdisciplinary matter.

Problems or Fragestellung

The source material and the methodology used are dictated by questions put by historians when starting their investigations. Two main streams can be discerned: interest in working-class food consumption and interest in macro-economic food consumption. The study of working-class food consumption has been integrated into the standard-of-living debate concerning the first industrial revolution as well as the second industrial revolution. National food consumption was examined within the framework of the study of national accounts, social policy and demographic development.

Thus, diet history, quite rightly, is continuously related to other 'histories' and other historical problems (otherwise historical food research has no meaning at all, save for 'antiquarians'). However, is this enough? The history of diet in the past would benefit greatly from explicitly asking a set of clear questions, related to broad theoretical concepts of historical development.[32] For instance, attention could be paid to the theory of the *régulationnistes*, who are suggesting a broad theory of capitalist

Figure 5.1 Meat consumption in the cities of Ghent and Antwerp and in Belgium in the 19th and 20th centuries

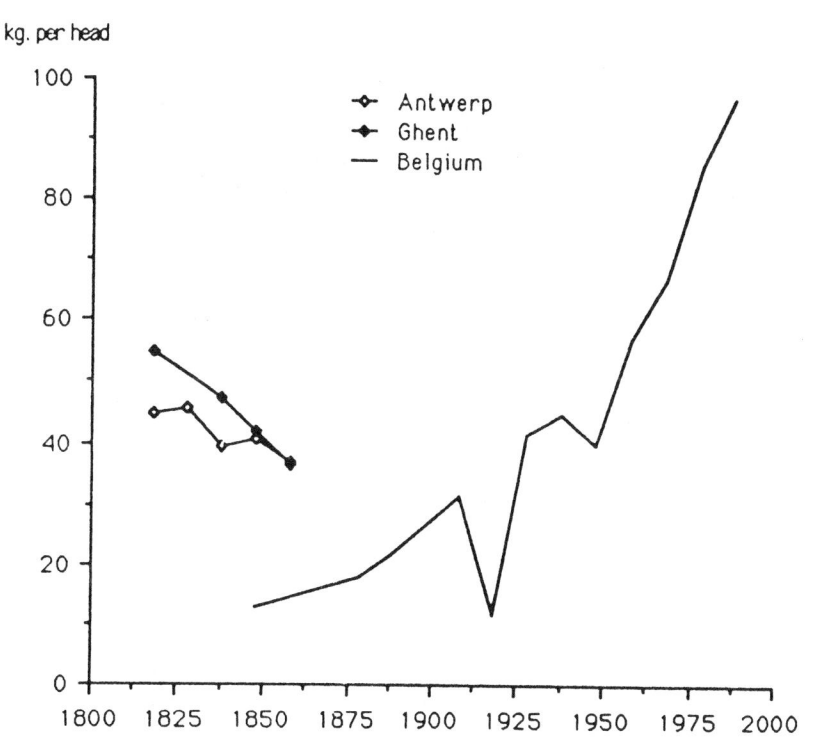

Sources: Lis and Soly (1977), p. 466; Vandenbroeke (1975b), p. 118; Vandenbroeke (1983), p. 242; Institut Économique Agricole (1988), p. 85.

development of the world where the 'workers' standard of consumption' plays an important role.[33] The theory of the so-called Budapest School, studying the concept of human needs from a Marxist starting point, is also worth looking at.[34]

Main results

Specific questions asked by historians lead, of course, to specific answers. Here, in presenting some results, these questions have been pushed aside. I will merely concentrate on the Belgian statistics of consumed food and drinks. The difficulty, then, is to combine the results achieved by means of various methods based on various source materials.

The per-capita statistics dealing with specific foodstuffs can be easily combined, as shown in Figure 5.1. Combining the yearly meat consumption figures for Ghent and Antwerp with the national averages for Belgium gives an overview from 1800 to

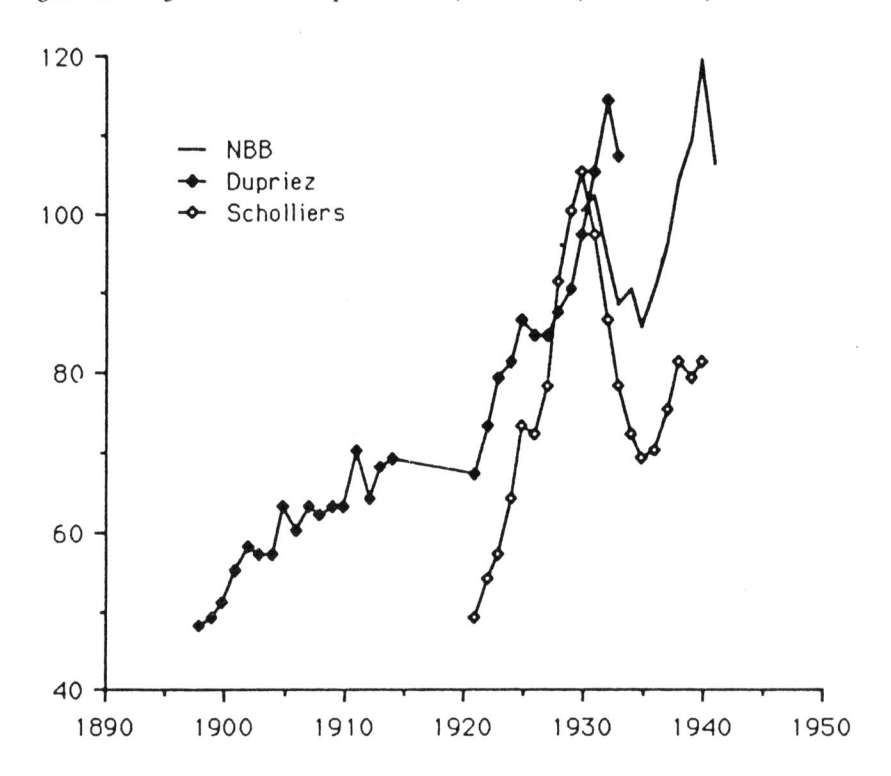

Figure 5.2 Belgian food consumption indices, 1896-1940 (1929-30=100)

Sources: Statistiques Économiques Belges (1942), p. 325; Dupriez and Bourboux (1933-34), p. 85; Scholliers (1982b), p. 851-869.

1980 of per-capita food consumption. A clear picture emerges: A distinct decrease during the first half of the 19th century, a slow recovery till the 1880s, and a marked growth in the last decades before the war is shown. War, of course, meant a sharp decline, but recovery occurred surprisingly fast. Again, the Second World War brought about a fall in average meat consumption which was not as significant as during the First World War. Growth was quite sensational from the 1950s onward, reaching an average of about 100 kg today.

The combining of results of other types of research is less easy. In Figure 5.2 an attempt is made to combine the figures of Dupriez (index of quantity of food consumed) with the results of the calculations by the Banque Nationale (retail sales index) and the calculations I did on food purchases in co-operative stores. These are data of different types. Nevertheless, a clear picture emerges: a rather slow increase in food consumption before the war, a marked growth during the 1920s (which was more important for the sales of co-operative stores than it was for the national average) and a decline during the 1930s which was more important for co-operative

Table 5.1 Development of per-capita calorie intake in 18th- and 20th-century Belgium (in kcal)
(a) National average and working-class families

	End 18th	1820	1843	1830	1853	1853	1850	1860	1891
Calorie intake	2580	2590	2040	2435	1810	2200	2267	2600	1910
Animal food (%)	16	28	4	23	2	4	23	8	22
Population concerned	A Flanders	A Antwerp	WC Brussels	A Ghent	WC Cities	WC Country-side	A Antwerp	WC Belgium	WC Brussels

	1891	1910	1921	1929	1948	1957	1970	1987
Calorie intake	3140	3570	3785	3370	2383	2531	2840	2940
Animal food (%)	25	31	34	36	27	30	32	36
Population Concerned	WC male	WC adults	WC (cities, Belgium)	WC	A all	A	A	A

(b) Middle-class families

	1846	1850	1870	1880	1910
Calorie intake	3608	2830	3410	3274	3472
Animal food (%)	28	44	62	46	39
Population concerned	College Melle	Bourgeoisie Brussels	Bourgeoisie Brussels	College Melle	College Melle

A: Average of the population
WC: Working class in towns or regions

Sources: Vandenbroeke (1975b), p. 140; Lis and Soly (1977), p. 475; van den Eeckhout (1980a), p. 27; Ducpétiaux (1855), pp. 268–385; Julin (1933), pp. 564–5; Gottschalk (1932), p. 838; Bauters (1983), p. 267; Scholliers (1987), pp. 85–6; Institut Économique Agricole (1988), p. 838.

sales.

Another opportunity for comparison is offered by the daily per-capita calorie intake and the share in this from animal foodstuffs which provide a reliable summary of both quantitative and qualitative changes. However, comparison is somewhat difficult because of the different standards (now adult males are considered, now total population; now the national average has been taken into account, now the working-class population of a city). Nevertheless, a summary of this kind of information provides a clear overview of the results reached by historical food research in Belgium since the 1930s (see Table 5.1).

A distinction has been made between data covering working-class families and national averages on the one hand, and middle-class families on the other. The differences in food consumption between classes are clear. The deterioration during the first half of the 19th century is obvious. Consider, for example, the calorie intake of working-class families in Antwerp in the 1820s and in the 1850s. A slow improvement in the second half of the 19th century is also evident (see the data for Brussels in 1843 and 1891 and the national data in 1853 and 1860). A marked improvement occurred between the 1890s and the 1920s (data only consider adult male workers!). Finally, official statistics only allow the daily per-capita calorie intake of the Belgians to be computed from the 1940s onwards. A significant quantitative increase occurred, but this slowed down from the 1970s, whereas the qualitative shifts (more animal-sourced calories and proteins) are still going on.

So, although based on different standards, these results do allow us to follow the general development of nutrition and to point to regional and class differences in development.

To sum up, it must be stressed that general food conditions worsened during the first half of the 19th century. Improvement occurred rather slowly during the last quarter of the century in spite of large imports of grain, but accelerated during the 1920s after the shaping of new class relations. The economic crisis of the 1930s as well as the present-day crisis has slowed improvements. Social differences with regard to food habits were extremely sharp in the 19th century, but decreased during the course of the 20th century without, however, being accompanied by a loss of cultural and social significance.

Refinements and further research

There is still an enormous amount of work to be done. I have already pointed to some aspects that urgently need more attention. As for the source material, more qualitative data should be used (e.g., literature, cookbooks, schoolbooks, appropriate legislation, etc.). More quantitative data dealing with both middle-class and working-class consumption patterns should also be considered. Abundant data dealing with the consumption of meat, milk, butter, cheese, sweets, chocolate, etc., should be collected. Although Belgium is a small country, more attention should be paid to regional differences. There is, for example, hardly any interest in the food habits of the Walloon part of the country in the 19th and 20th centuries.

As for methodology, nutritional values of food in the past should be reconsidered carefully. Qualitative and quantitative data should also be integrated in order to refine the general picture. Finally, there is need to have homogeneous data of per-capita protein and calorie intake, allowing fully reliable comparisons.

Perhaps most energy on further research should be devoted to the integration of food history with a broad *Fragestellung*, that is to say, the linking of food history to general historical theories and combining food history with such divergent topics as industrialization, trade relations, class antagonism and struggle, division of (household) labour, demographic development, social distinction and cultural aspirations. This, of course, suggests a very wide field of investigation.[35] I think that such an approach would allow us to leave behind the purely descriptive approach that has dominated not only Belgium's research, but also historical food research in general. Perhaps one should conceptualize a general theory putting food consumption at the centre of historical development and trying to understand and characterize this development including all possible economic, political, social and cultural aspects by means of the history of food. This aim fits in with the role of food and drink in society that has been outlined in the introduction to this paper.

A concluding note

A concern with the significance of food history has pervaded this paper, emphasizing the role of this particular research topic within the much broader field of historical and theoretical study. It is, indeed, not entirely satisfactory to link food history to just one other historical problem. Far better would be the contribution of historical food studies to large-scale theoretical concepts of society's development. The history of food and drink is quite capable of playing this role.

As for myself, I think that processes of capital accumulation, and the ensuing modes of production leading to specific class relations and state policies, are at the very beginning of food and drink habits. Therefore, the historical study of food habits should start by looking at modes of production, class relations and state policies. Such an approach is capable of providing explications and interpretations and of provoking debate.

References

* This contribution has benefited from remarks and comments by the participants of the International Symposium on Historical Diet Research (Münster, May 1989) and from comments by P. van den Eeckhout.
1 George (1846); Dauby (1863).
2 Squiller (1863); Denis (1887).
3 Engel (1895).
4 Henry (1925).
5 Results published in *Statistiques Économiques Belges* (1942, 1960, 1970, 1980).
6 Dupriez and Borboux (1933-4).
7 Gottschalk (1932); Gottschalk (1931); Julin (1933).
8 Neyrinck (1944).
9 Reuss (1960). Also, before the war, attention was paid to the consumption of dairy products (Cools, 1937). The year-to-year food consumption data were continued, see Baudhuin (1965-6) in *Recherches économiques de Louvain,* various issues in the 1950s and early 1960s.
10 Poelmans (1958-9); Poelmans (1980).
11 Braudel (1961); *Pour une histoire* (1970); and the special issue of *Annales E.S.C.* 30 (1975), pp. 402-632. The influence of the *Annales* is also obvious in other European countries; see Teuteberg (1987).

12 Amongst the many prominent studies are Craeybeckx (1958); Scholliers (1960); van der Wee (1966); Vandenbroeke (1971b); van Uytven (1973); Baetens (1977); Morsa (1978); Scholliers (1980a); Servais (1983); Koninckx (1983); Yante (1985); Schokkaert and van der Wee (1988).
13 Vandenbroeke (1971a); Vandenbroeke (1975b); Vandenbroeke (1975c).
14 Vandenbroeke (1975a).
15 For this source material, see Laurent (1956).
16 Lis and Soly (1977).
17 P. Eeckhout (1980b).
18 P. Eeckhout (1980a).
19 P. Scholliers (1980b); P. Scholliers (1982a).
20 P. Scholliers (1982b).
21 Scholliers and Vandenbroeke (1982).
22 Eeckhout and Scholliers (1983).
23 Gadisseur (1990).
24 Blomme (1986); Eeckhout and Scholliers (1986).
25 Goossens (1988).
26 Scholliers (1985); Scholliers and Daelemans (1988).
27 Scholliers (1986).
28 Bauters (1983).
29 Scholliers (1987).
30 See the contribution by Vandenbroeke (1983) on meat consumption.
31 Moulin (1988); Moulin (1975).
32 This was suggested by, among others, Baudet (1981), who pleads for an integration of food consumption with economic theory (Schumpeter) and, more particularly, for the study of consumption in the economic, social and cultural processes (Norbert Elias, David Felix, among others).
33 For this theory, see Boyer (1986).
34 For this type of approach, see Preteceille and Terrail (1986).
35 For the same finding, see Teuteberg (1987).

Literature

Baetens, Roland, 'De voedselrationen van zeevarenden [The food rations of seafarers]', *Bijdragen tot de geschiedenis*, 60 (1977), pp. 273-309.

Baudet, Hann, 'Problèmes et méthodes de l'histoire de la consommation', in Emmanuel le Roy Ladurie *et al.* (eds), *L' histoire et ses méthodes* (Lille, 1981), pp. 123-9.

Baudhuin, Fernand, 'Prix, consommation et revenu', *Recherches Économiques de Louvain*, 20 (1965), pp. 401-28; 32 (1966), pp. 281-313.

Bauters, Daniel, 'Voedingspatroon van een internaatspopulatie in het Josefietencollege te Melle 1837-1914 [Food patterns of a school community in the Josefietencollege at Melle]', *Tijdschrift voor sociale geschiedenis*, 9 (1983), pp. 258-72.

Blomme, Jan, 'De hoofdelijke broodgraanconsumptie in Belgie 1850-1939: een alternatieve benadering [Per-capita consumption of cereals in Belgium]', *Tijdschrift voor sociale geschiedenis*, 12 (1986), pp. 401-15.

Boyer, Robert, *La théorie de la régulation: Une analyse critique*, (Paris, 1986).

Braudel, F. 'Alimentation et catégories d'histoire', *Annales E. S. C.*, 16 (1961), pp. 723-8.

Cools, L.-J. 'Réactions réciproques des marchés de beurre, de la margarine et du saindoux en Belgique de 1920 à 1939', *Bulletin Institut Sciences Économiques*, 9 (1937), pp. 329-47.

Craeybeckx, Jan, 'Brood en levensstandaard [Bread and the standard of living]' in *Contribution à l'histoire des prix*, Vol. 3 (Leuven, 1958), pp. 133-62.

Dauby, J., *Les classes ouvrières en Belgique. Parallèle entre leur condition d'autrefois et celle d'aujourd'hui* (Brussels, 1863).

Degryse, Karel, 'Thee, koffie en cacaoverbruik tijdens de vroege 18e eeuw in de Zuidelyke Nederlanden [Consumption of tea, coffee and cocoa in early 18th century Southern Netherlands]', *Archiefkunde*, 4 (1989), pp. 75-80.

Denis, Hector, *L'alimentation et la force du travail* (Brussels, 1887).

Ducpétiaux, Edouard, 'Budgets économiques des classes ouvrières en Belgique', *Bulletin Commission Centrale des statistiques* 6 (1855), pp. 264-440.

Dupriez, Léon H. and M. Borboux, 'Indices de la consommation en Belgique de 1897 à 1933', *Bulletin Institut Sciences Économiques*, 5 (1933-4), pp. 3-39.

Eeckhout, Patricia van den, 'Onderzoek naar kwantitatieve en kwalitatieve wijzigingen in de consumptie 1840-1890 [Quantitative and qualitative analysis of consumption 1840-1890]' in J. Hannes (ed.), *Consumptiepatronen en prijsindices [Patterns of demand and price indices]* (Brussels, 1980), pp. 21-9.

Eeckhout, P. van den, '*Het 19e eeuws sociaal-economisch leven te Brussel [19th century socio-economic life in Brussels]*', (doctoral thesis, Brussels, 1980).

Eeckhout, Patricia van den and Peter Scholliers, 'De hoofdelijke voedselconsumptie in België 1831-1939 [The per-capita consumption of food in Belgium 1831-1939]', *Tijdschrift voor sociale geschiedenis*, 9 (1983), pp. 273-301.

Eeckhout, Patricia van den and Peter Scholliers, 'De hoofdelijke tarwe- en roggeconsumptie in België: een repliek [The per-capita consumption of wheat and rye: a rejoinder]', *Tijdschrift voor sociale geschiedenis*, 12 (1986), pp. 415-20.

Engel, Ernst, *Die Lebenskosten belgischer Arbeiterfamilien früher und jetzt* (Dresden, 1895).

Gadisseur, Jean, *Le produit physique de l'economie belge 1830-1913* (Brussels, 1991).

George, P. F., *Sur les aliments d'hiver qui peuvent remplacer la pomme de terre* (Brussels, 1846).

Goossens, Martine, 'Belgian agricultural output in 1812 and 1845' (unpublished ms. Leuven, 1988).

Gottschalk, Max, 'Budgets ouvriers en 1891 et en 1929', *Revue Institut de Sociologie*, 4 (1931), pp. 749-73.

Gottschalk, Max, 'Le pouvoir d'achat et la consommation des ouvriers belges à différentes époques', *Revue internationale du travail*, 19 (1932), pp. 823-41.

Henry, Albert, 'La consommation des produits alimentaires en Belgique avant et après la guerre', *Métron* (1925), pp. 134-52.

Institut Économique Agricole, *Annuaire de statistiques agricoles* (Brussels, 1988).

Julin, Armand, 'La condition des ouvriers en Belgique naguère et aujourd'hui', *Revue du travail*, 34 (1933), pp. 557-77.

Koninckx, Christiaan, 'L'alimentation et la pathologie des deficiences alimentaires dans la navigation au long cours au XVIIe siècle', *Revue histoire moderne et contemporaine*, 30 (1983), pp. 109-38.

Laurent, R., 'Une source: les archives d'octroi', *Annales E. S. C.*, 11 (1956), pp. 197-204.

Lis, Catherina and Hugo Soly, 'Food consumption in Antwerp between 1807 and 1859. A contribution to the standard of living debate', *Economic History Review*, 11 (1977), pp. 460-86.

Morsa, Denis, 'Consommation et crises de subsistance sous l'ancien régime. Permanences et discontinuités dans le budget des Ursulines de Huy 1732-1741', *Annales du Cercle Hutois des Sciences et Beaux-arts*, 5 (1978), pp. 169-201.

Moulin, Léon, 'L'Aventure des alcools et l'Europe', *Revue générale* 33 (1974-2), pp. 19-28.

Moulin, Léon, *L'Europe à table. Introduction à une psychologie des pratiques alimentaires* (Paris, Brussels, 1975).

Moulin, Léon, *L'Europe à table* (Antwerp, 1988).

Neirynck, Michel, *De loonen in Belgie sedert 1846 [Wages in Belgium since 1846]* (Antwerp, 1944).

Poelmans, Jacqueline, 'La consommation en Belgique, 1948-1958', *Cahiers économiques de Bruxelles*, 1 (1958-9), pp. 601-53.

Poelmans, Jacqueline, 'Un quart de siècle de consommation en Belgique. Evolution de la structure des dépenses' in J. Hannes (ed.), *Consumptiepatronen en prijsindices [Patterns of Demand and Price Indices]* (Brussels, 1980), pp. 61-73.

Pour une histoire d'alimentation, ed. Jean-Jacques Hémardinquer (Paris, 1970).

Preteceille, E. and J. P. Terrail, *Capitalism, Consumption and Needs* (Oxford, 1986).

Reuss, C., 'L'évolution de la consommation des boissons alcoolisées en Belgique 1900-1958', *Bulletin institut des recherches économiques et sociales*, 26 (1960), pp. 85-123.

Schokkaert, Eric and Herman van der Wee, 'A quantitative study of food consumption in the Low Countries during the sixteenth century', *Journal of European Economic History*, 17 (1988), pp. 131-58.

Scholliers, Étienne, *Loonarbeid en honger [Wage labour and hunger]* (Antwerp, 1960).

Scholliers, Étienne, 'Peilingen naar het consumptiepatroon in de pre-industriële samenleving [Consumption patterns in pre-industrial society]' in J. Hannes (ed.), *Comsumptiepatronen en prijsindices [Patterns of Demand and Price Indices]* (Brussels, 1980), pp. 9-20.

Scholliers, Peter, 'Arbeidersconsumptie in transitie 1890-1930 [Workers' consumption in transition]', in J. Hannes (ed.), *Consumptiepatronen en prijsindices [Patterns of Demand and Price Indices]* (Brussels, 1980), pp. 30-9.

Scholliers, Peter, 'Verschuivingen in het arbeidersconsumptiepatroon 1890-1930 [Shifts in the consumption patterns of workers]', *Revue Belge d'histoire contemporaine*, 13 (1982), pp. 273-312.

Scholliers, Peter, 'Regionale verschillen tussen consumptiepatronen tijdens het interbellum: een methodologische verkenning [Regional differences between patterns of consumption. Methodological notes]', *Revue Belge de philologie et d'histoire*, 60 (1982), pp. 312-38, 839-59.

Scholliers, Peter, 'Oorlog en voeding [War and food]', *Tijdschrift voor sociale geschiedenis*, 11 (1985), pp. 30-50.

Scholliers, Peter, 'Modes of production, social policy and nutrition in Belgium in the 19th and 20th centuries', in Robert W. Fogel, *Long Term Changes in Nutrition and the Standard of Living* (Berne, 1986), pp. 107-17.

Scholliers, Peter, 'Sociale ongelijkheid en voedselconsumptie sedert 1850 [Social inequality and food consumption since 1850]' in A. de Knecht (ed.) *Voeding in onze samenleving* (Alphen, Brussels, 1987), pp. 68-92.

Scholliers, Peter and Frank Daelemans, 'Standards of living and standards of health in wartime Belgium', in Richard Wall and Jay Winter (eds), *The Upheaval of War* (Cambridge, 1988), pp. 139-58.

Scholliers, Peter and Christiaan Vandenbroeke, 'The transition from traditional to modern patterns of demand in Belgium' in H. Baudet (ed.), *Consumer Behaviour and Economic Growth in the Modern Economy* (London, 1982), pp. 25-71.

Servais, Paul, 'La Consommation alimentaire à Liège au XVIIe siècle. Le cas de l'abbaye du

Val-Benoit', *Revue histoire moderne et contemporaine*, 30 (1983), pp. 84-108.
Squiller, Jean, *Traité populaire des denrées alimentaires et de l'alimentation (choix, falsification, manutention, conservation et utilisation)* (Brussels, 1863).
Statistiques économiques belges, 4 vols (Brussels, 1942, 1960, 1970, 1980).
Teuteberg, Hans J., 'Die Ernährung als Gegenstand historischer Analyse' in Hermann Kellenbenz and Hans Pohl (eds), *Historia socialis et oeconomica, Festschrift für Wolfgang Zorn zum 65. Geburtstag* (Stuttgart, 1987), pp. 180-201.
Uytven, Raymond van, 'De drankcultuur in de Zuidelijke Nederlanden tot de 18e eeuw [The culture of drinking in the Southern Netherlands]' in *Drinken in het verleden* (Leuven, 1973), pp. 15-49.
Vandenbroeke, Christiaan, 'Cultivation and consumption of the potato in the 17th and 18th Century', *Acta Historiae Neerlandica*, 5 (1971a), pp. 15-39.
Vandenbroeke, Christiaan, 'Bijdrage tot de studie van de voeding en de lonen van zeelui tijdens de tweede helft van de 18e eeuw [Nutrition and wages of sailors during the second half of the 18th century]', *Tijdschrift sociale wetenschappen*, 16 (1971b), pp. 403-24.
Vandenbroeke, Christiaan, *Agriculture et alimentation dans les Pays-Bas autrichiens* (Ghent-Louvain, 1975a).
Vandenbroeke, Christiaan, 'L'alimentation à Gand pendant la première moitié du XIXe siècle', *Annales E.S.C.*, 30 (1975b), pp. 584-91.
Vandenbroeke, Christiaan, 'Evolutie van het wijnverbruik te Gent (14e-19e eeuw) [Development of wine consumption in Ghent]' in *Album Charles Verlinden* (Gent, 1975c), pp. 369-411.
Vandenbroeke, Christiaan, 'Kwantitatieve en kwalitatieve aspecten van het vleesverbruik in Vlaanderen [Quantitative and qualitative aspects of meat consumption in Flanders]', *Tijdschrift voor sociale geschiedenis*, 9 (1983), pp. 221-57.
Wee, Herman van der, 'Voeding en dieet in het Ancien régime [Food and nutrition in the ancien régime]', *Spiegel Historiael*, 1 (1966), pp. 94-101.
Yante, Jean-Marie, 'Grains et vins des terroirs mosellans de Remich et Grevenmacher (XVe-XVIIe siècles)', *Revue belge philologie et histoire*, 63 (1985), pp. 272-309.

Addendum

Following the macro-economic approach, represented by Blomme (1986) and Goossens (1988), Geert Bekaert published a paper on 'Caloric consumption in industrializing Belgium' (in *Journal of Economic History*, vol. 51, (1991), pp. 633-655). The author found that the total supply of calories remained unchanged in Belgium during the first half of the 19th century, thus challenging accounts of an absolute pauperization, represented e.g. by Lis and Soly (1977), but stressing the fact that social inequality grew. This article was published after this survey was written and could therefore not be incorporated.

6 The history of diet as a part of the *vie matérielle* in France

Eva Barlösius

Diet research in France in the 1960s and 1970s viewed the history of nutrition primarily from the standpoint of the *vie matérielle*. It can only be recorded and interpreted within the theory and the tradition of the *Annales*, which characterizes its advantages and disadvantages. The determination of its subject and its limitations, as well as the formulation of its problems and questions, derive fundamentally from the concept of the *nouvelle histoire*, though the influences were no longer so direct in the 1980s.[1] This paper concentrates on this period, which was of great significance for historical diet research, and aims to demonstrate some of the changes in the approach to the history of eating and drinking.

In 1961 a systematic treatment of the history of nutrition was initiated through Braudel's 'Enquête' on the subject 'Vie matérielle et les comportements biologiques' in the journal *Annales E.S.C.* In this 'Enquête' diet became an independent subject of the science of history.[2] Braudel thus fulfilled a task first taken on by Lucien Febvre.[3] Diet previously had the status of a secondary subject, probably much as in other countries. It was regarded as suitable for illustrating general developments of history, such as rising cereal prices. The 'Enquête' made the history of nutrition itself a central part of history. A lot of essays and some *grandes thèses*, – for example, Louis Stouff's about diet in Provence in the 14th and 15th centuries – are dedicated to it.[4]

With the 'Enquête' on the *vie matérielle* Braudel deliberately referred to Marc Bloch's preceding 'Enquête' on *noblesse* and to Lucien Febvre's about techniques. This method was intended to offer the chance to integrate other sciences and foreign colleagues into a collective project. In particular, the subject of 'La vie matérielle et les comportements biologiques', which implies a great variety of aspects usually treated in different sciences, was intended to present the possibility of joining them together in a 'science des sciences de l'homme'.[5] There is no doubt that problems, methods and aims of the history of nutrition were strictly defined and collectively discussed with the help of the 'Enquête'. This concentrated joint research on a subject is impressive for external observers and readers, especially because the internal conflicts and debates between the scholars remain invisible to them.[6]

The history of diet as a part of the vie matérielle

In the following I will try to pursue three intentions at the same time. I hope to succeed in indicating each of them clearly.

1. I will describe the content and chronology of the history of nutrition by outlining the questions, methods and results of some key works.
2. It seems to be necessary to demonstrate the direct attachment of the history of nutrition to the *nouvelle histoire* and to analyse the changing and displacement of questions and methods on this basis.
3. The initial effect the 'Enquête' on the *vie matérielle* had on the history of nutrition entailed a certain limitation of the subject, and many aspects of this *phénomen totale* of diet were left out.[7] It was a theoretical view to regard food and drink as a part of the *vie matérielle*, a view which could hardly integrate other perspectives like Lévi-Strauss's and Roland Barthes's analyses, even if they were near to, or a part of the 'Enquête'.

In the first *bulletin* of the 'Enquête' Braudel presented a comprehensive and wide-ranging concept of the *vie matérielle*, comprising five spheres of life: diet, habitation and clothing, standard of living, techniques and biological realities.[8] These spheres of life have in common the fact that they are closely related to the physical needs and the natural possibilities of man.

The *vie matérielle* forms an unconscious infrastructure, in so far as its satisfaction and shaping is the basis of the *courte durée*. Braudel presumed the material basis of life to be long-lasting structures (*longue durée*). They block, disturb and determine the *courte durée* because they limit historical development. In 1959 he was already talking about the *longue durée* in his popular essay 'Histoire et sciences sociales. La longue durée'. He characterizes the *longue durée* as the core of the subject, which is scientifically richer than its scintillating surface and which could become a common focus of research for social and historical sciences.[9] On the basis of his theoretically formulated intention the 'Enquête' and its numerous *bulletins* are the realization, especially since Braudel had already defined the basic ideas for the common work of the different individual sciences in the cited articles: 'Mathématisation réductions à l'espace, longue durée'.[10] These ideas were fulfilled or at least aspired to in most of the treatises concerning the *vie matérielle*.

Referring directly to Braudel's introduction to the 'Enquête', Robert Philippe focused the subject of the inquiry on the sphere of diet. He demanded 'Commençons par l'histoire de l'alimentation' because this comprises such a great area which could open a lot of useful paths of research.[11] The most important argument for the choice of researching the sphere of life concerning food and drink was surely that 'l'histoire alimentation sous-tend toute l'histoire des hommes'.[12] The satisfaction of this fundamental need was indispensable, whereby it was able to limit and affect historical development.

Indeed, 15 of the 18 *bulletins* which appeared from 1961 to 1969 were devoted to the subject of diet, while the other sectors of life were reduced to marginal topics. This fact raises the question why it was just the history of nutrition which seemed to be suitable to exemplify the main theoretical arguments of the *nouvelle histoire* and why secondary importance was ascribed to the other sectors of life of the *vie matérielle*.

It is obvious that historians thought that in the modern science of physiological nutrition they had ideal instruments at their disposal for reconstructing the history of nutrition quantitatively because the new physiological methods rendered measurable results concerning whether a given group of people had had enough and well-balanced nutrition in the past. They presumed that the two variables, the calories and the nutritive value, would offer a measure which could be adapted to the whole history of food and drink. In this way Braudel's desire for quantification and mathematization had become easily practicable, and the obstacles and limits which nutrition had presented to the *courte durée* could be calculated in dividing the naturally necessary foodstuffs by the historically available ones. To write about the history of diet from the perspective of bodily necessities doubtless corresponds to the fact that the satisfaction of this fundamental need has been threatened in the past and even today by hunger and lack of food.

In pursuit of this interest it was necessary to continue with Bloch's fundamental differentiation of two systems of diet and to develop it so that it could be used to integrate historical and empirical research. In 1954 Bloch noticed that it was impossible to imagine previous societies without the antithesis 'le bas peuple des campagnes en état de perpétuelle sousalimentation, les riches suralimentés'.[13] Philippe continued this differentiation and characterized the diet of the lower classes as monotonous because it was mainly based on one type of food, mostly cereals such as rye, wheat or rice. In contrast, the diet of the dominant classes was varied and, because of its high cost, only available to privileged people.

Most historians agreed that it was the monotonous nutrition of the majority which had to be researched first. This kind of nutrition was largely determined by cyclical structures of *longue durée* such as biological, geographical and climatic conditions. The tables of the higher social classes only represent processes and structures of *courte durée*. Historical aspects of diet, which are subject to a form of *vraie longue durée* and which Braudel presented in the second *bulletin*, were already demonstrated in his book *La Méditérranée*.[14] There he regarded the biological, geographical and climatic conditions and relations as structures which were relatively independent from man and to which man had to adapt. Claudia Honegger made the criticism that Braudel's structures became cases of *longue durée* where people sit bound like prisoners. This illustrates the impression that in this case history is not interpreted as a process of man appropriating nature, but vice versa.[15]

The reception of the physiology of nutrition made bodily needs the main subject of the history of food. Philippe summarized its problems as follows: 'De quelles manières se combinent les éléments nutritifs et établissent, ou non, par suite, des équilibres biologiques propres à chaque société, variés à chaque groupe'.[16] The lowest limit of a satisfactory supply of food is marked by bodily deficiencies, which are produced by an insufficient supply of calories or by an imbalance of nutritional components. Philippe immediately used this method of the history of nutrition in an *opération pilote*. His proposed instruments are found in Lavoisier's writing about the situation of diet just before the revolution: 'donc le Parisien à la veille des 1789 mangeait bien'.[17] He reached this conclusion by dividing the total consumption of food according to Lavoisier by the estimated number of population. The next step was to calculate the total calorie content of the food available and to take into account the relative division of nutrition. Philippe compared these with the values established by nutritional physiology.

In the first *bulletin* Frank Spooner further systematized this method.[18] He intended to design 'une méthode uniforme de calcul qui permette les comparisions entre regimes alimentaires, dans le temps et dans l'espace'.[19] Therefore, to calculate their calorie values and nutritional distribution, he proposed to divide foodstuffs into four groups: cereals; meat and fish; dairy products and fats; and beverages. Only in this way could the physiological nutritional value of certain foodstuffs be compared.

It is surprising how uncritically the historians of diet accepted the results of the physiology of nutrition. They did not offer the criticism that these results, of course, do not have the character of natural laws, but that they always reflect the position and the interests of this discipline's research.[20] It was an undue simplification to measure the value of a foodstuff by its nutritious substances and calories, as Aymard said in 1975, because measurable deficiency symptoms always result from a deficiency of vitamins and minerals.[21] The fact that people do not eat raw food but prepared meals, not grains but bread, was completely neglected, although the composition of physiological nutrition undergoes essential changes through food preparation.

This outline of the history of nutrition was limited to statistically measurable material and biological factors of food and drink, and represented the results of a quantifying history. Furthermore, it succeeded in relating the sphere of life concerning food and drink to the question of sufficient supply of foodstuffs; a question which was very important for most people in the past, and besides, it was equipped with a criterion to judge the history of nutrition. The disadvantage of this concept of the history of nutrition was that it accepted uncritically the reference values of dietetics and thereby also tended to reduce eating and drinking to the physical reproduction function. Historical diet research therefore missed an opportunity to develop its own historical approach independent of that of natural science.

Historians devoted themselves to preliminary historical studies concerning the concept of the history of nutrition and neglected other traditions. With regard to the first phase, which began with the 'Enquête' and lasted until about 1980, it is noticeable that the works concerning the 'histoire de l'alimentation' were taken into consideration and partly used as a basis, whereas those concentrating on the 'histoire de la gastronomie ou la cuisine' were at first consciously ignored. Brillat-Savarin's work, *Physiologie du Goût*, Grimod de la Reynière's writings, Briffault's work on cuisine in mid-19th century Paris and also the works of Gottschalk and Guégan in the mid-20th century which are thematically very similar, belong to the latter group.[22] The history of the art of cooking and gastronomy, which is the basis of the reputation of French cuisine as a whole and which is probably first associated with food and drink in France, was regarded as negligible because it only elucidated the dietary patterns of some privileged people and only represented processes of *courte durée*.

In more general writings about the 'histoire de l'alimentation', aspects of the production of foodstuffs were described without limitation to the *grande cuisine*. One frequently mentioned work was the volume *Études d'histoire générale. Histoire de l'alimentation* by L. Bourdeau.[23] It can be compared to Alfred Lichtenfelt's *Die Geschichte der Ernährung* and Kurt Hintze's *Geographie und Geschichte der Ernährung*,[24] which are mentioned in other contributions to this volume, especially Chapter 7. Nevertheless, it was impossible to base a scientific work upon one of these books.[25] Adam Maurizio's *Die Geschichte der Pflanzennahrung von den Urzeiten bis zur Gegenwart* of 1927, which was translated into French in 1932, was referred to, especially by Braudel, in order to describe the history of plants.[26]

There were two German essays about changes in the consumption and the prices of meat since the end of the Middle Ages which were preliminary studies and which the food historians discussed explicitly: Gustav Schmoller's essay 'Die historische Entwicklung des Fleischkonsums, sowie die Vieh- und Fleischpreise in Deutschland' of 1871 and Wilhelm Abel's work 'Wandlungen des Fleischverbrauchs und der Fleischversorgung in Deutschland seit dem ausgehenden Mittelalter' of 1937.[27] But Abel's more significant writings explaining agrarian crises and famines were also included.[28] In the third *bulletin* Robert Mandrou presented Schmoller's and Abel's essays with the question 'Théorie ou hypothèse du travail?' and so brought them within the reach of a bigger audience.[29]

In his essay, Schmoller assumes widespread keeping of livestock and high consumption of meat until the 15th century.[30] He shows a direct relation between the shortage of meat in the following century and the rise in meat and cattle prices. He explains this rise in prices as due to the sharp increase of population which the agrarian production could not keep up with in comparison to the relative stagnation in the beginning of the 15th century.[31] Consequently, Schmoller explains the causes of the *grande crise* by the population growth which the production of food could not keep up with.

Abel mainly studied the fluctuations in grain prices. He demonstrated that the big crisis at the end of the Middle Ages had been caused by an agrarian crisis and that therefore Bloch's explanations such as the devastation of the Hundred Years' War or the counterfeiting of coins were not correct. In 1980 Abel again defined the term 'agrarian crisis', summarizing: 'Unter Agrarkrise des Spätmittelalters versteht man das langfristige Missverhältnis zwischen den Erlös- und Kostenpreisen des Landbaues, den Rückgang des Getreidebaues ... ' in combination with devastation.[32] In the 1930s Ernest Labrousse also developed a theory of crises in France. As Honegger writes, its influence on methodology can hardly be overestimated.[33] The reception of his theory of crises led to the breakthrough of 'cyclical history' in the *Annales*. Labrousse's thesis was that the development of the economic situation in the pre-industrial age was mainly determined by crop failures.[34] This thesis motivated Le Roy Ladurie to conduct extensive climate studies to examine whether the agrarian crises of the late Middle Ages were due to climatic fluctuations.

Having briefly described the more general and introductory questions of the 'Enquête', I will now try to summarize the different perspectives and results of research. This is necessary because the historical research in nutrition has not developed as homogeneously as one might assume by regarding the appeals to the 'Enquête', the first essays and the way in which large and heterogeneous subjects were divided.

First some words about the most important publications containing the essays on historical nutrition research. Most of them appeared in the *bulletins* of the 'Enquête' of the *Annales E.S.C.* until 1969 and were later separately published under the column 'savoir-faire-savoir-vivre'. In addition, two supplements to the *Annales* about the history of nutrition were published. The first had the title *Pour une histoire de l'alimentation*, written by Jean-Jacques Hémardinquer who essentially supported the 'Enquête' and often wrote inspiring essays.[35]

Many essays in the *bulletins* were reprinted in this supplement and some new ones were included. The second supplement of the *Annales*, *Histoire de la consommation*, appeared in 1975. It contained a selection of lectures which were held at the Congrès National des Historiens Économistes Français in 1973. They remained within the scientific tradition of the supplement. In addition, there are three outstanding congress reports. The first of these congresses on the theme *Les problèmes de l'alimentation* took place in 1968, the second, in Tours in 1979, had as its subject *Pratiques et discours alimentaires à la Renaissance*.[36] These two reports were mainly written by those authors who had also contributed to the 'Enquête'. The third congress, with the topic *Manger et boire au Moyen Age* already reflects the shift of emphasis from the 'histoire de l'alimentation' to the 'histoire de la cuisine'.[37]

In the following I will rely on the differentiations, essentially in agreement with each other, made by Jacques Revel, Jean-Jacques Hémardinquer and Maurice Aymard between the different subjects of the research of nutrition and its methods.[38] They distinguish between three perspectives: an economic and historical agrarian view with emphasis on agrarian and starvation crises; a quantitative reconstruction of the consumption of food with a view to the physiology of diet; a psycho-sociological consideration of food and drink. I add a fourth one, which cannot be traced back to the other three perspectives and in which a relatively independent view has been developed. Its point of departure is Jean-Louis Flandrin, who began to write the history of food and drink as 'histoire du goût' in the early 1980s.

The first group of historians is interested in the relationship between the density of population and the food produced. They want to analyse hunger crises and search for their causes in crop failures caused by the climate or in deficiency crises produced by the demographic situation.[39] The latter arises if the available techniques are not adequate for feeding a growing population. In their models of explanation for agrarian crises they refer critically to the preliminary studies of Labrousse, Schmoller and Abel, and examine them empirically. Aymard characterized the perspective of research as 'une approche macroéconomique, qui cherchait à atteindre ou de moins à encadrer statistiquement, par le détour de la consommation, de la population, du commerce extérieur et des prix, l'impossible production'.[40] The emphasis of food history was on agriculture, and research was not limited to the history of nutrition but searched for the 'naissance de capitalisme' as Le Roy Ladurie wrote in his book, *Les Paysans de Languedoc*.[41]

It mostly concerns regional studies in which agrarian production and its prices are reconstructed for a certain period. Materials are for instance, the *compoix*, as for Roy Ladurie, or account-books, as for Stouff. In these investigations the preferred timespan is from the 15th to the 18th century because the crises which are considered are doubtlessly pre-industrial agrarian crises. The production and prices of cereals and meat are often related to one another. Until the 19th century cereals were the main foodstuff and meat was a sign of prosperity and wealth because stock-farming did not exploit available methods of providing food. 'The choice between cereals and meat depends on the number of people', Braudel emphasized, because agriculture is ten to twenty times superior to stock-farming according to calorific counts.[42]

Work on the history of cultivated plants such as wheat, rice and corn are closely related to this subject. Work on these plants, which were the main foodstuff for the lower social classes, is concerned with the most important part of nutrition.

I would like to consider some of this work in detail. Le Roy Ladurie's famous work about *Les Paysans de Languedoc* (1966) was not directly related to the 'Enquête', but it has occupied a key position in the French nutrition research as well as in the whole *nouvelle histoire*. Le Roy Ladurie uses quantitative methods to describe an agrarian cycle for the Languedoc area lasting from the end of the 15th to the beginning of the 18th century. He adopts the Malthusian model of the hypothesis whereby changes in demographic structure are responsible for agrarian crises, because agricultural production does not increase in step with population increases. With this view he discarded the assumption that climate changes were the cause of agrarian crises as they would result in crop-failures of short duration. He subdivides the agricultural cycle into three phases: *étiage*, *essor* and *maturité*. This book has become a model because, as Iggers puts it, 'here perhaps for the first time a serious attempt has been made to write a history of material culture' called for by Braudel.[43]

The 'grande thèse' *Ravitaillement et alimentation en Provence aux XIVe et XVe siècles* written by Louis Stouff in 1970 is surely the most extensive and the most detailed regional study. In the introduction Stouff explains that he read the appeal of Braudel and Philippe some days after he had heard of the existence of the account-books of the Bishop of Arles and some time before he found the books of the butcher of Carpentras. This material goes back to the 15th century and it provided an opportunity to examine the production and the consumption of meat in the period of the *grande crise* and to consider the thesis of Schmoller and Abel in that light.

The historians of the second group adopted the concept of quantitative examination of the available food in calories and nutritive value, which had been proposed by Philippe and Spooner. They used records of town taxes, accounts of hospitals, monasteries and councils as their material. A large part of these works is concerned with the rations of sailors and workers and the food supplies of prisons and the army. In his introduction to the volume *Pour une histoire de l'alimentation*, Hémardinquer underlined this part of the historical research of diet as the 'plus originale et la plus austère, n'aura pas été sans retentissement'.[44] As the method of working has already been described in detail above, it is sufficient now to name the complex of subjects and the results and to discuss the criticism of this direction of research, particularly as it was formulated by Aymard.

The first works concentrated on isolated or fixed groups which were fed together, that is, on the earliest organization of common food supply. The demand for more involvement with the nutrition of the lower social classes and the consequences of the social differences had therefore been thrust into the background at first. The first results also seem quite inadequate; an example of this is Frederic C. Lane's examination of the food supply of Venetian sailors on board a ship at the beginning of the 15th century. He came to the conclusion that 'la nourriture à bord était largement suffisante'.[45] Here, the obvious question should have been asked why there were troubles and complaints again and again if the supply on board was sufficient. To answer this question, another theoretical approach would have been necessary – an approach which does not reduce the history of food and drink to the scientific perspective of the supply of nutritive values, but which regards the selection and the preparation of meals as a process in which first of all social and psychological motives become visible. Other examinations of the food supply of the upper social classes demonstrate the limitations of this concept. Works are in existence describing the households of ambassadors and that of Cardinal Mazarin. They reached astounding conclusions: every member of these households must have consumed 7000–8000 calories a day.[46]

In his essay 'Pour l'histoire de l'alimentation: quelques remarques de méthode', Aymard criticizes the fact that the questions posed by this direction of French nutrition research were too simple, 'les plus banales fort parfois pietiner l'enquête'.[47] One problem was that they took the physiological nutrition optimum established by the FAO/WHO as a status quo and used it as a measure. This was attained in industrial countries, but only seldom in the past and even today not yet in most non-industrial areas. The importance of minerals studied in connection with diseases of nutrition in the 19th century was underestimated. In the same volume Aymard published a study together with H. Bresc about 'Nourritures et consommation en Sicilie entre XIVe et XVIIIe siècles'.[48] In this essay the authors led their research in two main directions which can be transferred to other regions and periods. First, they determined the available foodstuffs for the whole population. Afterwards they examined the nutrition of certain limited and fixed groups.

This direction of historical nutrition research, which was regarded as the most original pursued by the 'Enquête' on the *vie matérielle*, has rapidly lost its importance since the special edition *Histoire de la consommation*, and it only played a subordinate or supplementary role in the 1980s.

The psycho-social orientation of historical nutrition research can be understood as a counter-movement to this kind of research. It was interested in the quality of the process of eating and drinking rather than in the quantity of food consumed. It was lost in the great number of writings of the other two directions, or at least it remained remarkably unnoticed in the research of nutrition which had been constructed as a collective enterprise. Possibly this was because the psycho-socially orientated group did not want to become merely a simple supplement to the quantitative research of nutrition. We can say that it differed essentially from this other group because its scientific starting-point was not the physical need for food, but the social and cultural development of food and drink. Therefore its subjects are the psycho-social dimensions of food and drink, the process of eating and drinking, and not the physical dimensions, the foodstuffs themselves.

The two most important representatives of this direction were Jean-Paul Aron and Roland Barthes, who had already presented their scientific thematization of this sphere of life in the third *bulletin*. This remained Roland Barthes's only contribution to the 'Enquête' which was not adopted by historical nutrition research, but which has found recognition within sociology.[49] In his essay 'Pour une psycho-sociologie de l'alimentation contemporaine' Barthes disclosed pictures and ideas which are connected with the foods and meals of the nutrition of today. On the one hand food and drink were physical needs, but on the other hand the particular character of their satisfaction was always structured by meanings and signs which determine the selection and the preparation of the meals. As the physical needs lose importance in modern society, the symbolic character of food and drink becomes more and more predominant.

The main representative of the structuralistic research of nutrition, Lévi-Strauss, whose 'triangle culinaire' and research about 'L'origine des manières de table' have become very well known in the social sciences, did not take part in the 'Enquête', although he often collaborated in the theoretical discussions of the *Annales E.S.C.*[50] In his essay 'Histoire et sciences sociales', already mentioned above, Braudel remarked that Lévi-Strauss 'reduced the language of cuisine to Gusteme just for the fun of it'.[51] Barthes's contribution to the subject of food and drink can be regarded as a 'passing interest', whereas nutrition was a central topic of research for Jean-Paul Aron. His first essay was published in the third *bulletin*. He became popular with his book, *Le mangeur du XIXe siècle*, which led to the development of the *grande cuisine*.[52] Aron's central figure is the eater himself, whose changing attitude to food and drink led to the development of a 'sensibilité alimentaire'. With this history of mentalité Aron succeeds in breaking from the traditional *courte durée*, which writes the history of the *grande cuisine* as a succession of famous cooks.

At the beginning of the 1980s a new direction of historical nutrition research developed around Flandrin. This differs in at least two ways from the themes and methods of historical work up to this time. First, it departed from the school of thought which regarded the history of nutrition as part of the *vie matérielle* in the centre of which were the available foodstuffs, as this placed limitations on historical development, and concentrated on the history of cooking the prepared foodstuffs. Second, eating and drinking were no longer regarded as bodily necessities with physiological nutritional aspects. Interpretation now centred on the meals eaten and drunk, whereby changes were also seen as subject to sensual and aesthetic criteria.

Like Pierre Bourdieu in *La Distinction*, Flandrin differentiates between bodily necessity – 'la nécessité' – and the cultural aspect of preparation – 'le goût'. Already in his first contribution to the *Annales*, 'Le goût et la nécessité: sur l'usage des graisses', he introduced what was for himself the basic difference: 'Dans le comportement alimentaire des peuples comme celui des individus, il faut distinguer la part du goût et la part de la nécessité.'[53] The selection and the preparation of meals, the changes in cooking cannot be traced back directly to bodily factors of nutrition. They are subject to a history of taste.

Flandrin sees the historical and social point at which the *bon goût* became important for the selection and the preparation of food in the development of the aristocratic *haute cuisine* from the 17th to the 18th century. Since the 17th century taste had attained a new importance in the sphere of life concerning food and drink and in other domains of life as well. Materials which show this change of habits in cooking are cookery-books, which had been left relatively untouched within the historical research of the 'Enquête', and the changing methods of combining the ingredients leading to conclusions as to changes in taste. As far as the quantitative examination of ingredients is concerned, this new concept of historical diet research remained within the tradition of the 'Enquête'.

A second centre of interest was the question when regional differences in taste and cooking developed and how to examine these. As regional cookery-books and manuscripts hardly exist up to the 16th century, at least in France, and as those which do exist cannot be definitely allocated to a place or period, Flandrin relies on travel books and reports. Together with Mary and Philipp Hyman, he discussed the frequently proposed thesis that cooking in Europe in the Middle Ages had been basically uniform.[54]

By making the cultural implications of certain diets the centre of interest, this direction has broken the theoretical limits of the *vie matérielle* and rendered the prepared meal a subject of research. Nevertheless, the way of thinking of the 'histoire du goût' has not yet been developed theoretically far enough to be used to trace cultural and social motives and orientations, which are the basis of the changes in taste. Social distinction, which is said to be a motive for the changes in taste in aristocratic cuisine, does not seem to be transferable to the various regional cuisines and does not explain the changes in taste in bourgeois cuisine. The task of the theoretical characterization of the *vie matérielle* through the socio-cultural dimension of food and drink makes a sociological theorization of food and drink of vital importance as this is the only way to reconstruct the cultural and sociological motives and orientations which materialize in the meals themselves and the methods of cooking.

References

1 In his idea of the concept of the *nouvelle histoire* Le Goff regards 'culture matérielle' as one of the key themes (see Le Goff *et al.* (1978), p.9). There is at present no French work which gives a comprehensive survey of historical nutrition research and its results. I would expressly mention Thomas Hamelmann's (1989) thesis whose intention was to 'fill this

gap and to describe the development which historical research into nutrition in France has gone through'.
2 See Braudel (1961a), pp. 421–4.
3 See Revel (1978), p. 25.
4 Stouff (1970).
5 See Braudel (1961a), pp. 421–4. This intention of Braudel's to bring together the various different cultural and social sciences and also to involve foreign colleagues is also expressed in the name of the scientific coordination centre 'Maison science de l'homme' which he founded in 1970. An example of the collaboration with other fields of research is the idea of the 'Enquête sur le sel dans l'histoire' (Le Goff, 1961, pp. 959–61). The results of this inquiry are summarized in Hocquet (1974), p. 393–424; Hocquet (1978–9); Hocquet (1984); Bergier (1982).
6 Iggers (1975); Iggers (1978).
7 This expression 'phénomén totale' originates from the French sociologist Marcel Mauss.
8 Braudel (1961b), p. 547.
9 Braudel (1958), pp.58, 60.
10 Ibid., p. 83. The quantification of the historical method became established in the *Annales* in the 1960s. See Bloch *et al.*, (1977).
11 *Pour une histoire* (1970).
12 Philippe (1961a), pp. 549–52.
13 Bloch (1970), pp. 40–5.
14 See the first part of Braudel (1949).
15 Bloch *et al.*, (1977), p.124.
16 Philippe (1961a), p. 551.
17 Philippe (1961b), p. 565.
18 Spooner (1961), pp. 568–74. Spooner had already collaborated with Braudel in 1955 on 'Les métaux monétaires et l'économie du XVIe siècle' (Braudel and Spooner (1955), pp. 233–64).
19 Spooner (1961), p. 558.
20 This is, for example, shown in the differences between the values laid down by the Deutsche Gesellschaft für Ernährung (DGE [German Society for Nutrition]) and the World Health Organization (WHO). The roughage debate is even more illuminating. Even in the 1970s roughage was regarded as superfluous as nutritional science only considered the foodstuffs digested. Today it is regarded as an important and necessary accompaniment to a healthy diet.
21 See Aymard (1979), pp. 431–44.
22 Brillat-Savarin (1825); Grimod de la Reyniere (1803–12); Guégan (1934); Gottschalk (1948); Briffault (1946).
23 Bourdeau (1894).
24 Lichtenfelt (1913); Hintze (1934).
25 Teuteberg (1987), pp. 181–202.
26 Maurizio (1927).
27 Schmoller (1871), pp. 284–362; Abel (1937), pp. 411–52.
28 Abel (1974); Abel (1973).
29 Mandrou (1961), pp. 965–71.
30 Schmoller (1871), p. 302.
31 Schmoller (1871), p. 343.
32 Abel (1980), p. 19.

33 See Bloch et al., (1977), p. 26.
34 See Abel (1978), p. 22. This thesis motivated Le Roy Ladurie (1967), among others, to conduct his extensive climate studies to examine whether the agrarian crises in the late Middle Ages were due to climate fluctuations.
35 *Pour une histoire de l'alimentation* (1970). Numerous essays on nutritional history have appeared in the *Cahiers des Annales* and *Revue d'histoire moderne et contemporaine*.
36 *Pratiques et discours* (1982).
37 Manger et boire (1984).
38 Revel (1978); *Pour une histoire de l'alimentation* (1970); Aymard (1975).
39 Hémardinquer collected the investigations of this group under the heading 'Études Regions. Villes et Campagnes' and in the above mentioned congress report of 1968 they are entitled 'Chertes et crises de subsistance'.
40 Aymard (1975), p. 481.
41 Le Roy Ladurie (1966).
42 Braudel (1949).
43 Iggers (1978), p. 77.
44 *Pour une histoire de l'alimentation* (1970), p. 11.
45 Lane (1963), pp. 133-8.
46 See Couperie (1963), pp. 1133-41.
47 Aymard (1979), p. 431.
48 Aymard and Bresc (1975), pp. 592-600.
49 This is shown by the fact that his works are frequently quoted and have been translated into German.
50 Lévi-Strauss (1969), pp. 19-26; Lévi-Strauss (1968).
51 Braudel (1958).
52 Aron (1973).
53 Flandrin (1983b), p. 369.
54 Mennell (1985), for example, is of the same opinion.

Literature

Abel, Wilhelm, 'Wandlungen des Fleischverbrauchs und der Fleischversorgung in Deutschland seit dem ausgehenden Mittelalter, *Berichte über Landwirtschaft*, 22 (1937), no. 3, pp. 411-52.
Abel, Wilhelm, *Massenarmut und Hungerkrisen im vorindustriellen Europa* (Hamburg, Berlin, 1974).
Abel, Wilhelm, *Agrarkrisen und Agrarkonjunktur* (3rd rev. edn, Hamburg, Berlin, 1978).
Abel, Wilhelm, *Strukturen und Krisen der mittelalterlichen Wirtschaft* (Stuttgart, New York, 1980).
Actes du 93ᵉ Congrès national des Sociétés savantes, Vol. 1: *Les problèmes de l'alimentation*, Vol. 2: *Histoire institutionelle religieuse, sociale et politique* (Tours, 1968).
Aliments et société (Paris, 1984).
André, Jacques, *L'Alimentation et la cuisine à Rome* (Paris, 1981).
Andries, Lise, 'Cuisine et littérature populaire', *18e siècle*, 15 (1983), pp. 33-52.
Aron, Jean-Paul, 'Biologie et alimentation au XVIIIe siècle et au début du XIXe siècle', *Annales E.S.C.*, 16 (1961), pp. 971-7.
Aron, Jean-Paul, *Essai sur la sensibilité alimentaire à Paris au 19e siècle* (Paris, 1967).

Aron, Jean-Paul, *Le mangeur du XIXe siècle* (Paris, 1973).
Aron, Jean-Paul, 'Sur les consommations arivées à Paris dans la deuxième moitié du XIXe siècle', *Annales E.S.C.*, 30 (1975), pp. 553–63.
Ashtor, E., 'Essai sur l'alimentation des diverses classes sociales dans l'occident médieval' (Bulletin no.16), *Annales E.S.C.*, 23 (1968), pp. 1017–53.
Audoin-Rouzeau, Frédérique, 'Medieval and early modern butchery: evidence from the monastery of Charité-sur-Loire (Nièvre)', *Food & Foodways*, 2 (1987), pp. 31–48.
Aymard, Maurice, 'The "Annales" and French historiography (1929–1979)', *Journal of European Economic History*, 1 (1972), pp. 491–510.
Aymard, Maurice, 'The history of nutrition and economic history', *Journal of European History*, 2 (1973), pp. 207–19.
Aymard, Maurice, 'Pour l'histoire de l'alimentation: quelques remarques de méthode', *Annales E.S.C.*, 30 (1979), pp. 431–44.
Aymard, Maurice, 'Dietary changes in Europe from the 16th to 20th century, with particular reference to France and Italy', in Henri Baudet and Henk van der Meulen (eds), *Consumer Behaviour and Economic Growth in Modern Economy* (London, Canberra, 1982), pp. 111–29.
Aymard, Maurice and H. Bresc, 'Nourritures et consommation en Sicilie entre XIVe et XVIIe siècles', *Annales E.S.C.*, 30 (1975), pp. 592–600.
Aymard, Maurice, Jean-Louis Flandrin and Steven L. Kaplan, 'French Editorial', *Food & Foodways*, 1 (1985), pp. iii–v.
Bahloul, Joelle, 'Nourritures de l'altérité: le double langage des juifs algériens en France', *Annales E.S.C.*, 38 (1983), pp. 325–40.
Barthes, Roland, 'Pour une psycho-sociologie de l'alimentation contemporaine' (Bulletin no.3), *Annales E.S.C.*, 18 (1961), pp. 977–86.
Baulant, Micheline, 'Niveaux de vies paysans autour de Meaux en 1700-1750', *Annales E.S.C.*, 30 (1975), pp. 505–19.
Benassar, Bartholomé, 'L'alimentation d'une ville espagnole au XVIe siècle. Quelques données sur les approvisionnements et la consommation de Valladolid' (Bulletin no.2), *Annales E.S.C.*, 6 (1961), pp. 728–40.
Bennassar, Bartholomé and J. Goy, 'Consommation alimentaire', *Annales E.S.C.*, 30 (1975), pp. 402–29.
Bergier, Jean-François, *Une histoire du sel* (Fribourg, Switzerland, 1982).
Bernard, René Jean, 'L'alimentation paysanne en Gévaudan au XVIIIe siècle', *Annales E.S.C.*, 24 (1969), pp. 1449–63.
Bertin, Jacques and Jean-Jacques Hémardinquer, 'Pour un atlas d'histoire de la vie matérielle: Cartes historiques des cultures vivières', *Annales E.S.C.*, 21 (1966), pp. 1012–25.
Bertin, Jacques *et al.* (eds), *Atlas des cultures vivières* (Paris, 1971).
Beutler, Corinna, 'Un chapitre de la sensibilité collective: la littérature agricole en Europe continentale au XVIe siècle', *Annales E.S.C.*, 28 (1973), pp. 1280–301.
Bloch, Marc, 'Les Aliments de l'ancienne France' in Jean-Jacques Hémardinquer (ed.), *Pour une histoire de l'alimentation* (Paris, 1970), pp. 231–5.
Bloch, M. *et al.*, *Schrift und Materie der Geschichte. Vorschläge zur systematischen Aneignung historischer Prozesse*, ed. Claudia Honegger (Frankfurt, 1977).
Blond, Georges and Germaine Blond, *Festins de tous les temps: Histoire pittoresque de notre alimentation* (Paris, 1976).
Bolens, Lucie, 'Pain quotidien et pain de disette dans l'Espagne muselmane', *Annales E.S.C.*, 35 (1980), pp. 462–76.

Bonnet, Jean-Claude, 'Le système du repas et de la cuisine chez Rousseau', *Poétique*, 6 (1975), no. 22, pp. 244–67.
Bonnet, Jean-Claude, 'Le réseau culinaire dans l'Encyclopédie', *Annales E.S.C.*, 31 (1976), pp. 891–914.
Bonnet, Jean-Claude, 'Les manuels de cuisine', *18e siècle*, 15 (1983), pp. 53–64.
Bonnet, Jean-Claude, 'L'écriture gourmande de Grimod de la Reynière', *L'Histoire*, 3 (1986), pp. 83–8.
Bourdeau, L., *Études d'histoire générale. Histoire de l'alimentation* (Paris, 1894).
Braudel, Fernand, *La Méditéranée et le monde méditéréen à l'époque de Philippe* (Paris, 1949).
Braudel, Fernand, 'Histoire et sciences sociales: La longue durée', *Annales E.S.C.*, 13 (1958), pp. 725–53.
Braudel, Fernand, 'Retour aux enquêtes', *Annales E.S.C.*, 16 (1961a) pp. 421–4.
Braudel, Fernand, 'Vie matérielle et comportements biologiques', (Bulletin no.1), *Annales E.S.C.*, 16 (1961b), pp. 545–9.
Braudel, Fernand, 'Alimentation et catégories de l'histoire', (Bulletin no.2), *Annales E.S.C.*, 16 (1961c), pp. 723–8.
Braudel, Fernand, 'Achats et ventes de sel à Venise (1587-1593)', (Bulletin no.3), *Annales E.S.C.*, 16 (1961d), pp. 961–5.
Braudel, Fernand and Frank Spooner, 'Les Métaux monetaires et l'économie du XVIe siècle', *Rapport au Congrès International de Rome*, 4 (1955), pp. 233–64.
Briffault, Eugène, *Paris à table* (Paris, 1946).
Brillat-Savarin, Jean-Anthelme, *La physiologie du goût* (Paris, 1825).
Brown, W. Norman, 'La vache sacrée dans la réligion hindue', *Annales E.S.C.*, 19 (1964), pp. 643–64.
Bruneton-Governatori, Ariane, 'Alimentation et idéologie: le cas de la Châtaigne', *Annales E.S.C.*, 39 (1984), pp. 1161–85.
Bruneton-Governatori, Ariane, *Le pain de bois: ethnohistoire de la châtaigne et du châtaignier* (Toulouse, 1984).
Bulletin Philologique et Historique du Comité des Travaux Historiques et Scientifiques (Paris, 1971).
Camporesi, Pietro, *Le pain sauvage. L'imaginaire de la faim de renaissance au XVIIIe siècle* (Paris, 1981).
Charbonnier, P., 'La Consommation des seigneurs auvergnats du XVe au XVIIIe siècle', *Annales E.S.C.*, 30 (1975), pp. 465–77.
Chaunu, Pierre, *Histoire, science sociale. La durée, l'espace et l'homme à l'époque moderne* (Paris, 1974).
Chiva, Maurice and Claude Fischler, 'Food likes, dislikes and some of their correlates in a sample of French children and young adults', in Jörg M. Diehl and Claus Leitzmann (eds), *Measurement and Determinants of Food Habits and Food Preferences* (Wageningen, 1986).
Claudian, Jean and Yvonne Serville, 'Aspects de l'évolution récente du comportement alimentaire en France: compositions de repas et urbanisation' in Jean-Jacques Hémardinquer (ed.), *Pour une histoire de l'alimentation* (Paris, 1970), pp. 174–87.
Couperie, Pierre, 'Régimes alimentaires dans la France du XVIIe siècle', *Annales E.S.C.*, 18 (1963), pp. 1133–41.
Couperie, Pierre, 'L'alimentation au XVIIe siècle: Les marchés de pourvoierie', *Annales E.S.C.*, 19 (1964), pp. 467–78.
Coutancier, Benoit, *L'administration des petites pêches, 1681-1896. Le cas du Bordelais* (Paris, 1985).

Dauphin, Cécile and Pierette Pézérat, 'Les consommations populaires dans la seconde moitié du XIXe siècle à travers les monographies de l'Ecole de Le Play', *Annales E.S.C.*, 30 (1975), pp. 537–53.

Davies, C.L.S., 'Les rations alimentaires de l'armée et de la marine anglaise au XVIe siècle' (Bulletin no.9), *Annales E.S.C.*, 18 (1963), pp. 139–41.

Derville, Alain, 'Dîmes, rendements du blé et 'révolution agricole' dans le nord de la France au moyen age', *Annales E.S.C.*, 42 (1987), pp. 1411–32.

Désert, Gabriel, 'Viande et poisson dans l'alimentation des français au milieu du XIXe siècle', *Annales E.S.C.*, 30 (1975), pp. 519–36.

Dion, Roger, *Histoire de la vigne et du vin en France des origines au XIXe siècle* (Paris, 1959).

Durand, Georges, *Vin, vigne et vignerons et Lyonnais en Beaujolais, XVIe-XVIIIe siècles* (Paris, 1979).

'Enquête national sur la consommation', *Annales E.S.C.*, 25 (1970), pp. 1492–3.

Erbe, Michael, *Zur neueren französischen Sozialgeschichtsforschung. Die Gruppe um die Annales* (Darmstadt, 1979).

Farge, Arlette, *Délinquance et criminalité. Le vol alimentaire à Paris au XVIIIe siècle* (Paris, 1971).

Fernoit, Jean and Jacques le Goff (eds), *La cuisine et la table. 5000 ans de gastronomie* (S.l. 1986).

Fink, Beatrice, 'L'avènement de la pomme de terre', *18e siècle*, 15 (1983), pp. 19–32.

Fischler, Claude, 'Diététique savante et diététique spontanée: la bonne nutrition enfantine selon des mères de famille française', *Culture technique*, 16 (1986), pp. 50–9.

Fischler, Claude, 'Gastro-nomie et gastro-anomie', *Communication*, 31 (1979), pp. 189–210.

Fischler, Claude, 'Food habits, social change and the nature/culture dilemma', *Information sur les sciences sociales*, 19 (1980), pp. 937–53.

Fischler, Claude, 'La formation des goûts alimentaires', in Dr. Lagardère (ed.), *La prévention et l'enfant* (Paris, 1987).

Fischler, Claude, 'La symbolique du gros', *Communication*, 46 (1987), pp. 255–77.

Fischler, Claude, 'Food, self and identity', *Information sur les sciences sociales*, 27 (1988), pp. 274–92.

Flandrin, Jean-Louis, *Différences et différenciation des goûts: Reflexions sur quelques exemples européens entre le 14e et le 18e siècle* (Oxford, 1981).

Flandrin, Jean-Louis, 'La diversité des goûts et des pratiques alimentaires en Europe du 16e au 18e siècle', *Révue d'histoire moderne et contemporaine*, 306 (1983a), pp. 66–83.

Flandrin, Jean-Louis, 'Le goût et la nécessité: sur l'usage des graisses dans les cuisines d'Europe occidentale (XIVe-XVIIe siècle)', *Annales E.S.C.*, 38 (1983b), pp. 369–401.

Flandrin, Jean-Louis, 'Internationalisme, nationalisme et régionalisme dans la cuisine du 14e et 15e siècle: Le témoignage des livres de cuisine', *Manger et boire au Moyen Age*, 2 (1984), pp. 75–91.

Flandrin, Jean-Louis, 'La distinction par le goût' in Philippe Ariés and Georges Duby (eds), *Histoire de la vie privée*, vol. 3 (1986), pp. 266–309.

Flandrin, Jean-Louis, 'Pour une histoire du goût', *L'Histoire*, 3 (1986), pp. 108–10.

Flandrin, Jean-Louis, Mary Hyman and Philip Hyman, *Le cuisinier français* (Paris, 1983).

Flandrin, Jean-Louis and Philip Hyman, 'Regional tastes and cuisines: problems, documents and discourses on food in southern France in the 16th and 17th centuries', *Food & Foodways*, 1 (1986), pp. 221–51.

Frijhoff, Wilhelm and Julia Dominique, 'L'alimentation des pensionnaires à la fin de l'Ancien Régime', *Annales E.S.C.*, 30 (1975), pp. 491–505.

Furet, François, 'Histoire quantitative et construction du fait historique', *Annales E.S.C.*, 26

(1971), pp. 63-75.

Garine, Igor de, and C. M. Hladik, *Anthropology of Food: Scope and Field Approaches. From Nonhuman Primates to Man* (Paris, Cambridge, s.a.).

Garine, Igor de, 'Culture et nutrition', *Communication*, 31 (1979), pp. 70–92.

Garine, Igor de, 'Les modes alimentaires: histoires de l'alimentation', in *Moeurs et usages*, vol. 1 (Paris, 1984), pp. 1–174.

Gaulin, Steven J. C., 'Choix des aliments et evolution', *Communication*, 31 (1979), pp. 33–52.

Gilet, Philippe, *Par mets et par vins. Voyages et gastronomie en Europe* (Paris, 1985).

Gottschalk, Alfred, *Histoire de l'alimentation et de la gastronomie depuis la préhistoire jusqu'à nos jours* (Paris, 1948).

Grimod de la Reynière, Alexandre Balthaser, *Almanach des gourmands* (Paris, 1803–12).

Grimod de la Reynière, Alexandre Balthaser, *Le manuel des amphitryons* (Paris, 1808).

Guégan, Bertrand, *Le cuisinier Français* (Paris, 1934).

Guy, Christian, *La vie quotidienne de la société gourmande du XIVe siècle* (Paris, 1971).

Heffer, Jean, 'Jacques Mairesse and Jean-Marie Chanut. La culture du blé au milieu du XIXe siècle: Rendement, prix, salaires et autres coûts', *Annales E.S.C.*, 41 (1986), pp. 1273–301.

Hémardinquer, Jean-Jacques, 'En France aujourd'hui: Données quantitatives sur les consommations alimentaires' (Bulletin no.1). *Annales E.S.C.*, 16 (1961a), pp. 553–64.

Hémardinquer, Jean-Jacques, 'Essai de cartes de graisses en France' (Bulletin no.2), *Annales E.S.C.*, 16 (1961b), pp. 747–9.

Hémardinquer, Jean-Jacques, 'Le thé à la conquête de l'Occident: Le cas marocain' *Annales E.S.C.*, 17 (1962a), pp. 1145–51.

Hémardinquer, Jean-Jacques, 'Notes bibliographiques 1', *Annales E.S.C.*, 17 (1962b), pp. 913–16.

Hémardinquer, Jean-Jacques, 'A propos de l'alimentation des marins' (Bulletin no.11), *Annales E.S.C.*, 18 (1963a), pp. 1133–41.

Hémardinquer, Jean-Jacques, 'A propos de l'alimentation des marins: a) sur les galères de Toscanes au XIVe siècle', *Annales E.S.C.*, 18 (1963b), pp. 1141–9.

Hémardinquer, Jean-Jacques, 'Un film inespéré: La création du mais' (Bulletin no.11), *Annales E.S.C.*, 18 (1963c), pp. 1150–2.

Hémardinquer, Jean-Jacques, 'Note sur l'alimentation à la fin du XVIIe siècle' (Bulletin no.15), *Annales E.S.C.*, 28 (1968), pp. 819–23.

Hémardinquer, Jean-Jacques, 'Faut-il démythifier le porc familial?', *Annales E.S.C.*, 24 (1969), pp. 1745–59.

Pour une histoire de l'alimentation, ed. Jean-Jacques Hémardinquer (Paris, 1970).

Hintze, Kurt, *Geographie und Geschichte der Ernährung* (Leipzig, 1934).

Histoire et géographie des fromages. Actes de colloque de géographie historique Caen 1985 (Caen, 1987).

Hocquet, Jean-Claude, 'Métrologie du sel et histoire comparée en Méditerranée', *Annales E.S.C.*, 29 (1974), pp. 393–424.

Hocquet, Jean-Claude, *Le sel et le fortune de Venise, 1200-1650*, 2 vols. (Lille, 1978–9).

Hocquet, Jean-Claude, *Le sel et le pouvoir: de l'an mil à la Révolution francaise* (Paris, 1984).

Hocquet, Jean-Claude, 'Le pain, le vin et la juste mesure à la table des moines carolingiens', *Annales E.S.C.*, 40 (1985), pp. 661–87.

Hyman, Philip and Mary Hyman, 'Les cuisines régionales à travers les livres de recettes', *18e siècle*, 15 (1983), pp. 65–74.

Iggers, Georg G., 'Die Annales und ihre Kritiker. Probleme moderner französischer Sozialgeschichte', *Historische Zeitschrift*, 219 (1975), pp. 578–608.

Iggers, Georg G., *New Directions in European History* (Middletown, 1975).
Katz, Soloman H., 'Anthropologie sociale/culturelle et biologie', in E. Morin and M. Piatelli-Palmarini (eds), *Pour une anthropologie fondamentale* (Paris, 1974), pp. 49–86.
Katz, Soloman H., 'Un exemple d'évolution bioculturelle: la feve', *Communication*, 31 (1979), pp. 53–69.
Kerblay, Basil, 'L'évolution de l'alimentation rurale en Russie, 1896-1960', *Annales E.S.C.*, 17 (1962), pp. 855–910.
Knabe, Peter-Eckard, 'Esthétique et art culinaire', *18e siècle*, 16 (1986), pp. 125–36.
Lane, Frédéric C. 'Salaires et régime alimentaire des marins au début du XIVe siècle', *Annales E.S.C.*, 18 (1963), pp. 133–8.
Laurioux, Bruno, 'Spices in the medieval diet: a new approach', *Food & Foodways*, 1 (1981), pp. 43–78.
Laurioux, Bruno, 'Les Premiers livres de cuisine', *L'Histoire*, 3 (1986), pp. 51–7.
Le Goff, Jacques, 'Une enquête sur le sel dans l'histoire' (Bulletin no.3), *Annales E.S.C.*, 16 (1961), pp. 959–61.
Le Goff, Jacques, Roger Chartier and Jacques Revel, *La nouvelle histoire* (Paris, 1978).
Le Grand d'Aussy, P. J. B., *L'histoire de la vie privée des Français*, 3 vols (Paris, 1782, repr. Paris 1967).
Le Roy Ladurie, Emanuel, *Les paysans de Languedoc* (Paris, 1966).
Le Roy Ladurie, Emanuel, *Histoire du clima depuis l'an mil* (Paris, 1967).
Le Roy Ladurie, Emanuel, 'L'aménorrhée de famine, XVIIe-XXe siècles', *Annales E.S.C.*, 24 (1969), pp. 1589–601.
Lehmann, Gilly, 'Les cuisiners anglais face à la cuisine française', *18e siècle*, 18 (1983), pp. 75–93.
Lévi-Strauss, Claude, *Mythologiques. L'origine des manières de table* (Paris, 1968).
Lévi-Strauss, Claude, 'Le triangle culinaire', *L'Arc*, 26 (1969), pp. 19–26.
Lichtenfelt, Alfred, *Die Geschichte der Ernährung* (Berlin, 1913).
Lisanti, Louis, 'Sur la nourriture des 'Paulistes' entre XVIIe et XIXe siècles' (Bulletin no. 10), *Annales E.S.C.*, 18 (1963), pp. 522–40.
Mahias, Marie-Claude, 'Milk and its transmutations in Indian society', *Food & Foodways*, 2 (1988), pp. 265–88.
Mandrou, Robert, 'Les consommations des villes françaises (viandes et boissons) au milieu du XIXe siècle' (Bulletin no. 2), *Annales E.S.C.*, 16 (1961), pp. 740–4.
Mandrou, Robert, 'Théorie ou hypothèse de travail?', (Bulletin no. 3), *Annales E.S.C.*, 16 (1961), pp. 965–71.
Mandrou, Robert, 'Histoire allemande de produits alimentaires' (Bulletin no. 7), *Annales E.S.C.*, 17 (1962), pp. 916–9.
Manger et boire au Moyen Age. Actes du colloque de Nice s.l., s.a. (Paris, 1984).
Maurizio, Adam, *Die Geschichte unserer Pflanzennahrung von den Urzeiten bis zur Gegenwart* (Berlin, 1927).
Maurizio, Adam, *Geschichte der gegorenen Getränke* (Berlin, 1933).
Menell, Stephen, *All Manners of Food* (Oxford, 1985).
Mollat, Michel (ed.), *Le rôle du sel dans l'histoire*, (Paris, 1968).
Morineau, Michel, 'Rations militaires et rations moyennes en Hollande du XVIIe siècle' (Bulletin no.10), *Annales E.S.C.*, 18 (1963), p. 5.
Morineau, Michel, 'Rations de marins (Angleterre, Hollande, Suède, Russie)', *Annales E.S.C*, 290 (1965), pp. 1150–60.
Morineau, Michel, 'Histoire sans frontiére: Prix et "Révolution agricole"', *Annales E.S.C.*, 24

(1969), pp. 403–23.

Morineau, Michel, 'La pomme de terre au XVIIIe siècle', *Annales E.S.C.*, 25 (1970), pp. 1767–85.

Moulin, Léo, *Europe à table: Introduction à une psychosociologie des pratiques alimentaires* (Paris/Brussels, 1975).

Mulliez, Jacques, 'Du blé "malnécessaire". Réflexions sur les progrès de l'agriculture 1750-1850', *Revue d'histoire moderne et contemporaire*, 29 (1979), pp. 3–47.

Mulon, Marianne, 'Recettes médievales', *Annales E.S.C.*, 19 (1964) pp. 933–7.

Paruto, N. T., 'Les famines dans l'ancienne Russie (X-XIVe siècle)', *Annales E.S.C.*, 25 (1970), pp. 185–91.

Pereira, M. Holperin, 'Niveaux de consommation, niveaux de vie au Portugal, 1874-1922', *Annales E.S.C.*, 30 (1975), pp. 610–32.

Perles, Catérine, 'Les origines de la cuisine', *Communications*, 31 (1979), pp. 4–14.

Pfister, Christian, 'Fluctuation climatique et prix céréaliers en Europe du XVIe en XXe siècle', *Annales E.S.C.*, 43 (1988), pp. 25–54.

Philippe, Robert, 'Commençons par l'histoire de l'alimentation' (Bulletin no. 1), *Annales E.S.C.*, 16 (1961a), pp. 549–52.

Philippe, Robert, 'Une opération pilote: L'étude du ravitaillement de Paris au temps de Lavoisier' (Bulletin no.1), *Annales E.S.C.*, 16 (1961b), pp. 564–7.

Piuz, Anne-Marie, 'Alimentation populaire et sous-alimentation au XVIIe siècle', in Jean-Jacques Hémardinquer (ed.), *Pour une histoire de l'alimentation* (Paris, 1970), pp. 129–45.

Piuz, Anne-Marie, 'Le marché du détail et la consommation de la viande à Genève au XVIIIe siècle', *Annales E.S.C.*, 30 (1975), pp. 575–84.

Poitrineau, Abel, 'L'alimentation populaire en Auvergne au XVIIe siècle' (Bulletin no.5), *Annales E.S.C.*, 17 (1962), pp. 323–31.

Pratiques et discours alimentaires à la Renaissance. Actes du Colloque de Tours 1979, ed. Jean-Claude Margolin and Robert Sanzet (Paris, 1982).

Revel, Jacques, 'Les privilèges d'une capitale: l'approvisionnement de Rome à l'époque moderne', *Annales E.S.C.*, 30 (1975), pp. 563–75.

Revel, Jacques, 'Alimentation', in Jacques le Goff and Jacques Revel (eds), *La nouvelle histoire* (Paris, 1978), pp. 24–6.

Revel, Jacques, *Un festin en paroles: histoire littéraire de la sensibilité gastronomie de l'antiquité à nos jours* (Paris, 1979).

Roche, Daniel, 'Cuisine et alimentation populaire à Paris', *18e siècle*, 15 (1983), pp. 7–18.

Roche, Daniel, 'Le ventre des Parisiens au XVIIIe siècle', *L'Histoire*, 3 (1986), pp. 121–3.

Rochefort, René, 'Le livre noir de la faim' (Bulletin no. 7), *Annales E.S.C.*, 17 (1962), pp. 914–20.

Roel, A. Eiras and M. J. Enriquez Morales, 'La consommation alimentaire d'Ancien Régime: Les collèges de Saint-Jacques de Compostelle', *Annales E.S.C.*, 30 (1975), pp. 454–64.

Rosenberger, Bernard, 'Cultures complémentaires et nouritures de substitution au Maroc, XVe-XVIIIe siècle', *Annales E.S.C.*, 35 (1980), pp. 477–503.

Rouche, Michel, 'Le banquet des moines au Moyen Age', *L'Histoire*, 3 (1983), pp. 71–3.

Ruggiero, Romano, 'A propos du commerce du blé dans la Méditerranée des XIVe et XVe siècles', *Hommage à Lucien Febvre*, II (1954), pp. 149–56.

Sabban, Françoise, 'Le système des cuissons dans la tradition culinaire chinoise', *Annales E.S.C.*, 38 (1983), pp. 341–68.

Schmoller, Gustav, 'Die historische Entwicklung des Fleischconsums sowie der Viehpreise in Deutschland', *Zeitschrift für die gesamte Staatswirtschaft*, 27 (1871), pp. 284–362.

Soler, Jean, 'Sémiotique de la nourriture dans la Bible', *Annales E.S.C.*, 28 (1973), pp. 943–55.
Spooner, Frank, 'Régimes alimentaires d'autrefois: proportions et calculs en calories' (Bulletin no.1), *Annales E.S.C.*, 16 (1961), pp. 568–74.
Stoianovich, Troian, 'Le Maïs dans le Balkans' (Bulletin no.14), *Annales E.S.C.*, 20 (1965), pp. 1026–40.
Stouff, Louis, 'La viande. Ravitaillement et consommation à Carpentras au XIVe siècle', *Annales E.S.C.*, 24 (1969), pp. 1444–8.
Stouff, Louis, *Ravitaillement et alimentation en Provence aux XIVe et XVe siècles* (Paris, 1970).
Stouff, Louis, 'Y avait-il à la fin du Moyen Age une alimentation et une cuisine provenale originales?', *Manger et boire au Moyen Age*, 2 (Paris, 1982), pp. 93–9.
Teleki, G., 'Primate subsistence patterns: collector-predators and gatherer-hunters', *Journal of Human Evolution*, 4 (1975), pp. 125–84.
Teleki, G., 'The omnivorous chimpanzee', *Scientific American*, January 1979, pp. 38–42.
Teuteberg, Hans Jürgen, 'Die Ernährung als Gegenstand historischer Analyse', in Hermann Kellenbenz and Hans Pohl (eds), *Historia socialis et oeconomica. Festschrift für Wolfgang Zorn zum 65. Geburtstag* (Stuttgart, 1987), pp. 181–202.
Thouvenot, Claude, *Le pain d'autrefois: chroniques alimentaires d'un monde qui s'en va* (Nancy, 1987).
Thuillier, Guy, 'L'alimentation au XIXe siècle au Nivernais' (Bulletin no.13), *Annales E.S.C.*, 20 (1965), pp. 1170–84.
Thuillier, Guy, 'Note sur les sources de l'histoire régionale de l'alimentation pour la France du XIXe siècle' (Bulletin no.17), *Annales E.S.C.*, 23 (1968), pp. 1301–18.
Tits-Dieuade, Marie-Jeanne, 'Les Campagnes flamandes du XVIIe au XVIIIe siècle au les succès d'une agriculture traditionelle', *Annales E.S.C.*, 39 (1984), pp. 590–610.
Tits-Dieuade, M.-J., 'L'évolution du prix du blé dans quelques villes d'Europe occidentale du XVe au XVIIIe siècle', *Annales E.S.C.*, 42 (1987), pp. 529–48.
Toussaint-Samat, Maguellone, *Histoire naturelle et morale de la nourriture* (Paris, 1987).
Valensi, L., 'Consommations et usages alimentaires en Tunisie aux XVIIIe et XIXe siècles', *Annales E.S.C.*, 30 (1975), pp. 600–10.
Van der Stegen, Judith, *L'évolution des réserves de grains au XVIIe et XVIIIe siècle. L'exemple d'une province du sud* (s.l.1980).
Vandenbroeke, Christiaan, 'L'alimentation à Gent pendant la première moitié du XIXe siècles', *Annales E.S.C.*, 30 (1975), pp. 584–92.
Vedel, Jacques, 'La consommation alimentaire dans le Haut Languedoc aux XVIIe et XVIIIe siècle', *Annales E.S.C.*, 30 (1975), pp. 478–91.
Verdier, Yvonne, 'Pour une ethnologie culinaire', *L'Homme*, 9 (1969), pp.49–59.
Vincent, Bernard, 'Consommation en Andalousie', *Annales E.S.C.*, 30 (1975), pp. 445–54.
Wyczański, Andrzej, 'La consommation alimentaire en Pologne au XVIe siècle' (Bulletin no. 15), *Annales E.S.C.*, 17 (1962), pp. 318–23.
Zabinski, Zbigniew, 'L'Indice biologique du pouvoir d'achat de la monnaie' (Bulletin no. 15), *Annales E.S.C.*, 23 (1968), pp. 808–18.
Zanetti, Dante, 'Contribution à l'étude des structures économiques: L'approvisionnement de Pavie au XVIe siècle', *Annales E.S.C.*, 18 (1963), pp. 44–62.

7 The diet as an object of historical analysis in Germany

Hans J. Teuteberg

As far as is known, it was in the 18th century that the first attempts were made by medical and mercantilist writers to write comprehensively about the *antiquitates culinariae*, but these publications were merely simple compilations of all available information displayed in an unchecked and disconnected way to the reader.[1] The focal points of these tracts were individual foodstuffs and luxury foods, whose value to the prolongation of human life in the sense of transmitted dietetic regimens was discussed.

At the beginning of the 19th century, some gourmand writers began to bring more order to this mass of facts: notably Carl Friedrich von Rumohr, Gustav Blumroeder and Eugen Baron Vaerst.[2] These friends of culinary art founded a lively literary group, mainly focusing on recipes and cooking techniques but also dealing with definitions of taste, appetite, the origins of all foodstuffs and delights of the table, and even with restaurants and table etiquette, great feasts, and hospital provisions in the past.

Certainly these kinds of historical digression, similar to the works of Jean-Anthelme Brillat-Savarin[3] in France and Alexis Soyer[4] in England, were a necessary adjunct to a gourmand philosophy (*'gastrosophy'*), but they bespeak earnest study of historical sources, especially of authors of antiquity. The books were intended for the reading middle class, which was supposed to be educated to a higher 'art of eating'. In contrast to the encyclopaedists of the age of the Enlightenment, whose main interest was focused on technological and dietetic aspects, research now dealt with the pleasure of eating and with socio-cultural implications. In the opinion of these gastrosophers, eating and drinking meant more than the unthinking consumption of food: they considered eating as an act of creating culture. For the first time, eating habits appeared as an expression of human civilization and at the same time as an integrated part of history. These witty and ingenious authors tried to trace the changes in the art of eating of all civilized nations; travel reports, moralizing sermons and poetry were among the sources used. After the mid-19th century these summarizing examinations increased. A certain Eduard Reich, a medical instructor at the University of Berne, published two volumes under the title *Nahrungs- und*

Genussmittelkunde in which medical, scientific, hygienic, and cultural factors were examined for the first time in all the literature then available.[5] As the author emphasized, he sought to look simultaneously at natural and cultural history as well as health care. He used as his sources historical, geographical, ethnological and mercantilistic works. The rich library holdings of the famous University of Göttingen, where Reich had earlier been a senior lecturer, provided the main base of his research. The voluminous compendium he produced was a strange mixture of the humanities and natural sciences, and it tried to do justice to the 'double nature' of nutrition. Reich not only dealt with human diet and the physiological, aetiological and hygienic problems connected with it, but also with the cuisines of several nations. The sum of European knowledge of nutrition since the late 17th century was collected in this learned work. With it, Reich created the first provisional overview of the development of nutrition, although the organization of his ideas is not always helpful or useful to modern scholars.

German cultural history, which began to flourish after 1850 in the wake of historicism, continued the historical research into eating habits but lost contact with the natural sciences. The first attempts to write the history of eating and drinking manners were made in a belletristic and eclectic manner. Through the analysis of city archives scholars tried to gain insight into the eating habits of the late Middle Ages and early modern times. Central to this approach were the culinary habits of the upper-middle class, but the banquets of renowned men and of the nobility were also examined. Johannes Scherr, Karl Biedermann, Gustav Friedrich Klemm, Gustav Freytag, Georg Ludwig Kriegk, Johann Janssen and, last but not least, Karl Lamprecht were interested in the eating and drinking habits of the 'Old Germans'.[6] Other cultural historians followed them.[7] All this can be interpreted as a documentation of the German middle class which was gaining strength and self-confidence, and trying to give an account of its accomplishments in the course of history. The structure of these portrayals was oriented for the most part towards material culture: table and kitchen implements, dining rooms and table decoration, main courses, appetizers and desserts, the order of meals, drinks, and big feasts. They were always concerned with banquets or Sunday dining; the simple porridge of the common people was not mentioned.[8] Since cooking belonged primarily to the female sphere of activities, the everyday life of the woman and her work in the kitchen became the focus of historical attention for the first time. Cultural history, which developed independently alongside state history, initiated true social history research from today's point of view because it undertook scientific analysis of sources, though the outlook remained quite one-sided in factual as well as in temporal terms. It is worth mentioning that the same kind of historio-cultural study of diet got off the ground in France and England at the same time.[9]

In close connection with these historio-cultural efforts, works were created which can be regarded as precursors of modern ethnology and folklore. An early empirical survey of meals and drinks was begun in 1865 by Wilhelm Mannhardt (1831–80).[10] He was the publisher of the *Zeitschrift für deutsche Mythologie und Sitten [Magazine of German Mythology and Custom]*, and he was particularly interested in Germany's rural customs and legends. But his book was mainly oriented towards folkloric customs, with the result that detailed descriptions of nourishment and food only rarely come to the surface. It is indeed interesting that Mannhardt, in contrast to cultural historians, recorded for the first time the eating behaviour of the lower social classes. From the viewpoint of linguistic history, the ethnologist and cultural historian, Moriz Heyne, created a work in 1901 which remains unsurpassed, *Das deutsche Nahrungswesen von den ältesten Zeiten bis zum Ende des 16. Jahrhunderts [The German Diet from the Oldest Times until the 16th Century]*, which unfortunately was subsequently not continued.[11] Fritz Eckstein, in various articles in his *Handwörterbuch des deutschen Aberglaubens [Handbook of German Superstitions]*, also pursued similar intentions concerning linguistic history. Relevant references in Jacob and Wilhelm Grimm's *Deutsches Wörterbuch [German Dictionary]*, published from 1852, served as an important source.[12] Finally, the ethnologist Martin Wähler tried to formulate a general idea of German regional cuisines and the traditions on which they are based.[13] He differentiated between food and cultural areas in order to highlight the various developments.

The empirical study of rural eating habits, investigated by Wilhelm Mannhardt in 1865, was continued more methodically and extensively at the beginning of the 20th century. A number of records from different parts of the country were thus collected in Württemberg around 1900 and in Bavaria around 1909–10. These reporters gave relatively free accounts structured only by the most important features. They spoke of subjects like main courses and drinks for special occasions or for working days and Sundays, table and kitchen implements, but also the sequence of meals, special ways of cooking, serving and eating. After further inquiries in German states and Prussian provinces and the drafting of linguistic dictionaries, extensive work on an *Atlas der Deutschen Volkskunde [Atlas of German Ethnology]* was done between 1930 and 1935. It covered mainly German-speaking areas all over Europe, and dealt with the subject of food, though not exhaustively.[14] The answers to the precisely and uniformly preformulated questions provided a superb base of sources for a temporal comparative cross-section. With the help of between 15,000 and 20,000 answer sheets, which have been kept in storage, important elements of the nutritional culture of the early 20th century could now be described. Unfortunately, only a small fraction have been analysed so far. This early form of 'oral history' was continued through further inquiries in 1951 and 1970.[15]

Compared to these very considerable preliminary studies of older cultural history and ethnology the contributions of economic historians to the history of the changes in the consumption of food were at first quite modest. Although, as is evident in the works of, for instance, Johann Heinrich Gottlieb von Justi, Friedrich List, and Johann Heinrich von Thünen, and later Robert Mohl, Johann Gottfried Hoffmann, Lorenz vom Stein, Wilhelm Roscher, Georg von Below, Max Sering and Gustav Schmoller, the problems of production, commerce, price formation, transport costs and consumption tax, and questions concerning food legislation were definitely in the foreground of scientific interest, the real questions of consumption were not scientifically analysed. Up to the mid-19th century this group of authors, who reacted to the frequent increases in prices, famine, and bread riots with practical proposals and solutions, did not provide readers with extensive empirical descriptions.[16] Only Karl Biedermann, economist and historian of the University of Leipzig and one of the founding fathers of German cultural history, described the food supply in 18th-century Germany in its context, taking information from early husbandry literature, encyclopaedias, and medical topographies.[17]

Since the rise of statistics has provided rough records about per-capita consumption in the early 19th century, particularly in Prussia, attention turned to concrete records of consumption in the form of household budgets.[18] This kind of quantitative recording of food consumption in economic terms represented a considerable methodical step forward. It led some political economists who were working on a historical basis to make the first comprehensive comparisons with the past. Thus, Gustav Schmoller in 1870 dealt with the changes in German meat consumption since the late Middle Ages, while Johannes Conrad contrasted the nutritional situation in Berlin in the late 18th century with that of his time to show the consequences of urbanization and the increased standard of living in a more favourable light. Both of these works can be considered to be pioneering works in this field.[19] But as in other agrarian-historical treatises, the authors did not go beyond the comparison of food quantities with prices, and on this basis, rather naively, they deduced structural changes. As many articles in the then representative *Handwörterbuch der Staatswissenschaften [Handbook of Political Sciences]* from the first to the third edition around 1900 show, people were already very well informed about the production and marketing of the most important foodstuffs and luxury goods in the German economy. Even the food laws and food technology, which had been summarized in handbooks, could now look back on a vivid research history.[20] But there were hardly coherent reports about the temporal and spatial development of domestic consumption and only fragmentary information from the present.

Then, during the first decades of the 20th century, some surprising monographs were published under the extremely pretentious title *Geschichte der Ernährung [History of Nutrition]*.[21] The authors of these monographs were a physician and a geographer, who understandably could not meet the demands of a scientific historiography. Naively they tried to encompass every aspect of human nutrition from primeval times to the present in every country of the world. However, because of the lack of preliminary studies these works were inevitably unsuccessful. The individual chapters were not well planned with respect to their division into epochs, and amounted to nothing more than card indexes turned upside down full of random historical notes lined up like pearls on a string. In most cases concise bibliographical data were missing; neither had the material been checked against further reference nor had the authors attempted to put it within its historical context. So the usefulness of these first historiographies of nutrition was negligible; they deceptively reflected a store of knowledge which could not have been achieved at that time.

The studies on the history of vegetable nutrition and fermented drinks by the Polish botanist, Adam Maurizio, who published also in the German language, Edmund O. von Lippmann's *Geschichte des Zuckers [History of Sugar]*, and the detailed historical investigations on bread by Walter von Stokar were of more value.[22] These monographs were not only more meaningfully arranged with respect to history, but were also reliably supported by references. Lippmann's work reached beyond the subject of sugar, as he also dealt with the history of the gathering of honey and the introduction of hot drinks like coffee, tea, and cocoa, which were sweetened in most cases. Nevertheless, even these books lacked a reference to the historical context.

Rudolf Häpke, who was appointed economic historian at the newly founded University of Hamburg, was the first to realize the deficient work done by historians on the changes in popular nourishment following the First World War. He thus felt obliged to draft a suitable treatise.[23] Because of the lack of sufficient studies he unfortunately could not realize the full range of these problems, so he only outlined his thoughts in an inspiring essay to which he subsequently did not return. Summaries of historical diet research during the period of the Weimar Republic only go to show that relatively poor research work was done in the German history of nutrition up to that time.[24] On the whole, the eating habits of the late Middle Ages and of early modern times were known far better than was 19th-century nutrition. The Third Reich did not bring any progress in these studies. The research which was important was that in rural customs from which the folklore studies profited most of all, as was mentioned earlier.

During the two decades following the Second World War, investigations in the history of human nutrition developed as outlined above. Historically interested physiologists of nutrition, botanists and economic geographers, apart from dealing with folklore and cultural history, continued to publish occasional studies with the imperfections already shown.[25] A comparative study proves that the individual disciplines did not take much notice of each other and that they did not consider the changes in nutrition with regard to other disciplines. There were no historical surveys and no general attempts at work on a larger scale, as had already been undertaken by that time in England, France, the Netherlands and the United States.[26]

The mid-1960s saw a sea-change in dealing with the history of nutrition when historians, economists, and social scientists again moved close to each other and when problems and methods concerning political economy, sociology, psychology, folklore, anthropology and geography were dealt with by historians on a larger scale. A final displacement of the earlier cultural history set in, the terms and methods of which had already been found to be obsolete in the 1950s. In particular, there were impulses by historians who had gathered around the Parisian journal *Annales* and by interdisciplinary conferences at Queen Elizabeth College in London, where, in contrast to Germany, the traditional scientifically oriented science of nutrition and history had entered into an early productive symbiosis. But these impulses were also shown by the close cooperation of folklore and social history in Münster. All these impulses led to a discussion of the basic problems of the historical science of nutrition, especially by new methodical aspects, and they led to new contributions to a history of nutrition. Although the areas and centuries in question had been tackled differently, there was agreement on the fact that this important field of research had been neglected for too long a time and that it would be profitable to work it through. The discussion of the problem of world famine, which was actively being engaged in at this time, doubtlessly accelerated the intensification of the research work. Scientists from other European countries also took up these research impulses after some delay and started to work on the history of nutrition at a more far-reaching level. In the 1970s the ethnologists/folklorists and anthropologists who were interested in food research began to come together at regular international conferences, and since that time interested scientists have convened regularly in special sections of the international congresses of economic historians.[27] Also the first shy approaches of a special psychology and sociology of nutrition were seen: however, there was still little interest in historical problems.[28] It is not possible on this occasion to analyse the literature on historical food research in particular, as it has been fed by many sources and has seen exponential growth during the last 15 years. Only individual titles of great merit and some general research trends can be referred to here.[29]

Today in nearly all countries one of the main areas of research in the explanation of the connections between industrialization, population growth (or rather urbanization), and the revolutionary changes in everyday food seems to be the period from the late 18th century to the First World War. Nutrition is regarded as a decisive factor for measuring the average standard of living, and the most diverse conditions between rural and urban life but also between cultural and economic areas and the social classes (or rather occupational groups) are worked out quantitatively and qualitatively. In doing so one is interested in the changes in consumption of different kinds of food and drink, the quantity of which is registered on a macro- and microeconomic level and, if possible, converted into nutritive value units. Furthermore, there is a growing interest in the influences of the rising food industry, whose innovative character and formation of capital had up to that time largely been underestimated. The new methods of preservation, the extension of new urban networks of transportation and commerce, and finally the considerable improvements in the quality of food under new laws are also of interest.

In addition, scholars remained interested in the older nutritional state of the *ancien régime*. The methods of supplying grain to big cities and the typical correlations between price increases and food riots were studied most intensively of all. National and municipal welfare benefits, the consumption of food, the changes in meal patterns and the actual deficits of nutrition were also studied.[30] Fernand Braudel's detailed studies on food as a part of the *civilisation matérielle*, especially in the Mediterranean regions from the 15th to the 18th century, and his fundamental studies on the subject and methods of a history of nutrition have also been given attention beyond the borders of France. It is remarkable that the debate over methodological problems has been fuelled almost solely by French historians during the last twenty years.[31]

Scientists of the French *Annales* school correlate the history of nutrition with the elucidation of collective behaviour, or the structures of consciousness that direct daily consciousness.[32] Unlike the case earlier, it is no longer sufficient to work up economic and demographic data alone; rather an exploration of the changing attitudes to marriage, family, sexuality, and death is attempted, which all entailed particular rules of behaviour manifested in myths, religious symbols, feasts, etc. In this case nutrition habits serve as an additional mirror to reflect long-term changes in behaviour. With good reason it is thought that by way of dietary customs demographic, economic, political-judicial, sociocultural and even climatic and ecological phenomena can be combined in homogeneous categories which can be compared to each other outside the bounds of time and space. Nutritional habits seem to be an always reliable guide in the web of time, as eating and drinking have necessarily existed at all times and places. Human food is used as an indicator for the analysis of larger structural changes; it supports a better understanding of behavioural patterns and changes in behaviour that are expressed in trends and the *Zeitgeist* of the period. There are only a few German investigations which follow this French research direction.[33]

Furthermore, influential scientists dealing with the history of nutrition agree that changes in nutrition have to be analysed in their economic, psycho-social, cultural, and ethnological, but also in their physiological, medical, and demographic aspects. It is no longer regarded as sufficient to describe the food situation by correlating food prices and population statistics. It has become more and more apparent that the composition of nutrition has by no means always adjusted to the trends of market prices. Besides the differing prices of individual foods and the low scope of the money economy, it is important to analyse the meal patterns, which are very different in their respective cultural surroundings, and the recipes characteristic of their respective regions. This analysis can only be done with the assistance of ethnology and geography. Up to now, economic historians have underestimated the influential regional differences in food, and have thus made erroneous assumptions from time to time. The substitution of one general or luxury foodstuff by another, especially in times of famine, has been recognized as an important desideratum of research. The conversions from quantities of food into today's nutritive value units, sometimes done too hastily, have turned out to be full of methodological pitfalls; one must know not only the actual quality of dishes at the time (there are, for instance, more than a dozen kinds of meat, with different calorie values!) but also weight, height, workload, climate, and other things. Furthermore, the utilization of stored food and meals and the supply of essential vitamins, trace elements, and fibre must be considered. As recent research work has convincingly shown, it seems that famine alone does not cause a significant increase of the death rate; much more influential are deficiency diseases that emerge from malnutrition and the susceptibility to epidemics, which, of course, are not always the result of nutritional problems. According to Maurice Aymard, one object of historical food research has to be to find which part of the population at a given period of time was undernourished according to today's criteria and was particularly prone to nutritional diseases. This means a closer cooperation between medical history and social history, or rather demography, as it is practised by Thomas McKeown, Arthur E. Imhof, and Reinhard Spree.[34] A collection of essays done by the American historians, Robert I. Rotberg and

Theodore K. Rabb, on the subject of *Hunger and History* has been devoted to this complex of questions.[35]

Although the majority of the population between the 16th and the early 19th centuries probably lived close to subsistence level and, except on holidays, lived entirely on food that was monotonous and rich in carbohydrates, historical food research is conscious of the important part that predominating tastes had on the choice and composition of meals. The preferences and dislikes appearing at this point were by no means limited to the rich minority; they were also expressed by the manifold, religiously influenced, national customs of nutrition. Therefore, besides availability and calorie value, the world hierarchy connected with food has to be described according to cultural surroundings and social classes. Thus it is well known that the eating of white bread had the same social rank as the use of table silver and that the spread of the drinking of coffee can by no means be explained by economic reasons alone: as is well known, the developing coffee houses were focal points for the gradual emancipation of the middle classes.[36] Lately, Jean-Louis Flandrin has pursued changes in taste on the basis of French cookery-books throughout the centuries. He intends to juxtapose 'landscapes of taste', which had their own styles in meals, with the styles of art, architecture, and literature.[37]

As far as one can see up to now, a division of the European history of diet into periods runs, for the time being, into many difficulties. As nutrition can be classed with the biological as well as the psycho-social nature of man, the physical needs are always inseparably mixed with mental and social vital interests. A division of the changes in nutrition has to consider this characteristic double-sided nature and must include findings of the natural sciences and the humanities as well. This is, of course, easier said than done. As a part of everyday life food and nutrition were never subject to real revolutionary changes. The changes in eating customs always took place imperceptibly, beneath the surface of events. Breaks in the course of nutritional conditions can hardly be found because innovations in nutrition were only gradually adopted before the beginning of the industrial age. All exact datings are misleading; they reflect a precision which cannot exist.

At present it cannot be foreseen whether the double-sided nature of nutrition, which is located equally strongly in physical and social areas, can be systematized by conventional theories dividing evolutions into historical stages, forms of nutrition or meal-patterns, or by actual or ideal types of dishes without regard to time and space. The daily intake of food is, of course, necessary for all people at all times and all places, but the particular customs associated with it are quite different. It can be said that these differences in meal customs alone have played the decisive part in the relations between peoples and nations which made the differences in culture patterns possible. The preferences for and dislikes of certain foods and dishes, which arose from taste, smell, and appearance, have become stereotyped conceptions of the culture of other peoples. In a nutshell, one can say that the national character of a people was often judged by its cuisine. Observing what and how people eat contributed to the positive and negative judgements on alien peoples. The intrusion of Europeans into the ancient American civilization and later into Japan, which had up to this point been inaccessible, constituted great turning points in both their histories of nutrition. Both cultures became to different degrees 'westernized'. But it may be doubted whether such events, which have come from outside, can be pressed into a logical scheme of division into periods, as within societies all over the world there have been people who actively made norms of behaviour and people who accepted these norms more or less passively. As is shown by existing studies, even in culturally less differentiated times and places food circumstances were always so manifold that they always had different means of expressing eating customs. Nobility and clergy in ancient Europe, on the one hand, had certain uniform kinds of consumption which reached beyond national borders and contrasted with the consumption habits of peasants and craftsmen. In times of religious asceticism, in the widespread fasting periods, but also in the sufferings of recurrent famine and in incredible price increases for grain there developed, on the other hand, socially standardizing elements in nutrition habits, since in certain circumstances even money cannot prevent food shortages. But comparisons of social classes must in any case be added to the analyses of cultural surroundings. These few references may show that all attempts at a division into periods remain highly simplifying abstractions in contrast to the reality of nutrition.

Mainly orienting himself by the fluctuation of grain prices, the German agrarian historian, Wilhelm Abel, compiled the following stages of central European nutrition:

1. As a result of great epidemics (especially the plague) and the huge death toll resulting from them, the components of nutrition changed drastically during the 14th and 15th century, and a large improvement in quality was achieved. This must be related to the radical changes in the economy and the society of the later Middle Ages.
2. During the following centuries of early modern times there was a general impoverishment in food in Europe. In particular, there was a decrease in meat consumption, or rather an increase in the contribution of vegetable nutrition. This is demonstrated by the food expenditure of an artisan's family.
3. In the 19th century again there was a radical change in the supply of food. To judge by meat prices and wages, the first advances towards the modern affluent society were made in the developing industrial states of Europe around 1850.

However, Abel's thesis of the comparatively high meat consumption in the later Middle Ages, which had already been put forward by Gustav Schmoller and Wilhelm Roscher, increasingly questioned the opinions of medievalists.[38] They doubt the representativeness of his calculations, which form the foundations for his first stage. But the great breakthrough to mass consumption after the mid-19th century is confirmed again and again by detailed statistics. The rapid quantitative and qualitative improvement of the national diet in Germany was, as in some other comparable neighbouring countries, connected with a chain of innovations in food as well as with the decreased use of certain former basic foodstuffs. Since the 1960s

Günter Wiegelmann, in his studies on the ethnology of nutrition, has been trying to impose a division into periods on socio-cultural aspects beyond economic problems of the market for the first time.[39] Criticizing earlier divisions into stages, he put the main stress on innovations in nutrition and pursued their effects on the menus and meals of the lower social classes. Above all, he pointed out that actual turning-points occurred when a change in the ingredients of nutrition and its preparation took place. Typical examples are the change-over from porridge to coffee breakfast with sandwiches or in the replacement of milk and grain nutrition at lunch by meat and vegetable dishes. By means of cross-sections of cultural areas, the folklorist from Münster has formed the opinion that besides the great turning-points around 1770 and the First World War, the times around 1850 and 1880 are to be considered as divides for the structural changes of the 19th century.

Furthermore, he pointed out that, contrary to earlier assumptions, eating and meal patterns already came into being in the 18th century, and not for the first time, through industrialization and urbanization. Here the older, much trusted thesis of the transition from a primary immobile way of living in pre-industrial times to the more dynamic living conditions of the industrial age comes into doubt, and attention is drawn to certain trends of consolidation in the later 19th century. A regular correlation between rapid changes in nutrition and economic fluctuations, as is stated by Wilhelm Abel and the cultural fixation theory of the Swedish folklorist, Sigurd Erixon, seems to him not to be valid in this precise form. Using maps showing the dissemination of certain foodstuffs Wiegelmann points out how, for instance, potatoes, bread and chicory coffee gained a foothold as the essence of the worker's diet already during the extension of the rural home industry in the later 18th century. The year 1830 is shown to be a turning-point by the rapid increase in the consumption of brandy. In a nutshell, Wiegelmann takes the view that the decisive innovations in the nutritional system since the Middle Ages are to be placed – with regard to the temporal shifting of stages which is typical of cultural innovations – between 1680 and 1830, mainly however during the late 18th century. This would coincide with other theories of modernization.

Building on this time-frame, I have some time ago proposed an extended scheme of stages which posits the following stages of development in nutrition in central Europe:

1. The pre-historical nomadic hunter-gatherer economy.
2. Transition to settled agriculture and cattle-breeding after 8000 BC (Neolithic Revolution).
3. The intensification of the agricultural food production of Greco-Roman antiquity from 800 BC to AD 500.
4. The nutrition during the medieval dominion from the great migrations to the establishment of cities, 500–1300.
5. The structural change in food production as a result of the decrease in population caused by the epidemics during the later Middle Ages and early modern times, 1300–1500.

6. The end of the medieval nutrition and the refinement of eating customs by courtly culture, world trade, and natural sciences from 1500 to 1680.
7. The introduction of new general and luxury foods from 1680 to 1770.
8. The reception of food innovations by the rural population from 1770 to 1850.
9. The beginning of the 'diet revolution' from 1880 to 1930.
10. The onset of the age of the 'affluent society' from 1960 onwards.

We will refrain from a detailed explanation of this scheme of division into periods, as an explanation has lately been published.[40]

Finally, some hypotheses and theses on the history of nutrition are propounded which have emerged from 20 years of studying German food history and which may stimulate further research. First, the development of man's food habits is in many respects similar to the changes in sexual behaviour: in the course of history there has obviously occurred a gradual loss of instincts and a simultaneous increased excess of drives. The natural 'biological clock' for the satisfaction of the need for food, which any animal is equipped with, became lost. In addition to the original animal thirst and hunger pangs there was now appetite, which had quite different sources; thus more food could be consumed than was necessary for supplying the calories needed. The food habits, which originally were only determined by physical needs, became more and more standardized. The absolute physiological requirements and individual psychic urges of the daily form of nutrition in the course of the centuries became tied up with social conventions, trends and habits, which established fixed customs and rules and sometimes were raised to the level of magic-religious taboos. As Norbert Elias has shown, the refinement of table manners is connected with the advancement of certain thresholds of awkwardness which contributed to the establishment of European civilization.[41] Indeed, the atrophy of the original food instinct of man led to new risks of eating improperly (most of all, of overfeeding); at the same time, however, there was the possibility, which animals do not have, of the constant refinement of food and an increase in the range of choices. Natural products were accommodated more and more to the wants of man. Thus the history of nutrition has to serve a dual informative purpose: on the one hand, it has to inquire into the satisfaction of the natural satiation instinct and into a psychological basic need; on the other hand, there is the inquiry into the influences which the rules of nutrition had on the establishment of culture and civilization. Up to now these aspects have rarely been correlated with each other; in most cases one or the other aspect has been tackled in isolation.

Second, as far as one can see, at no point in history could man really dispose of his nutrition independently and unrestrainedly. Everywhere he met with ethical and social obstacles. In earlier centuries and before the beginning of mass affluence the majority of the population had never possessed enough economic means to satisfy all emerging nutrition wants simultaneously and completely. Thus, early on human abilities were developed to reduce nutritional requirements enormously and not to give in to every desire at once. Many institutional barriers helped to limit man's freedom of decisions to a tolerable level and to ease the satisfaction of wants and to be economical with respect to food. The development and decline of such behavioural patterns gives without doubt deeper insights into the changes in nutrition.

Third, the structural characteristics of an epoch can best be reconstructed by socially accepted models. Such socio-cultural value systems, which condition the scope of individual behaviour practically from birth, are obviously regularly imparted by certain social opinion leaders. He who puts such socially accepted thresholds of restraint to his fellow men, which the individual oversteps at his peril, must be regarded as the holder of ruling status. The history of nutrition, which focuses on such standardizing groups and classes as well as on their inner motivations and outer justifications, renders a considerable service to the understanding of cultural systems and of social change in general.

Fourth, in his well-known cultural lag theory, William F. Ogburn maintained that material culture, or the sum of all scientific-technical experiences, knowledge and methods, regularly changes faster than immaterial culture, the sum of all institutions, values and norms. According to this model discrepancies must emerge again and again because the immaterial range lags behind the material one. The existing results of the historical ethnology of nutrition, as well as those of the modern sociology of nutrition, show that actually the respective socio-cultural behavioural patterns for one system of nutrition change much more slowly than the outer material circumstances. The changes in socio-cultural nutritional habits, especially of meals, respond to this by delayed reaction to changes in food supply. Therefore it seems to be wrong to judge behavioural changes in daily eating and drinking by outer technical-scientific structural changes. Surely economic situations and crises have had far-reaching effects on the human form of nutrition, as agricultural goods have indeed always been limited. However, it is one of the most exciting questions to find out when changes in nutritional habits which had been triggered by these outer events occurred. As the first appearance of an innovation in nutrition should not be confused with its immediate social acceptance in general, simple linear reactions of economic changes are obviously historically not generally valid.

Finally, nutrition in historical research up to now has too often merely been regarded as a substratum of material culture: one inquired into food, cooking techniques, kitchen and dining-room furnishings, recipes, tableware, etc. For most people, however, the meal in earlier times meant more than just an assembly of prepared food and drinks; it was also always a means of communication with others. Through the act of consumption a simultaneous exchange of information is always institutionalized. Meals signal or substitute for certain forms of behaviour which might be played out in quite different spheres of life. A meal expresses certain living conditions – common social interests as well as social differences. Every history of nutrition that intends to be far-reaching has to consider such coded symbols and potential meanings in which nutritional habits are concealed, and must decode them. Then it can be shown that the importance of nutrition in the field of social communication has to be measured by quite different means. As has already been shown by these studies on individual foods and dishes, these in many cases pass through temporally clearly recognizable rises and declines of social esteem, which help explain the substitution of one food or dish by another in the food and meal patterns.

As this short survey has shown, historical nutrition research in Germany may indeed look back on an amazing history. However, only during the last two decades has it become a real target of closer economic and social research under the impulses of neighbouring disciplines and monographic studies of neighbouring countries. Now it can be seen that we are not dealing with just a short flaring-up of a fashionable interest, but with a certain reorientation of the whole field to the hitherto neglected questions of the private sphere of consumption and to new forms of interdisciplinary cooperation.

References

1 Leidenfrost (1768, 1780); Zückert (1775); Frank (1783); Danz (1806); Becker (1810, 1812); Aramanthes (1715); Marperger (1716); Engelbrecht (1730); von Plenck (1784); Krünitz (1796); Beckmann (1783–1805).
2 König (1823); Anthus (1838, 1962); Vaerst (1851).
3 Brillat-Savarin (1825).
4 Soyer (1853).
5 Reich (1860–1). See also Grotjahn (1902); Hartwich (1911).
6 Scherr (1852; 1948); Biedermann (1854, 1880); Klemm (1854–5); Klemm (1854–9); Freytag (1859, 1859–67); Kriegk (1868); Janssen (1879–94); Lamprecht (1886).
7 Weber (1882); Goetz (1882); Morgenstern (1862, 1886); Specht (1887); Schranka (1890); Fuhse (1891); Schulz (1890); Schulz (1903); Steinhausen (1903); Gollmer (1909); Bauer (1920, 1967); Reichmann (1925); Gleichen-Russwurm and Wenker (1929–30); Gutkind (1929); Hussong (1937); Hartmann (1941); Treue (1942); Döbler (1972); Rosenfeld and Rosenfeld (1978).
8 Exceptions are Delbrück (1903); and Eccardus (1907).
9 Franklin (1880–91). There the author deals with the time between the 12th and 18th century and with the focus on the *grand siècle* of Louis XIV. See also Bordeau (1894); Crespi (1891); Brothwell (1919, 1969).
10 Mannhardt (1865); Mannhardt (1868); Mannhardt (1875–1877). On his and other early ethnological enquiries in the 19th and 20th centuries, see Weber-Kellermann (1965), 520; Jacobeit (1965).
11 Heyne (1901).
12 Eckstein (1936–7); Eckstein (1927); Eckstein (1927). See also Grimm.
13 Wähler (1938), pp. 140–55. Detailed descriptions of ethnological diet research in Germany in *Ethnological food research* (1971), pp. 99–108.
14 For the 'Atlas' the following details were solicited among others: time and terms for meals, breakfast food, beverages for main dishes, methods for the production of butter, terms for buttermilk and sour milk, special dishes for Christmas, New Year, marriages and funerals, ways of baking bread and of eating out of one common bowl, etc.
15 In the 1951 and 1970 surveys which registered, among other things, the rural culture of nutrition before 1914, questions were directed towards the contents of midday, afternoon, and evening meals, emergency food and the buying and storage of food. Only part of the

material gained has so far been analysed by the folklorist, Günter Wiegelmann, from Münster. See *Atlas der deutschen Volkskunde* (1959–79); and *Erläuterungen* (1959ff.).
16 See Jantke and Hilger (1965).
17 Biedermann (1854, 1958).
18 For more details about the great literature on early nutritive statistics and its calculation method, see Teuteberg and Wiegelmann (1972), p. 44; Teuteberg and Wiegelmann (1986), pp. 225–80. To avoid repetition we will not give an account of the development of nutritional statistics in here.
19 Schmoller (1871); Conrad (1881); Apelt (1898, 1899).
20 Uffelmann (1893), pp. 2–8; Karmarsch (1872).
21 Lichtenfelt (1913); Hintze (1934).
22 Maurizio (1927); Maurizio (1933); Lippmann (1890, 1929); Lippmann (1934); Stokar (1951).
23 Häpke (1921), pp. 507ff.
24 See, for example, the corresponding paragraphs in Kulischer (1929, 1958), pp. 25–33 and Oldenberg (1923).
25 Glatzel (1955); Deutsch-Renner (1947); Schiedlausky (1956, 1959); Schmitthenner (1960); Bickel (1949); Bickel (1959); Schrämli (1960).
26 Drummond and Wilbraham (1969, 1958); Cummings (1940, 1970); Curtis-Bennett (1949); Salaman (1985); Moss (1958); Gottschalk (1948); Burema (1953).
27 *Ethnological Food Research* (1971); *Ethnologische Nahrungsforschung* (1975); *Food in Change* (1986); *Food in Perspective* (1977, 1981); *Long-Term Changes* (1986).
28 All the relevant literature on sociology and psychology of nutrition up to 1979 in Neuloh and Teuteberg (1979); See *The Digest. A Newsletter for the Interdisciplinary Study of Food* (1977ff.); Diehl (1978); *Nutritional Behavior* (1983); Logue (1986).
29 Abel (1966); Abel (1974); Wiegelmann (1967); Wiswe (1970); Teuteberg and Wiegelmann (1972); Schmauderer (1975); *Ernährung und Ernährungslehre* (1976); Teuteberg and Wiegelmann (1986).
30 Woodham-Smith (1962, 1975); Sheldon (1973); Abel (1974); Abel (1966, 1978); Clarkson (1975); Dowe (1981); Thompson (1980); Kaplan (1976); Post (1985); *Hunger* (1986); *Hunger and History* (1986).
31 Thuilliet (1968); Depuis (1970); *Pour une histoire* (1970); Aymard (1973).
32 Reichhardt (1978); Iggers (1978).
33 Barlösius (1988); Teuteberg and Wiegelmann (1986).
34 McKeown (1979); McKeown (1976); *Leib und Seele* (1983); Imhof (1981); Imhof (1984); *Mensch und Gesundheit* (1980); Imhof and Larsen (1976); Spree (1981).
35 *Hunger and History* (1985).
36 Teuteberg (1981).
37 Flandrin (1984); Flandrin (1983); Flandrin and Hyman (1986).
38 Teuteberg and Wiegelmann (1972), pp. 94–132.
39 Wiegelmann (1967), pp.27–75.
40 Teuteberg (1986).
41 Elias (1978), chapter 2.

Literature

Abel, Wilhelm, *Agrarkrisen und Agrarkonjunktur* (2nd rev. edn, Hamburg, Berlin, 1966; 3rd rev. edn, Hamburg, Berlin, 1978).
Abel, Wilhelm, *Der Pauperismus am Vorabend der Industriellen Revolution* (Göttingen, 1966).
Abel, Wilhelm, *Massenarmut und Hungerkrisen im vorindustriellen Europa* (2nd edn, Göttingen, 1974).
Anthus, A. [Gustav Blumroeder], *Vorlesungen über Esskunst* (Leipzig, 1838; new edn, Berne, Stuttgart, Vienna, 1962).
Apelt, Kurt, *Die Konsumtion der wichtigsten Kulturländer in den letzten Jahrzehnten* (doctoral thesis, Halle a.S., 1898; Berlin, 1899).
Aramanthes [Gottlieb Wilhelm Corvinius], *Nutzbares, galantes und curiöses Frauenzimmer-Lexikon...* (Leipzig, 1715).
Atlas der deutschen Volkskunde, ed. Heinrich Harmjanz and Erich Röhr (Leipzig, 1937–9), new series ed. Matthias Zehnder (Marburg, 1959–1979), *Erläuterungen* (Marburg, 1959ff.).
Aymard, Maurice, 'The history of nutrition and economic history', *The Journal of European Economic History*, 2 (1973), pp. 207–18.
Barlösius, Eva, 'Essgenuss als eigenlogisches soziales Gestaltungsprinzip. Zur Soziologie des Essens und Trinkens, dargestellt am Beispiel der grande cuisine Frankreichs', (doctoral thesis, Hanover, 1988).
Bauer, Hans, *Tisch und Tafel in alten Zeiten. Aus der Kulturgeschichte der Gastronomie* (Leipzig, 1920; new. edn, 1967).
Becker, Johann Hermann, *Versuch einer allgemeinen und besonderen Nahrungsmittelkunde*, vol I, *Litteratur und Geschichte der Nahrungsmittelkunde*, 3 parts (Stendal, 1810–12).
Beckmann, Johann, *Beyträge zur Geschichte der Erfindungen*, 5 vols (Leipzig, 1780–1805).
Bickel, Walter, *Der Menschheit grösste Leidenschaft: Gastronomische Plaudereien* (Stuttgart, 1959).
Bickel, Walter, *Deutsche Landesküchen* (Nordhausen, 1949).
Biedermann, Karl, *Deutschland im 18. Jahrhundert*, 2 vols (Leipzig, 1854; reprint 1958).
Bordeau, Louis, *Histoire de l'alimentation* (Paris, 1894).
Brillat-Savarin, Jean-Anthelme, *La Physiologie du goût* (Paris, 1825).
Brothwell, Don R. and Patricia Brothwell, *Food in Antiquity. A Survey on the Diet of Early People* (London, 1919; new. edn, London, 1969).
Burema, L., *De voeding in Nederland van de middeleeuwen tot de twingtigste eeuw [Nutrition in the Netherlands from the Middle Ages to the 20th century]* (Assen, 1953).
Clarkson, Leslie A., *Death, Disease and Famine in Preindustrial England* (Dublin, 1975).
Conrad, Johannes, 'Der Konsum an notwendigen Nahrungsmitteln in Berlin vor einhundert Jahren und in der Gegenwart', *Jahrbücher für Nationalökonomie und Statistik*, 37 (1881), pp. 509–24.
Crespi, Alfred John Henry, *The Diet of Great Men* (London, 1891).
Cummings, Richard Osborne, *The American and His Food. A History of Food Habits in the U.S.A.* (Chicago, 1940; repr. New York, 1970).
Curtis-Bennett, Sir Noël, *The Food of the People. Being the History of Industrial Feeding* (London, 1949).
Danz, Johann Traugott Leberecht, *Versuch einer allgemeinen Geschichte der menschlichen Nahrungsmittel*, 2 vols (Leipzig, 1806).
Delbrück, Max, *Beiträge zur Geschichte des Bieres und der Brauerei* (Berlin, 1903).
Depuis, Jacques 'Coutumes alimentaires, sociéte et économie', *Annales de Geographie*, 79 (1970), pp. 529–44.

Deutsch-Renner, Hans, *Ernährungsgebräuche. Ursprung und Wandel* (Vienna, 1947).
Diehl, Joerg M., *Ernährungspsychologie* (Frankfurt am Main, 1978).
Döbler, Hans-Ferdinand, *Kultur- und Sittengeschichte der Welt*. vol. II: *Kochkünste und Tafelfreuden* (Gütersloh, Berlin, Munich, Vienna, 1972).
Dowe, Dieter, 'Methodologische Überlegungen zum Problem des Hungers in Deutschland in der ersten Hälfte des 19. Jahrhunderts' in Werner Conze and Ulrich Engelhardt (eds), *Arbeiterexistenz im 19. Jahrhundert. Lebensstandard und Lebensgestaltung deutscher Arbeiter und Handwerker* (Stuttgart, 1981), pp. 202–34.
Drummond, Jack Cecil and Anne Wilbraham, *The Englishman's Food. A History of Five Centuries of English Diet* (London, 1939; 2nd rev. edn, London, 1958; new edn, 1969).
Eccardus, *Geschichte des niederen Volkes in Deutschland*, 2 vols (Stuttgart, 1907).
Eckstein, Fritz, 'Bier' in *Handwörterbuch des deutschen Aberglaubens*, vol. I (Berlin, Leipzig, 1927a), pp. 1255–82.
Eckstein, Fritz, 'Brot' in *Handwörterbuch des deutschen Aberglaubens*, vol. I (Berlin, Leipzig, 1927b), pp. 1590–659.
Eckstein, Fritz, 'Speise' in *Handwörterbuch des deutschen Aberglaubens*, vol. 8 (Berlin, Leipzig, 1936–7), pp. 156–234.
Elias, Norbert, *Über den Prozess der Zivilisation. Soziogenetische und psychogenetische Untersuchungen* (6th edn Frankfurt am Main, 1978).
Engelbrecht, Martin, *Des Menschen Zung und Gurgel Weid. Zur Notturft und Ergötzlichkeit vorgestellet durch die unterschiedlichsten Arten der Geträncke* (Augsburg, 1730).
Ernährung und Ernährungslehre im 19. Jahrhundert, ed. Edith Heikschel-Artelt (Göttingen, 1976).
Ethnological Food Research in Europe and USA. Reports from the First International Symposium for Ethnological Food Research, ed. Nils-Arvid Bringéus and Günter Wiegelmann (Lund, 1971; Göttingen, 1971).
Ethnologische Nahrungsforschung. Vorträge des zweiten internationalen Symposiums für ethnologische Nahrungsforschung, Helsinki August 1975, ed. Niilo Valonen and Juhani and E. Lehtonen (Helsinki, 1975).
Flandrin, Jean-Louis and Philip Hyman, 'Regional tastes and cuisines: problems, documents and discourses on food in southern France in the 16th and 17th centuries', *Food and Foodways*, 1 (1986), pp. 1–31.
Flandrin, Jean-Louis, 'Internationalisme, nationalisme et régionalisme dans la cuisine des XIVe et XVe siècles: Le témoignage des livres de cuisine', in *Actes du Colloque des Nice (15–17 octobre 1982)*, vol. II, *Cuisine, manières des tables, régimes alimentaires* (Nice, 1984), pp. 74–94.
Flandrin, Jean-Louis, 'La diversité des goûts et des pratiques alimentaires en Europe du XVIe au XVIIIe siècle', *Revue d'Histoire Moderne et Temporale* 30 (1983), pp. 56–83.
Food in Change. Eating Habits from the Middle Ages to the Present Day, ed. Alexander Fenton and Eszter Kisbán (Edinburgh, 1986).
Food in Perspective. Proceedings of the Third International Conference on Ethnological Food Research Cardiff, Wales, 1977, ed. Alexander Fenton and Trefor Owen (Edinburgh, 1981).
Frank, Johann Peter, *System einer vollständigen medicinischen Polizey*, vol. III: *Von Speise, Trank und Gefässen...* (Mannheim, 1783).
Franklin, Alfred, *La Vie privée d'autrefois*, Vol. I: *La Cuisine*. Vol. II: *La Repas*, Vol. III: *Variétes Gastronomiques* (Paris, 1880–91).
Freytag, Gustav, *Bilder aus deutscher Vergangenheit*, 2 vols (Leipzig, 1859).

Fuhse, Fritz, *'Sitten und Gebräuche der Deutschen beim Essen und Trinken von den ältesten Zeiten bis zum Schluss des XIV. Jahrhunderts*, (doctoral thesis, Göttingen, 1891, Wolfenbüttel, 1891).

Glatzel, Hans, *Nahrung und Ernährung. Altbekanntes und Neuerforschtes vom Essen* (Berlin, Göttingen, Heidelberg, 1955).

Gleichen-Russwurm, Alexander von and Friedrich Wenker, *Kultur- und Sittengeschichte aller Zeiten und Völker*, 16 vols (Hamburg, 1929–30).

Goetz, Wilhelm, *Speise und Trank vergangener Zeiten in deutschen Landen* (Basel, 1882).

Gollmer, Richard, *Die vornehme Gastlichkeit der Neuzeit* (Leipzig, 1909).

Gottschalk, Alfred, *Histoire de l'alimentation et de la gastronomie depuis la préhistoire jusqu'à nos jours*, 2 vols (Paris, 1948).

Grimm, Jacob and Wilhelm, *Deutsches Wörterbuch* 13 vols (Leipzig, 1852 ff.).

Grotjahn, Alfred, *Über Wandlungen der Volksernährung* (Leipzig, 1902).

Gutkind, Curt Sigmar, *Das Buch der Tafelfreuden* (Leipzig, 1929).

Häpke, Rudolf, 'Das Ernährungsproblem in der Geschichte', *Jahrbuch für Gesetzgebung, Verwaltung und Volkswirtschaft im Deutschen Reich*, 45 (1921), pp. 507 ff.

Hartmann, W., *Gastmahl der Völker* (Stuttgart, 1941).

Hartwich, Carl, *Die menschlichen Genussmittel, ihre Herkunft, Verbreitung, Geschichte, Anwendung, Bestandteile und Wirkung* (Leipzig, 1911).

Heyne, Moriz, *Das deutsche Nahrungswesen von den ältesten geschichtlichen Zeiten bis zum 16. Jahrhundert* (Leipzig, 1901).

Hintze, Kurt, *Geographie und Geschichte der Ernährung* (Leipzig, 1934).

Hunger and History. The Impact of Changing Food Production and Consumption Patterns on Society, ed. Robert I. Rotberg and Theodore K. Rabb (Cambridge, Mass., 1985).

Hunger. Quellen zu einem Alltagsproblem seit dem Dreissigjährigen Krieg, ed. Ulrich-Christian Pallach (Munich, 1986).

Hussong, R., *Der Tisch der Jahrhunderte* (Berlin, 1937).

Iggers, George G., *Neue Geschichtswissenschaft* (Munich, 1978).

Imhof, Arthur E. and Oivind Larsen, *Sozialgeschichte und Medizin* (Stuttgart, 1976).

Imhof, Arthur E., *Die gewonnenen Jahre. Von der Zunahme unserer Lebensspanne seit 300 Jahren oder von der Notwendigkeit einer neuen Einstellung zu Leben und Sterben* (Munich, 1981).

Imhof, Arthur E., *Die verlorenen Welten. Alltagsbewältigung durch unsere Vorfahren und warum wir uns heute so schwer damit tun* (Munich, 1984).

Jacobeit, Wolfgang, *Bäuerliche Arbeit und Wirtschaft. Ein Beitrag zur Wissenschaftsgeschichte der deutschen Volkskunde* (East Berlin, 1965).

Janssen, Johannes, *Geschichte des deutschen Volkes seit dem Ausgang des Mittelalters*, 8 vols (Freiburg, 1879–94).

Jantke, Carl and Dietrich Hilger, *Die Eigentumslosen. Der deutsche Pauperismus und die Emanzipationskrise in Darstellungen und Deutungen der zeitgenössischen Literatur* (Freiburg/Munich, 1965).

Kaplan, Steven Laurence, *Bread, Politics and Political Economy in the Reign of Louis XV* (The Hague, 1976).

Karmarsch, Karl, *Geschichte der Technologie seit der Mitte des 18. Jahrhunderts* (Munich, 1872).

Klemm, Gustav Friedrich, *Allgemeine Kulturwissenschaft*, 2 vols (Leipzig, 1854–5).

Klemm, Gustav-Friedrich, *Die Frauen*, 6 vols (Leipzig, 1854–9).

König, Joseph, *Geist der Kochkunst*, rev. and ed. Carl Friedrich von Rumohr (Stuttgart, Tübingen, 1823).

Kriegk, Georg Ludwig, *Deutsches Bürgertum im Mittelalter* (Frankfurt am Main, 1868).

Krünitz, Johann Georg, 'Kochen', in Johann Georg Krünitz, *Oeconomisch-technologische Encyclopädie, oder allgemeines System der Tausch-, Stadt-, Haus- und Landwirthschaft* vol.42 (Berlin, 1796).
Kulischer, Josef, *Allgemeine Wirtschaftsgeschichte des Mittelalters und der Neuzeit*, vol. II (Munich, 1929; 2nd edn, Munich, 1958).
Lamprecht, Karl, *Deutsches Wirtschaftsleben im Mittelalter. Untersuchungen über die materielle Kultur des platten Landes aufgrund der Quellen zunächst des Mosellandes* (Leipzig, 1886).
Le Goff, Jacques, Roger Chartier and Jacques Revel (eds), *La nouvelle histoire* (Paris, 1978).
Leidenfrost, 'Revolution der Diät von Europa seit 300 Jahren', *Wöchentliche Duisburger Anzeigen*, vol.1768, part 21–26. New edn in August Wilhelm Schlözer, *Briefwechsel meist historischen und statistischen Inhalts*, part 8, no. 44 (Göttingen, 1780), pp. 93–130.
Lichtenfelt, Hans, *Die Geschichte der Ernährung* (Berlin, 1913).
Lippmann, Edmund O. von, *Geschichte des Zuckers von den ältesten Zeiten bis zum Beginn der Rübenzuckerfabrikation* (Leipzig, 1890; 2nd edn, 1929).
Logue, Alexandra Woods, *Psychology of Eating and Drinking* (New York, 1986).
Long-Term Changes in Nutrition and Standard of Living. 9th Congress of the International Economic History Association, Research Topics, Section B 7, ed. Robert W. Fogel (Berne, 1986; Chicago, 1986).
Mannhardt, Wilhelm, *Die Korndämonen. Beitrag zur germanischen Sittenkunde* (Berlin, 1868).
Mannhardt, Wilhelm, *Mythologische Forschungen aus dem Nachlass*, ed. Hermann Patzig (Strasbourg, 1884).
Mannhardt, Wilhelm, *Roggenwolf und Roggenhund. Beitrag zur germanischen Sittenkunde* (Danzig, 1865).
Mannhardt, Wilhelm, *Wald und Feldkulte*, 2 vols (1875–77; 3rd edn, Darmstadt, 1968).
Marperger, Paul Jakob, *Vollständiges Küchen- und Keller- Dictionarium...* (Hamburg, 1716).
Maurizio, Adam, *Die Geschichte unserer Pflanzennahrung von den Urzeiten bis zur Gegenwart* (Berlin, 1927).
Maurizio, Adam, *Geschichte der gegorenen Getränke* (Berlin, 1933).
McKeown, Thomas, *The Modern Rise of Population* (London, 1977).
McKeown, Thomas, *The Role of Medicine: Dream, Mirage or Nemesis?* (Princeton, N.J., 1979).
Mensch und Gesundheit in der Geschichte, ed. Arthur E. Imhof (Husum, 1980).
Morgenstern, (Bauer) Lina, *Die menschliche Ernährung und die kulturhistorische Entwicklung der Kochkunst* (Berlin, 1862; 2nd edn, Berlin, 1886).
Moss, Peter, *Meals through the Ages* (London, 1958).
Neuloh, Otto and Hans J. Teuteberg, *Ernährungsfehlverhalten im Wohlstand. Ergebnisse einer empirisch-soziologischen Untersuchung heutiger Familienhaushalte* (Paderborn, 1979).
Nutritional Behaviour as a Topic of Social Sciences, ed. Hans J. Teuteberg and Johanna P. Edema (Frankfurt am Main, 1983).
Plenck, Josephus Jacobus von, *Bromatologie oder Lehre von den Speisen und Getränken* (2nd edn, Vienna, 1785).
Oldenberg, Karl, 'Die Konsumtion', in *Grundriss der Sozialökonomik*, vol. II, part 1 (2nd edn, Tübingen, 1923), pp.188–263.
Post, John D., *Food Shortage, Climatic Variability and Epidemic Diseases in Preindustrial Europe. The Mortality Peak in the Early 1740s* (London, Ithaca, N.Y., 1985).
Pour une histoire de l'alimentation, ed. Jean-Jacques Hémardinquer (Paris, 1970).
Reich, Eduard, *Die Nahrungs- und Genussmittelkunde, historisch, naturwissenschaftlich und hygienisch begründet*, 2 vols (Göttingen, 1860–1).
Reichhardt, Rolf, 'Histoire des mentalités', *Internationales Archiv für Sozialgeschichte der*

deutschen Literatur, 3(1978), pp. 130–66.
Reichmann, Johannes W. and Walter Hofstaetter, *Ein Jahrtausend deutsche Kultur. Quellen von 800–1800*, vol. 1: *Die äusseren Formen des deutschen Lebens* (3rd edn, Leipzig, 1925).
Rosenfeld, Hans Friedrich and Helmut Rosenfeld, *Deutsche Kultur im Spätmittelalter 1250–1500* (Wiesbaden, 1978).
Salaman, Redcliffe Nathan, *The History and Social Influence of the Potato* (Cambridge, 1985).
Scherr, Johannes, *Geschichte der deutschen Kultur und Sitte* (Leipzig, 1852; 11th edn, Stuttgart, 1948).
Schiedlausky, Georg, *Essen und Trinken. Tafelsitten bis zum Ausgang des Mittelalters* (Munich, 1956; 2nd edn, Munich, 1959).
Schlözer, August Ludwig, *Briefwechsel meist historischen und statistischen Inhalts*, vol. VIII, no. 44 (Göttingen, 1780), pp. 93–130.
Schmauderer, Eberhard, *Studien zur Geschichte der Lebensmittelwissenschaft* (Wiesbaden, 1975).
Schmitthenner, Erika and Heinrich, 'Speise und Trank in Europa', *Wissenschaftliche Veröffentlichungen des Deutschen Insituts für Medizinische Länderkunde*, new series, 17–18 (1960), pp. 109–65.
Schmoller, Gustav, 'Die historische Entwicklung des Fleischconsums sowie der Viehpreise in Deutschland', *Zeitschrift für die gesamte Staatswissenschaft*, 27 (1871), pp. 284–362.
Schranka, Eduard Maria, *Die Suppe. Ein Stückchen Kulturgeschichte* (2nd edn, Berlin, 1890).
Schrämli, Harry, *Der Koch als Fackelträger der Kultur* (Lucerne, 1959).
Schultz, Alwin, *Alltagsleben einer deutschen Frau zu Anfang des 18. Jahrhunderts* (Leipzig, 1890).
Schultz, Alwin, *Das häusliche Leben der europäischen Kulturvölker vom Mittelalter bis zur zweiten Hälfte des 18. Jahrhunderts* (Berlin, 1903).
Sheldon, Walther, *English Hunger and Industrial Order* (London, 1973).
Soyer, Alexis, *The Pantropheon; or History of Food and its Preparation from the Earliest Ages of the World* (London, 1853).
Specht, Franz Anton, *Gastmähler und Trinkgelage bei den Deutschen von den ältesten Zeiten bis ins 19. Jahrhundert* (Stuttgart, 1887).
Spree, Reinhard, 'Zu den Veränderungen der Volksgesundheit zwischen 1870 und 1913 und ihren Determinanten in Deutschland, vor allem in Preussen' in Werner Conze and Ulrich Engelhardt (eds), *Arbeiterexistenz im 19. Jahrhundert. Lebensstandard und Lebensgestaltung deutscher Arbeiter und Handwerker* (Stuttgart, 1981), pp. 235–92.
Steinhausen, Georg, *Geschichte der deutschen Kultur* (Leipzig, 1903).
Stokar, Walter von, *Die Urgeschichte des Hausbrotes* (Leipzig, 1951).
Teuteberg, Hans J., 'Kaffeetrinken sozialgeschichtlich betrachtet', *Scripta mercaturae*, 14 (1981), pp. 27–54.
Teuteberg, Hans J. and Günter Wiegelmann, *Unsere tägliche Kost. Geschichte und regionale Prägung* (2nd edn, Münster, 1986).
Teuteberg, Hans J. and Günter Wiegelmann, *Der Wandel der Nahrungsgewohnheiten unter dem Einfluss der Industrialisierung* (Göttingen, 1972).
Teuteberg, Hans J., 'Periods and turning-points in the history of European diet: preliminary outline of problems and methods', in Alexander Fenton and Eszter Kisbán (eds), *Food in Change. Eating Habits from the Middle Ages to the Present Day*, (Edinburgh, 1986), pp. 11–23.
Thompson, Edward P., *The Moral Economy of the English Crowd in the 18th Century* (London, 1971).
Thuilliet, G., 'Les Sources de l'histoire regional et l'alimentation', *Annales E.S.C.*, 23 (1968), pp. 1301–19.

Treue, Wilhelm, *Kleine Kulturgeschichte des deutschen Alltags* (Potsdam, 1942).
Uffelmann, 'Nahrungsmittelpolizei' in *Handwörterbuch der Staatswissenschaften*, vol. 5 (1st edn, Jena, 1893), pp. 2–8.
Vaerst, Eugen Baron, *Gastrosophie oder Lehre von den Freuden der Tafel*, 2 vols (Leipzig, 1851).
Wähler, Martin, 'Die deutsche Volksnahrung' in Wilhelm Pessler (ed.), *Handbuch der deutschen Volkskunde*, vol. 3 (Potsdam, 1938), pp. 140–55.
Weber, Felix, *Gastronomische Bilder* (Leipzig, 1882).
Weber-Kellermann, Ingeborg, *Erntebrauch in der ländlichen Arbeitswelt des 19. Jahrhunderts aufgrund der Mannhardt-Befragung in Deutschland von 1865* (Marburg, 1965).
Wiegelmann, Günter, *Alltags-und Festtagsspeisen. Wandel und gegenwärtige Stellung* (Marburg, 1967).
Wiswe, Hans, *Kulturgeschichte der Kochkunst* (Munich, 1970).
Woodham-Smith, Cecil, *The Great Hunger. Ireland 1845–1849* (London, 1962; 4th edn, London, 1975).
Zückert, Johann Friedrich, *Allgemeine Abhandlung von Nahrungsmitteln* (Berlin, 1775).

8 Food research from the viewpoint of ethnology, economic and social history in the former German Democratic Republic, 1949–1989

Rudolf Weinhold

Hitherto there has been a lack of bibliographical surveys like that presented in this paper. Although titles concerned with historical-ethnological food research are occasionally found in regional bibliographies, there has not been a systematic and comprehensive survey, perhaps because this subject has not been the focus of attention for a long time. Therefore, in order to compile historical and, in a broader sense, cultural studies for the period covered by this paper we had to start from scratch. With an ever widening view of the subject we soon became aware that, besides the papers covering the fields included in the title, we also had to consider regional, local historical and agrarian-historical investigations in the field of food production. Without this wider view, there would have been enormous gaps in this paper.

It should be emphasized, though, that in the former GDR, as everywhere else, food researchers have made great efforts focused on the practical aspects of nutrition, that is, on physiology, biology and chemistry, on the analysis and technology of foodstuffs, and on the science of their preparation. Proof of the approaches, methods and results of these studies can be found in a concentrated form in the periodical *Ernährungsforschung*,[1] issued since 1956 by the Institute for Food Research and the Centre of Vitamin Research in Potsdam-Rehbrücke, later merged into the Central Food Institute of the GDR Academy of Sciences. Those interested primarily in history and ethnology will be pleased to find in this periodical frequent articles of a generally scientific orientation that are concerned with the history of food and nutrition.[2]

The subjects of most of these articles are closely related to those papers which approach food research from a historio-cultural position, that is, one based on the history of civilization in a broad sense. They include both ethnological and historical studies of widely varying depth and scope, ranging from well-grounded monographic analyses to local historical and geographical approaches. These papers make up the main part of the material considered in this bibliography, and they are presented below according to their subjects and complex of questions.

Many of these studies deal with bread, its preparation and the equipment required for it. The first and most important of these is Walter von Stokar's *Urgeschichte des Hausbrotes*, published in Leipzig in 1951. In the importance of its findings, this monograph reaches far beyond the scope of archaeology into interdisciplinary realms. In this respect it can therefore still be considered as a standard work from a methodological standpoint.

Elisabeth Tornow's monograph on the advances in the field of cereals, flour and bread chemistry and of milling and baking technology[3] traces important lines of this development up to the present day. There are several local historical and geographical studies from Thuringia, Saxony, the Harz mountains, the March of Brandenburg and Lower Lusatia describing baking activities and equipment.[4] The oven, whether private or communal property, has been an object of particular interest.[5]

The attention of ethnology has furthermore been directed to special kinds and shapes of baked goods, which is mainly due to the fact that they used to be of importance in folklore and festivities. Examples are the gingerbread and similar sweetmeats[6] baked around Christmas, as well as *Klemmkuchen*,[7] a pastry baked in a clamping iron which was very popular in the Elbe and Oder region, and finally *Naute*,[8] dainties almost fallen into oblivion and once highly enjoyed by children mainly made of honey or syrup, grits, flour and poppy, completed with cream and spices or vinegar. They were very popular in Berlin, the Oderbruch region and the Uckermark, as well as around Magdeburg and in Mecklenburg. The etymology of the word *Naute* is uncertain. Earlier publications derive it from the Hebrew word *naut* which is the name of a pastry prepared for the Sabbath and other festivities. But it is also possible that this word came from the French word *nougat*.

Potato-based food is the subject of a number of further papers and reports. The majority of these discuss this subject from a historical standpoint. Among topics discussed are the introduction and propagation of the potato, in particular its cultivation in the Vogtland,[9] which was a very early innovator, in Thuringia,[10] Brandenburg,[11] and Lower Lusatia.[12] Other studies also discuss its preparation,[13] not excluding, of course, the famous Thuringian and Vogtlandian dumplings. The well-researched study by Ingeborg Müller on the part played by the potato and its cultivation in the Vogtland in the course of the changes in the feeding habits which took place in the 18th and in the early 19th centuries,[14] is especially worth mentioning because of its interdisciplinary approach which connects ethnological and socio- and economic-historical points.

Compared to the papers on vegetable-based foodstuffs, the papers on meat-based food are smaller in number and less comprehensive. They concentrate upon the slaughtering day and associated customs and meals.[15] In some cases regionally specific sausages and meat dishes are also presented.[16] We should not forget to mention the well-informed description of the so-called 'Leipzig larks',[17] a type of wild fowl practically extinct today, and its culinary utilization. Up to the second third of the 19th century 10,000 of these birds, various species of which inhabited Northern Saxony and Saxony-Anhalt, were caught and eaten every year. The largest species, the Calandra lark, up to 21 cm long and with a 43 cm wingspan, was also taken to the markets of neighbouring regions to be sold as a highly sought after delicacy.

Some of the studies are dedicated to milk and dairy products. Renate Winter's study of milk and its processing in the former province of Pomerania[18] is the most comprehensive and outstanding in its content. It is based on philological inquiries but also takes into consideration the underlying product and its utilization. Further papers describe rural milk storage and cooling equipment,[19] a butter-churn[20] and cheese production.[21] Finally, a historio-economically orientated study which considers the whole territory of the former GDR also includes the historical basis of milk production and utilization.[22]

Beekeeping and its products have found scant coverage in the papers referred to here. This subject is dealt with in a regional linguistic study of honey[23] and more broadly in a world-wide study of the economic importance of beekeeping.[24]

A subject mainly popular in local and regional historical descriptions and sketches is the brewing industry and its products. An exception is Herbert Langer's well-researched treatise on modern times.[25] The author describes production volumes, beer qualities, beer trade, the license to brew beer and the resultant controversies between town and country, the brewing equipment and process, wage work in the breweries as well as the cooperation in the brewing trade as a primeval form of capitalist beverage production. The majority of papers on this subject are confined to the description of local conditions, mainly seeking to work up historical material.[26] Two concise reports refer to special top-fermented types of beer with a long tradition: the 'Leipziger Gose'[27] and the 'Berliner Weisse'.[28] The list of alcoholic drinks is completed by information on former and present-day wine-growing. There is a monograph[29] on its history and the processing of its vintages in changing times. Regional studies describe the origin of viniculture in the Brandenburg territories,[30] which ceased to exist a long time ago. Stronger alcoholic drinks are dealt with in papers on Nordhäuser corn brandy,[31] the beginnings and consequences of the distilling of potato-spirits[32] and, going largely beyond the borders of the former GDR, on the history of rum.[33]

The authors of papers which are dedicated to the subjects of food preparation and consumption, eating habits and associated customs, but also to economically and socially dependent and differentiated eating patterns, seek a synthesis of the partial findings mentioned above. Methodical starting-points for this were marked by Martin Wähler in a paper published in the three-volume *Handbuch der deutschen Volkskunde* by Wilhelm Pessler.[34] However, the application of more recent knowledge as well as that gained by evaluating the material in the *Atlas der deutschen Volkskunde* by Teuteberg and Wiegelmann,[35] for instance, is neglected by most of the regional and, in particular, the locally orientated investigations. There is still a lack of historical-ethnological descriptions of the feeding habits and dietary condition of the GDR as a whole. But a short look at the literature on the subject shows that we are not alone in Europe with respect to this deficiency. Surveys and investigations which cover small territories prevail. The first attempts at a farther-reaching collection and incorporation of the material into the whole historical and cultural process are found in the work *Zur Geschichte von Kultur und Lebensweise der werktätigen Klassen und Schichten des deutschen Volkes*,[36] published for the first time in 1972. These intentions are continued in the chapter 'Volksnahrung' by Ingeborg Müller and Ulrich Bentzien in *Mecklenburgische Volkskunde*,[37] published in 1988.

The feeding habits and diets of other parts of the former GDR have also been the subject of research, not only by ethnologists. An example is the former Brandenburg-Prussia, where both ethnologists and nutritional scientists worked in our field. Helmut Haenel, one of the most prominent of the latter and director of the Institute for Nutritional Sciences of the Academy of Sciences in Potsdam-Rehbrücke, contributed substantially to the increase of our historio-cultural knowledge on this subject by making some comparisons of the bills of fare of poor people in the town of Potsdam with those of the royal Prussian court in the 18th century.[38] Also noteworthy are the results of his analysis of Prussian troop catering in 1813. He stated that the daily ration of the rank and file came, in the main, up to our modern standards of a reasonable diet as to its protein, fat and carbohydrate content, calorie value and basic nutritive substances as well as to the percentage of vitamin B_1, iron and fibre. He only criticizes the overly high salt ration and the overly low vitamin C and calcium content.[39] One can only hope that such rations were standard in those days. As we know, military campaigns have their specific problems in this respect.

Further studies cover other regions, such as the Lower Harz mountains,[40] Altmark[41] and south-eastern Thuringia,[42] and more or less specifically the food in some towns.[43] Genuinely ethnological approaches are found in two studies dedicated to the popular fare in Saxon Switzerland (mountainous area around Dresden) and surrounding territories before the introduction of the potato,[44] that is, during the second half of the 19th and the beginning of the 20th centuries.[45] Finally, the booklet *Schlüsselhecht und nackter Barsch. Vom Kochen an Bord und von Fischgerichten der Küstenbevölkerung an Ostsee und Nordsee [Pike and Naked Perch: Cooking on Board Ship and Fish Dishes of the Inhabitants of the Baltic and North Sea Coast]*[46] links research into food history and cooking recipes.

With a sketch on the weekly bill of fare in a Hessian village[47] around 1920-30 published in the periodical *Ernährungsforschung*, we leave the territory of our report. We are taken further afield by the 'Fragebogen zu einer Volkskunde des Nahrungswesens'[48] by Ingeborg Weber-Kellermann, which served as the basis for part of her research among Germans living in Hungary. Her goal was to reveal and interpret interethnic relations in this field, which were an important factor of the mutual cultural give-and-take between diverse national groups in the Hungarian part of so-called Swabian Turkey, that is, the districts of Tolna, Somogy and Baranya, as well as northern Bácska, and can still be found in a number of villages today.

A treatise on the kitchens in the Arnstadt doll city of 'Mon Plaisir'[49] refers to a remarkable piece of historical evidence of which hitherto too little notice has been taken. This great historio-cultural and ethnological source from the 18th century, which has not yet been evaluated, occupies the rooms of a whole house. It also includes well-equipped kitchens, whose furnishings and utensils are considered to be perfect miniature reproductions of the noble and middle-class originals.

Food and its preparation have also attracted the interest of various dialectologists. The paper on milk and milk processing written by Renate Winter in a Low-German dialect has already been referred to (see note 18 above). She is the author of an essay that presents the wide spectrum of common answers which used to be given to the question 'Wat gifft to eten?'[50] [What's for dinner?] in Pomerania. Short studies of menus from the Vogtland[51] as well as some descriptions of the most popular dishes in that region,[52] written in the local dialect, and an excursion on the food and drink of those inhabitants of southern Thuringia who speak an eastern Franconian dialect,[53] refer to the southern and south-western border regions of the former GDR.

The subject of food preparation and eating would be incomplete if we did not consider table manners and seating plans. Concerning the former, there are two miscellanea which also attack the often rather crude behaviour of the feudal nobility.[54] In contrast, Karl Baumgarten's treatise on the seating plan in old Mecklenburg farmhouses[55] elucidates historical and underlying social processes in the villages in the 19th and early 20th centuries: at the beginning of this development the farmer's seat was at the head of the table where people ate separated by sex (one bench each for men and women). In the second half of the 19th century and along with the increasing differentiation between the farmer and his servants, this patriarchal lifestyle began to disappear. This led in the 20th century to the separate taking of meals in two different rooms, the final breach with the traditional seating plan.

A variety of studies are concerned with the study of basic food constituents. Methodically they combine procedures of agrarian and economic history, occasionally also of primeval and early history. The latter applies to two major papers which show the wide range of today's food research. A Leipzig postdoctoral thesis is dedicated to the important subject of the beginnings of cereal-growing in the Middle East, its material and social preconditions and the consequences of that qualitative economic change for the history of mankind.[56] A Berlin thesis investigates a more recent period of cereal production. One of the main aspects of this study is the development of the equipment required for processing cereals. It discusses different types of porridge as well as the history of baking techniques since the Middle Ages and various kinds of food eaten during war and famines.[57] Finally, the periodical *Ernährungsforschung*,[58] already cited, offers a comprehensive survey of a great number of sources on the growing and consumption of corn since prehistoric times, drawn from specific literature on the subject. The relation between plant cultivation and biological science is analysed in a Jena thesis.[59]

Various food plants have been given special attention, some, such as manna grass,[60] because they were wild-growing plants whose fruits were collected in times of famine and also because of their flavour, others because they are grown rarely if at all in the GDR, among them buckwheat and common millet.[61] In addition spices,[62] above all garlic, merited special consideration, not only because of their appetizing and digestive properties, but also because of their importance for a wholesome lifestyle.[63]

Two studies from the Berlin region describe the cultural history of sugar. While one of them, with its museological orientation, mainly describes sugar-producing equipment,[64] the other takes a more comprehensive approach. Besides beet-sugar from the March of Brandenburg and tropical cane-sugar, synthetic glucose preparations are also discussed.[65]

Salt, with its particular importance to nutrition, has been highly appreciated by scientists of the Freiberg Mining College. A historical monograph traces its extraction and utilization from prehistoric times to the present day.[66] The production of evaporated salt in Germany between 1500 and 1900 is the subject of a postdoctoral thesis.[67]

Economic-historical inquiries predominate in a good dozen papers on food and nutrition; these are now presented chronologically. Problems with the supply of meat, milk and dairy products in antiquity are discussed in a treatise on the history of stock-farming in the Roman Empire.[68] An economic-historically orientated study on the food production of the Teutons[69] can in certain respects be considered as a supplement to that paper, although written 15 years earlier.

An important aspect of German–Slavic relations in the early Middle Ages is characterized by an investigation of the beginning and volume of German grain exports to pre-Mongolian Rus.[70]

The Hanseatic working group and the Commission on Agrarian History incorporated into the former GDR Society of Historians held two conferences in the early 1980s where our subject played an important part. Unfortunately, only abstracts of these events have appeared so far. One of the conferences was concerned with the customs, culture and ideology of medieval townspeople, in particular in the Hanseatic region.[71] Among other subjects, the change in the feeding habits of the Danzig middle class during the 16th century was raised: the rapid growth of the rich was also reflected in an increasing fat content and an unbalanced diet, which finally had an adverse effect on public health. The illustrative potential of middle-class wills and testaments in Austria from the 14th and 15th centuries with regard to urban food of that epoch was also demonstrated.

The subject matter dealt with at the other conference was the food situation of late feudalism.[72] The subjects discussed can be cited here only in brief: the correlation between food production and the resulting food spectrum; food demand, production and trade in the 16th century; the provision of ducal and electoral German courts with food during the 16th century; the food problem as a reason for conflicts between the urban and rural population in Thuringia in the 16th century;[73] the food situation of the lower classes in the western Saxon mining region in the 15th and 16th centuries; the food of ordinary people in late feudal Mecklenburg; the food of clerical and secular feudal lords in the Netherlands in the 15th and 16th centuries; food problems in Hungary and Hungarian agrarian exports between 1711 and 1848; the peasant's food situation in late feudal Hungary; urban food consumption (in particular in Vienna) in the late 18th century; food problems in Lower Saxony from 1770 to 1830; the prosperity of Altenburg peasants in the 17th and 18th centuries; the food of textile manufacturers in the Ore mountains; and food and drink in the late Middle Ages as based on archaeological sources (primarily on excavations in Magdeburg, Neuss and Lübeck).

Two studies concerned with facts and processes that are typical of the period from the 16th to the 18th centuries are also based on agrarian- and economic-historical inquiries. The points in question are the corn markets in Saxony and Thuringia as estimated in grain measures[74] as well as trends in Brandenburg stock-farming before the introduction of bourgeois farming methods.[75]

Two of the papers focused on the 19th and 20th centuries are concerned with trends in vegetable farming. A Berlin thesis discusses this subject for the whole of Germany, special attention being drawn to the processes taking place in the Weimar Republic.[76] A regional study describes the expansion of Spreewald vegetable gardening, well known far beyond its provincial boundaries since the 1870s.[77] There is another locally orientated paper which presents extracts from the history of the Saxon food and semi-luxury goods industry.[78] A comprehensive monograph on food production and the productivity of agriculture in Germany, France, Great Britain and the USA, however, is of world-wide breadth, particularly in its description of foreign trade and imports.[79] A study published in the *Yearbook of Economic History* is concerned with the increasing consumption of butter and margarine since the 1950s – a phenomenon much discussed not just in the former GDR. Due to its consequences, it has to be controlled as part of a reasonable food policy.[80]

Let me conclude this bibliographical survey by taking a look at papers which describe gastronomy and, in particular, culinary art from an ethnological and historio-cultural point of view, and at reprints of old cookery-books. Two books embrace the subject of hospitality, feasting and drink[81] in Europe. They address a wide public and, accordingly, are intended more as popular works than to satisfy scientific demands. Almost nostalgic in nature is a booklet on *Deutsche Landesküchen*[82] published in 1947 – for broad sectors of the population practically equivalent to provocation in that period of famine – which presented selected dishes whose basic constituents and ingredients were only available to those privileged by fate or on the black market. A cookery-book which 25 years later recalled the recipes of popular dishes from regions between the Thuringian Forest and Lusatia, Baltic Sea and Ore mountains has most likely found more interested users.[83] Since the late 1970s this book has been accompanied by regionally orientated recipe collections and booklets on spices from Thuringia, Saxony and Mecklenburg.[84] They were supplemented by the reprint of two north German cookery-books from the second half of the 19th century,[85] which, no doubt, were welcome not only to those interested in the popular fare.

A remarkable project which should also be mentioned here are the new editions of older works of culinary art.[86] The publishing house Verlag Edition Leipzig in particular deserves praise for its part in the project. The twenty or so documents on the history of and changes in food habits range from the cookery-book by Philippine Welser through the works of Egenolff and Rumpolt to the recipe collection of Johanne Wilhelmine Cotta.

This paper has given a survey of the literature on food history which has been available to me. We have learned from similar projects, however, that this is not everything which has been written on this subject. But it is hoped that the basics have been covered and, thus, that a picture of the current level of research has been provided.

What conclusions should be drawn now for further work, in particular in the field of ethnology, needs a paper to itself. This should state first of all whether the available material, as well as earlier findings, of course, is sufficient for a historical-ethnographical survey of particular periods of development of food production and food habits which evaluates already existing knowledge. This is possibly true of the 19th and 20th centuries. This material could also offer sufficient subject matter for separate topics, such as the introduction of potato cultivation and the associated change or extension of basic foods in some segments of the population.

For a verification of Günter Wiegelmann's discovery of innovative processes in dietary conditions and feeding between the late 17th century and the mid-19th century, especially in the territory discussed here, the data hitherto put together still seem to be incomplete. This is surely due to the fact that the underlying aspects of Wiegelmann's studies have hardly been considered, if at all, in most of our work. Many subjects, in particular those of a local or regional nature, have been too restricted in their methodological and theoretical approach to offer epoch-making findings. They are valuable in providing facts for the answers to such questions. But the argument that the territorial frame which was set here for quite pragmatic reasons has been restricted too much in some cases, i.e. only allows specific phenomena or processes to be considered in part, cannot be rejected. Central Europe presents itself as another field of reference whether one investigates the specific food habits of separate classes and strata or the reasons for regionally characteristic food. And, last but not least, it should be stated that there is still a great lack of scientific analysis in the field. It remains to be seen if future studies pay increased attention to these and further problems as well as to the further development of interdisciplinary food research through new findings.

References

1 *Ernährungsforschung*, 1(1956)ff.
2 See Haenel (1976); Haenel (1984); Pilz (1985); Pilz (1987); Geschichte (1976); Sitten (1976); Knapp (1979); Rothe (1978); Strübing (1967).
3 Tornow (1958).
4 Gill (1983–4); Klocke (1967); Müller (1983); Starkloff (1976); Weiden (1983–4); Zahmel (1984).
5 Fiedler (1963); Friedrich (1969, 1970); Lommatz (1966); Kretschmann (1980); Richter (1984).
6 Nickel (1961); Reitz (1957); Schmidt (1975); Beranek (1961).
7 Bastine (1980–1b); Kühne (1981); Ohnesorge (1964).
8 Schmidt (1967).
9 Richter (1961).
10 Edler (1973); Edler (1984).
11 Krausch (1976).
12 Krausch (1975).
13 Speerschneider (1976); Speerschneider (1984).

Food research from the viewpoint of ethnology, economic and social history   137

14 Müller (1976).
15 'Alte Bräuche' (1973); Giesecke (1976); Wüstefeld (1978).
16 Erfurth (1976); Von Fliesenwurst (1977).
17 Pilz (1987).
18 Winter (1963).
19 Fiedler (1963–4).
20 Zeun (1965).
21 Holstein (1973).
22 Fischer (1971).
23 Barthel (1966).
24 Güntzel (1975).
25 Langer (1979).
26 Bellin (1956); 'Von der Blütezeit' (1975); Gust (1981/82); Heddergott (1968); Horalek (1976); Humbsch (1981); Leister (1972); Ludwig (1977); Oehlandt (1981); 'Rathenower Bier' (1976); Saegler (1983); Stürzebecker (1980); Thoss (1968); Wagner (1973); Wagner (1961); Weisse (1962).
27 Pilz (1985).
28 Meidow (1959).
29 Weinhold (1973).
30 Fellin (1973); Gutjahr (1957).
31 Grutz (1981); Heber (1978).
32 Weinhold (1986).
33 Geschichte (1976).
34 Wähler (1934).
35 See Teuteberg and Wiegelmann (1972); Teuteberg and Wiegelmann (1986); Teuteberg (1987).
36 *Zur Geschichte von Kultur* (1972).
37 *Mecklenburgische Volkskunde* (1988).
38 Haenel (1976); Haenel (1984). More information on this topic in the following newspaper articles: Mehlhardt (1983); Paepke (1981).
39 Haenel (1987).
40 Ludwig (1973).
41 Hagen (1962).
42 Rosenkranz (1957).
43 Becker (1957).
44 Schober (1980).
45 Schober (1982).
46 *Schlüsselhecht und nackter Barsch* (1985).
47 Knapp (1979).
48 Weber-Kellermann (1958).
49 Roselt (1964).
50 Winter (1961).
51 Barthel (1970).
52 Barthel (1984).
53 Braungart (1983).
54 'Rauhe Sitten' (1976); Stieler (1983).
55 Baumgarten (1965).
56 Hoffmann (1979).

57 Reimann (1974).
58 Rothe (1973).
59 Zirnstein (1977).
60 Dräger (1960).
61 Bastine (1980–1a); Hanelt (1981).
62 Rothe (1978).
63 Strübing (1967).
64 Stengel (1952).
65 Schmidt-Berg-Lorenz (1963).
66 Emons and Walter (1984).
67 Walter (1985).
68 Parain (1971).
69 Schrot (1955–6).
70 Widera (1963).
71 Schattkowsky (1982).
72 Kagel (1985).
73 Held (1985).
74 Mielczarksi (1969).
75 Müller (1966).
76 Puls (1981).
77 Lange (1984).
78 Pönicke (1974).
79 Helling (1977).
80 Roesler (1988).
81 Schmitthenner (1967).
82 Bickel (1947).
83 Drummer (1982).
84 Fraass (1983); Ilgenstein (1984); *Sagenhafte Thüringer Rezepte* (1984); Itterheim *et al.* (1979); Becker (1976); 'Rezepte aus Mühlberg' (1983); '*Alte Rezepte*' (1980); *Rezepte zu Festen und Feiern* (1981); *Rezepte nach Jägerart* (1982); *Rezepte für Pottkiekers* (1984); Becker and Milbert (1985).
85 Ritzerow (1868, 1985); Hammerl (1898, 1985).
86 *Kochbuch der Phillippine Welser* (1983); Egenolff (1531, 1984); Rumpolt (1581, 1976, 1977, 1980); Rontzier (1589, 1979); Elsholtz (1682, 1984); *Vollständiges Nürnbergisches Kochbuch* (1691, 1979, 1986); Rosalia (1709, 1978); Sincerus (1713, 1982); Hagger (1719, 1977); Schellhammer (1984); Schellhammer (1989); *Der Geschickte und Wohlerfahrene Engelländische Koch* (1742, 1986); Eger (1745, 1983, 1984); *Textor-Kochbuch* (1980); *Das allerneueste Pariser Kochbuch* (1752, 1981); *Vollständiges Koch- Back- und Konfitürenlexikon* (1786, 1986); *Kochbuch der Johanne Wilhelmine Cotta* (1984); Goullon (1829, 1984); Hamm (1865, 1983, 1984).

Literature

Das allerneueste Pariser Kochbuch (Strasbourg, 1752; new edn, Leipzig, 1981).
'Alte Bräuche auf dem Eichsfeld. Das große Fest, wenn wir schlachten. Von Fetthäuten, Felgieker und Hülfenbergwürsten', *Thüringer Tageblatt*, (November 1973), Nr. 296.
Barthel, Friedrich, 'Rund um den Honig. Eine sprachliche Betrachtung', *Kulturspiegel für den*

Kreis Auerbach/Vogtland, (1966), pp. 43-5.

Barthel, Friedrich, 'Speisekarte auf Vogtländisch', *Kulturspiegel für den Kreis Auerbach* (1970), pp. 45-8.

Barthel, Friedrich, 'Lieblingsspeisen der Vogtländer im Spiegel der Mundartdichtung', *Vogtländische Heimatblätter*, 22(1984), no. 4, pp. 24-5.

Bastine, Werner, 'Verschwundene Kulturpflanzen unserer Heimat. 1. Der Buchweizen', *Gubener Heimatkalender*, 24(1980-1a), pp. 80-7.

Bastine, Werner, 'Klemmkuchen — einfach vergessenes Niederlausitzer Gebäck', *Luckauer Heimatkalender*, 12/13(1980-1b), pp. 72-8.

Bauer, Hans, *Tisch und Tafel in alten Zeiten. Aus der Kulturgeschichte der Gastronomie* (s. l. 1920; 2nd new edn, Leipzig, 1967).

Baumgarten, Karl, 'Die Tischordnung im alten mecklenburgischen Bauernhaus', *Deutsches Jahrbuch für Volkskunde*, 11(1965), pp. 5-15.

Becker, Fritz, *Das Kochbuch aus Thüringen, Sachsen und Schlesien / gesammelt, aufgeschrieben und ausprobiert* (Münster, 1976).

Becker, Hanns, 'Über Nahrungsmittel, Bekleidung, Unterkunft und Trinkwasserversorgung der Stadt Pegau in der Vergangenheit', *Heimatkundliche Blätter des Bezirks Dresden*, 3(1957), pp. 255-61.

Becker, Ursula and Lisa Milbert, *Mecklenburgische Rezepte* (Rostock, 1985).

Bellin, R., 'Das Neuruppiner Bier und die Bierziese' in *Neuruppin. 700 Jahre Stadtrecht* (Neuruppin, 1956), pp. 47-51.

Beranek, Josef, '"Salzwedeler Baumkuchen". Die Geschichte eines leckeren Baumes', *Der Altmarkbote*, 6(1961), pp. 354-60.

Bickel, Walter, *Deutsche Landesküchen. Ein Buch von deutscher Speise. Eine Auswahl der besten Rezepte der regionalen Küche nebst neuen Anweisungen für süsse Speisen, Salate, Gemüsegerichte und Eintöpfe nebst einer Physiologie des Essens* (Leipzig, Nordhausen/Harz, 1947).

Braungart, Margarethe, 'Was Leib und Seele zusammenhält. Kleine Betrachtung über Speise und Trank in unserer Sprache nebst einigen alten Rezepten mit wunderbaren Namen', *Almanach für Kunst und Kultur im Bezirk Suhl*, 4(1983), pp. 80-6.

Dräger, G., 'Mannagras — einst ein Leckerbissen', *Natur und Heimat*, 9(1960), pp. 544-6.

Drummer, Kurt and Käthe Muskewitz, *Von Apfelkartoffeln bis Zwiebelkuchen: Volkstümliche Gerichte aus der DDR zwischen Thüringer Wald und Lausitz, Ostsee und Erzgebirge* (Leipzig, 1982).

Edler, Wolfgang, 'Von anmuthigem Geschmack. Aus der Geschichte des Kartoffelanbaus in Thüringen', *Thüringer Tageblatt*, (December 1973), no. 302.

Edler, Wolfgang, 'Thüringer Kartoffelgeschichte: Die schmackhafte Erdknolle wurde um 1750 bei uns eingebürgert', *Das Volk*, 40(October 1984), no. 272.

Egenolff, Christian, *Von Speisen, Natürlichen und Kreuter Wein, aller verstandt* (Frankfurt, 1531; new edn, Leipzig, 1984).

Eger, Susanne, *Leipziger Kochbuch* (Leipzig, 1745; new. edn, Leipzig, 1983; 2nd edn, 1984).

Elsholtz, Johann Sigismund, *Diaeteticon* (Cölln/Spree, 1682; new edn, Leipzig, 1984).

Emons, Hans-Heinz and Hans-Henning Walter, *Mit dem Salz durch die Jahrtausende: Geschichte des weissen Goldes von der Urzeit bis zur Gegenwart* (Leipzig, 1984).

Ernährungsforschung. Ed. Zentralinstitut für Ernährungs Potsdam-Rehbrücke, vol. 1 (1956) ff.

Erfurth, Helmut, 'Zwiebelwurst als Festtagsschmaus: überlieferte Bräuche in Anhalt', *Liberal-Demokratische Zeitung, Ausgabe Anhalt/Dessau*, 31(1976), no. 306, p. 8.

Erfurth, Helmut, ' Von Fliesenwurst und schmackhafter Pottsuse', *Liberal-Demokratische*

Zeitung, Ausgabe Altmark/Stendal, 32(1977), no. 1, p. 5.

Fellin, H., 'Potsdamer Wein ... ', Brandenburgische Neueste Nachrichten, 23(1973), no. 167, p. 6.

Fiedler, Alfred, 'Zur Frage des kommunalen Backens in den Dörfern Sachsens während des 18. und zu Beginn des 19. Jahrhunderts', *Abhandlungen und Berichte des Staatlichen Museums für Völkerkunde Dresden*, 22(1963), pp. 181–201.

Fiedler, Alfred, 'Die Milchaufbewahrungsorte der bäuerlichen Wirtschaften in den sächsischen Bezirken der DDR', *Ethnographica*, 5/6(1963–4), pp.60–7.

Fischer, Heinz, *'Die Entwicklung der Milchwirtschaft in der DDR unter besonderer Berücksichtigung der historischen Traditionen'* (doctoral thesis, Berlin, 1971).

Fraass, Ulla, *Thüringer Koch- und Backrezepte* (Erfurt, 1983).

Friedrich, Dieter, 'Die Gemeindebacköfen im westlichen Fläming', *Zerbster Heimatkalender*, 11(1969–70), pp. 52–4.

'Die Geschichte des Rums', *Ernährungsforschung*, 21(1976), pp. 93–4.

Der Geschickte und Wohlerfahrene Engelländische Koch (Leipzig 1742; new edn, Leipzig, 1986).

Giesecke, Fritz, 'Echte Bördewurst – die schmeckt am besten: Von der Kunst des guten Altmärker Hausschlachtens', *Der neue Weg*, 31(Februar 1976), no. 42, p. 6.

Gill, Manfred, 'Das Backen in Letschin', *Heimatkalender für die Gemeinde Letschin*, (1983–4), pp. 83–7.

Goullon, François de, *Der neue Apicius oder die Bewirtung vornehmer Gäste* (Weimar, 1829; new edn, Leipzig, 1984).

Grutz, Helmut, *Nordhäuser Weinbrand* (Wiesbaden, 1981).

Güntzel, Alfons, *'Die weltwirtschaftliche Bedeutung der Bienenzucht. Eine ökonomischgeographische Untersuchung'* (doctoral thesis, Potsdam, 1975).

Gust, Franz-Ferdinand, 'Brauereigeschichte (von Potsdam)', *Märkische Volksstimme*, 36(1981), no. 302, 8; no. 306, 8; 37(1982), no. 7, 8; no. 17, 8; no. 31, 8, 55; no. 43, 8; no. 72, 8.

Gutjahr, R., 'Rathenower Rebensaft', *Heimatkalender Rathenow*, (1957), pp. 78–9.

Haenel, Helmut, 'Speisenkarte in Preussen vor 200 Jahren', *Ernährungsforschung*, 21(1976), pp. 89–93.

Haenel, Helmut, 'Essen und Trinken in Preussen im 18. Jahrhundert', *Ernährungsforschung*, 29(1984), pp. 18–25.

Haenel, Helmut, 'Preussische Truppenverpflegung 1813 im Vergleich', *Ernährungsforschung*, 32(1987), pp. 146–9.

Hagen, Fritz, 'Pelktüffeln, Stipp und Salzhering. Bauernkost in alter Zeit', *Der Altmarkbote*, 7(1962), pp. 293–4.

Hagger, Conrad, *Neues Saltzburgisches Koch-Buch*, 2 vols (Augsburg, 1719; new edn, Leipzig, 1977).

Hamm, Wilhelm, *Das Weinbuch. Wesen, Cultur und Wirkung des Weins; Statistik und Charakteristik sämtlicher Weine der Welt; Behandlung der Weine im Keller* (Leipzig, 1865; new edn, Leipzig, 1983; 2nd edn, 1984).

Hammerl, Traugott, *Norddeutsches Kochbuch für herrschaftliche sowie für die feinere bürgerliche Küche* (1898; new edn, Rostock, 1985).

Hanelt, Peter, 'Zur Geschichte des Anbaus von Buchweizen und Rispenhirse in der Lausitz', *Abhandlungen und Berichte des Naturkundemuseums Görlitz*, 55(1981), no. 4, pp. 1–13.

Heber, Bodo, 'Das Brennereiwesen und die Tabakfabrikation in der Stadt Nordhausen bis zum Beginn des 20. Jahrhunderts', *Beiträge zur Heimatkunde aus Stadt und Kreis Nordhausen*, 2/3(1978), pp. 120–5.

Heddergott, Berthold, 'Vom Brauwesen in Worbis', *Eichsfelder Heimatstimmen*, 2(1968), pp. 44–8.

Held, S. Wieland, 'Die Sicherung der Ernährung als bedeutsame Komponente der Beziehungen zwischen Stadt und Land in Thüringen im 16. Jahrhundert', *Jahrbuch für Wirtschaftsgeschichte*, (1985), no. 2, pp. 119–30.

Helling, Gertrud, *Nahrungsmittel. Produktion und Weltaussenhandel seit Anfang des 19. Jahrhunderts* (Berlin, 1977).

Hoffmann, Edith, *'Untersuchungen zur agrarischen Revolution der Produktivkräfte im Vorderen Orient'* (doctoral thesis, Leipzig, 1979).

Holstein, Günther, 'Gar manches über den Käse', *Das Volk*, 28(1973), no. 154.

Horalek, Horst, 'Historisches ums altmärkische Bier', *Altmärkischer Heimatkalender*, 6(1976), pp. 89–90.

Humbsch, Christian, 'Eine mittelalterliche Stadt der Brauerei', *Neuer Tag*, 30(1981), no. 20, 8; no. 32, 8; no. 37, 6; no. 44, 6.

Ilgenstein, Erhard, *Bier- und Rezeptbüchlein: Ausgesuchte Tafelfreuden* (Jena, 1984).

Itterheim, Roland, Christa Höfer and Robert Schmalwasser, *Thüringer Gewürzfibel* (Erfurt, 1979).

Kagel, Wolfgang, 'Das Ernährungsproblem im Spätfeudalismus', *Jahrbuch für Wirtschaftsgeschichte*, (1985), no. 4, pp. 249–52.

Klocke, Fritz, 'Backen und Aufbewahren des Brotes im Harz', *Nordharzer Jahrbuch*, 3(1967), pp. 145–7.

Knapp, A., 'Die Ernährung in einem hessischen Dorf vor 50 Jahren', *Ernährungsforschung*, 24(1979), pp. 61–3.

Kochbuch der Johanne Wilhelmine Cotta. Facsimile (Leipzig, 1984).

Kochbuch der Philippine Welser. Facsimile, 2 vols (new edn, Leipzig, 1983).

Krausch, Heinz-Dieter, '250 Jahre Kartoffelanbau in der Niederlausitz', *Geschichte und Gegenwart des Bezirks Cottbus*, 9(1975), pp. 97–112.

Krausch , Heinz-Dieter, 'Zur Geschichte des Kartoffelanbaus in Brandenburg', *Rathenower Heimatkalender*, 20(1976), pp. 30–6.

Kretschmann, Kurt, 'Romantik um alte Feldbacköfen und Backhäuser', *Heimatkalender für den Kreis Bad Freienwalde*, 24(1980), pp. 70–3.

Kühne, Heinrich, 'Von alten sächsischen Klemmeisen und Klemmkuchen', *Sächsische Heimatblätter*, 27(1981), no. 6, pp. 261–6.

Lange, Albrecht, 'Die territoriale Ausweitung des Spreewaldgemüseanbaus von den siebziger Jahren des 19. Jahrhunderts bis zur Gegenwart', *Letopis, Reihe C, Volksunde*, 27(1984), pp. 58–72.

Langer, Herbert, 'Das Braugewerbe in den deutschen Hansestädten der frühen Neuzeit', *Hansische Studien*, 4(1979), pp. 65–81.

Leister, G., 'Als man noch in Lengenfeld und Stein Bier braute', *Eichsfelder Heimatstimmen*, 4(1972), pp. 107–8.

Lommatz, F., 'Bauernbacköfen im Kreis Rochlitz', *Sächsische Heimatblätter*, 11(1966), pp. 330–4.

Ludwig, Otto, 'Bäuerliche Mahlzeiten im Unterharz', *Unser Harz*, 21(1973), pp. 114–15.

Ludwig, Otto, 'Bemerkungen zum Bier', *Thüringische Landeszeitung*, 33(1977), nos. 73, 84, 90, 126.

Mehlhardt, Dieter, 'Essen und Trinken im alten Preussen', *Brandenburgische Neueste Nachrichten*, 33(January 1983), p. 3.

Meidow, Werner, 'Ober, 'ne Weisse. Streifzug durch die Geschichte eines Berliner Getränks',

Berliner Heimat. Zeitschrift für die Geschichte Berlins, (1959), pp. 114–18.

Mielczarski, Stanislaw, 'Die Untersuchung des Getreidemarktes mit Hilfe der Kornmasse und der Versuch einer Anwendung auf den Getreidemarkt in Sachsen und Thüringen im 16. und 17. Jahrhundert', *Wissenschaftliche Zeitschrift des Pädagogischen Instituts Magdeburg*, 6(1969), no. 3, pp. 49–69.

Müller, Gerd, 'Gubener "Nationalgerichte"', *Gubener Heimatkalender*, 24(1980), pp. 78–9.

Müller, Gerhard, 'Brotbacken dunnemals', *Gubener Heimatkalender*, 27(1983), pp. 53–5.

Müller, Hans-Heinrich, 'Entwicklungstendenzen der Viehzucht in Brandenburg vor den Agrarreformen von 1807', *Jahrbuch für Wirtschaftsgeschichte* (1966), pp. 137ff.

Müller, Ingeborg, *Kartoffelnahrung im Vogtland: Zum Nahrungswandel in der Zeit des Manufakturkapitalismus* (Plauen, 1976).

Nickel, Johanna, 'Winterliches Festgebäck', *Kultur, Gesellschaft, Heimat. Oranienburger Heimatzeitschrift*, 31(1961), pp. 21–4.

Oehlandt, 'Der Eberwalder "Fuhrmatz" [Brauwesen]', *Heimatkalender für den Kreis Eberswalde*, (1981), pp. 95–6.

Ohnesorge, H., 'Ein längst vergessener Brauch im Oderland', *Heimatkalender Bad Freienwalde*, 8(1964), pp. 92–3.

Paepke, Karola, 'Vom Essen und Trinken in der ehemaligen Mark Brandenburg', *Märkische Union*, 191(1981), supplement 4;197, p. 3; 262, p. 3.

Parain, Charles, 'Zur Problematik der Geschichte der Viehzucht im römischen Reich', *Jahrbuch für Wirtschaftsgeschichte*, (1971), no. 2, pp. 165ff.

Pilz, Herbert, 'Gose und Gosenschänken', *Ernährungsforschung*, 30(1985), pp. 62–4.

Pilz, Herbert, 'Die Geschichte der Leipziger Lerchen', *Ernährungsforschung*, 32(1987), pp. 61–2.

Pönicke, Herbert, 'Brot – Schokolade – Zigaretten. Aus der Geschichte der Nahrungs- und Genussmittelindustrie', *Sächsische Heimat*, 20(1974), no. 7/8, pp. 262–8.

Puls, Uta, *'Die Entwicklung der Gemüseproduktion in Deutschland (1878 bis 1933/34) unter besonderer Berücksichtigung der Zeit der Weimarer Republik'* (doctoral thesis, Berlin, 1981).

'Rathenower Bier schon seit 1295', *Brandenburgische Neueste Nachrichten*, 26(1976), no. 81, p. 8.

'Rauhe Sitten bei Tisch. Als "Kavaliere" noch ins Tischtuch schnaubten und sich mit Knochen bewarfen', *Ernährungsforschung*, 21(1976), p. 159.

Reimann, Horst, *'Die geschichtliche Entwicklung und Bedeutung der Getreideproduktion und – verarbeitung unter besonderer Beachtung der Produktivkräfte'* (doctoral thesis, Berlin, 1974).

Reitz, Günther, 'Formschönes Weihnachtsgebäck', *Natur und Heimat*, 6(1957), pp. 360–2.

Alte Rezepte von Mudder Schulten (Neubrandenburg, 1980).

Rezepte zu Festen und Feiern von Mudder Schulten (Neubrandenburg, 1981).

Rezepte nach Jägerart, Fischerbrauch und Sammlersitte von Mudder Schulten (Neubrandenburg, 1982).

'Rezepte aus Mühlberg', *Die schwarze Elster*, (1983), no. 11, pp. 6–8; no. 12, pp. 6–8; no. 13, pp. 6–8; no. 14, pp. 7–10.

Rezepte für Pottkiekers, Schöttelkiekers un Naschkatten von Mudder Schulten (Neubrandenburg, 1984).

Richter, J. M., 'Zum Beginn und zur Ausbreitung des Kartoffelfeldbaus im Vogtland', *Sächsische Heimatblätter*, 7(1961), pp. 511–17.

Richter, Johannes, 'Zur Entwicklung und Verbreitung von Gemeinschaftsbackhaus und Privatbackofen im Erfurter Gebiet', *Veröffentlichungen zur Stadtgeschichte und Volkskunde/ Museen der Stadt Erfurt*, 1(1984), pp. 37–44.

Ritzerow, Frieda, *Mecklenburgisches Kochbuch. Ein Ratgeber für Alle, welche der Kochkunst beflissen sind, speciell für mecklenburgische Hausfrauen und solche, die es werden wollen* (1868; new 5th edn, Leipzig, 1985).
Roesler, Jörg, 'Butter, Margarine und Wirtschaftspolitik. Zu den Bemühungen um die planmässige Lenkung des Butter- und Margarineverbrauchs zwischen 1950 und 1965', *Jahrbuch für Wirtschaftsgeschichte* (1988), no. 1, pp. 33–47.
Rontzier, Franz de, *Kunstbuch von mancherley Essen* (Wolffenbüttel, 1598; new edn by Manfred Lemmer Halle, Leipzig, 1979).
Rosalia, Eleonora, *Freywillig aufgesprungener Granat-Apffel* (Leipzig, 1709; new edn, Leipzig, 1978).
Roselt, J. Christoph, 'Küchen und Küchengerät in der Arnstädter Puppenstadt "Mon Plaisier"', *Die Witte*, 1(1964), pp. 54–65.
Rosenkranz, Heinz, 'Zur Geschichte der Volksnahrung in Südostthüringen', *Thüringer Heimat*, 2(1957), pp. 65-7, 148–54.
Rothe, M., R. Schneeweis and R. Ehrlich, 'Zur historischen Entwicklung von Getreideverarbeitung und Getreideverzehr' *Ernährungsforschung*, 18(1973), pp. 249–84.
Rothe, M., 'Zur Geschichte von Verbreitung, Verarbeitung und Verbrauch von geschmacks- und aromareichen Würzmitteln, Genussmitteln und Lebensmitteln', *Ernährungsforschung*, 23 (1978), pp. 145–51.
Rumpolt, Marx, *Ein new Kochbuch*, (Frankfurt am Main, 1581; new edn, Leipzig, 1976; 1977; 3rd new edn, 1980).
Saegler, Helmut, 'Das Brauwesen in beiden Städten Brandenburgs', *Brandenburger Kulturspiegel*, (1983), no. 6, pp. 11–13; no. 7, pp. 15–17.
Sagenhafte Thüringer Rezepte zum Wandern, Kochen und Würzen (Suhl, 1984).
Schattkowsky, Martina, 'Mittelalterliche Lebensweise, Kultur und Ideologie der Stadtbevölkerung, vornehmlich im hanseatischen Raum', *Jahrbuch für Wirtschaftsgeschichte* (1982), no.3, pp. 235–7.
Schellhammer, Maria Sofia, *Das Brandenburgische Koch-Buch oder die wohlunterwiesene Köchinn: das ist: Unterricht, wie man allerley wohlschmeckende Speisen auffs füglichste zubereiten ... solle* (new edn, Rostock, 1984).
Schellhammer, Maria Sofia, *Das Brandenburgische Koch-Buch oder die wohlunterwiesene Köchinn...Der wohl-unterwiesenen Köchin zufällige Confect-Taffel* (2nd edn, Berlin, 1989).
Schlüsselhecht und nackter Barsch: Vom Kochen an Bord und von Fischgerichten der Küstenbevölkerung an Ostsee und Nordsee (Rostock, 1985).
Schmidt, Hanns F., 'Das Glanzstück war der Honigkuchen: Weihnachtliches aus der Altmark', *Liberal-Demokratische Zeitung, Edition Altmark/Stendal*, 30(1975), no. 287, p. 8.
Schmidt, Maria, 'Naute' in *Europäische Kulturverflechtungen im Bereich der volkstümlichen Überlieferung. Festschrift zum 65. Geburtstag von Bruno Schier* (Göttingen, 1967), pp. 241–4.
Schmidt-Berg-Lorenz, S., 'Zur Kulturgeschichte des Zuckers in Berlin und der Mark Brandenburg. Zucker aus Kaulsdorf, Rohr in Tahiti, Traubenzucker synthetisch', *Jahrbuch für brandenburgische Landesgeschichte*, 14(1963), pp. 34–52.
Schmitthenner, Erika and Heinrich Schmitthenner, *Speise und Trank in Europa* (Leipzig, 1967).
Schober, Manfred, 'Die Volksnahrung in der sächsischen Schweiz und den angrenzenden Gebieten vor der Einführung der Kartoffel in der Mitte des 18. Jahrhunderts', *Letopis Reihe C, Volkskunde*, 23(1980), pp. 64–77.
Schober, Manfred, *Wie die kleinen Leute lebten: Lebenserinnerungen, Gesprächsprotokolle und*

Briefe zum Leben der Arbeiter, Bauern und Handwerker im Raum Sebnitz während der 2. Hälfte des 19. und zu Beginn des 20. Jahrhunderts (Sebnitz, 1982).

Schrot, Gerhard, 'Die Nahrungsmittelproduktion der Germanen — ein Beitrag zur Wirtschaftsgeschichte der Germanen', *Wissenschaftliche Zeitschrift der Karl-Marx-Universität Leipzig. Gesellschafts- und Sprachwissenschaftliche Reihe*, 5(1955/56), pp. 295–303.

Sincerus, Alexius, *Der curiose ... Wohlerfahrne und allezeit wohlerstehende Becker* (Nuremberg, 1713; new edn, Leipzig, 1982).

Speerschneider, Heinz, 'Kartoffel und Kartoffelgerichte: Ein Beitrag zur Geschichte der Volksnahrung', *Mitteilungen des Staatlichen Heimat- und Schlossmuseums Burgk/Saale*, 8(1976), no. 4, pp. 64–71.

Speerschneider, Heinz, 'Dann gab es Thüringer Klösse: Um 1750 hielten die Kartoffeln bei uns Einzug', *Thüringer Neueste Nachrichten, Unsere Heimat*, 34 (October 1984), no. 213.

Starkloff, Helge, '*Backen im Kreis Sangerhausen*', mimeo, (Leipzig, 1976).

Stengel, Walter, *Zucker und Zuckergerät* (Berlin, 1952).

Stieler, Christoph, 'Tafelsitten der Schwarzburger: Eine Ausstellung der Staatlichen Museen Heidecksburg', *Rudolstädter Heimathefte*, 29(1983), no. 3/4, pp. 49–51.

Stokar, Walter von, *Die Urgeschichte des Hausbrotes* (Leipzig, 1951).

Strübing, E., Knoblauch in alten Zeiten. Zur Diätetik und Ernährung des Menschen, *Ernährungsforschung*, 12 (1967), pp. 589–623.

Stürzebecker, Horst, 'Vom Bierbrauen in Zossen', *Heimatkalender für den Kreis Zossen*, 23(1980), pp. 84–6.

Teuteberg, Hans J. and Günter Wiegelmann, *Der Wandel der Nahrungsgewohnheiten unter dem Einfluss der Industrialisierung* (Göttingen, 1972).

Teuteberg, Hans J. and Günter Wiegelmann, *Unsere tägliche Kost. Geschichte und soziale Prägung* 2nd edn (Münster, 1986).

Teuteberg, Hans J., 'Die Ernährung als Gegenstand historischer Analyse' in *Historia socialis et oeconomica. Festschrift für Wolfgang Zorn zum 65. Geburtstag* (Stuttgart, 1987), pp. 180–202.

Textor-Kochbuch. Das Kochbuch von Goethes Grossmutter Anna Margaretha Textor, geborene Lindheimer (new edn, Leipzig, 1980).

Thoss, Alfred, 'Vom Greizer Bierbrauen in alter Zeit', *Heimatbote*, 14(1968), no. 9, pp. 199–200.

Tornow, Elisabeth, *Vom Korn zum Brot* (2nd edn, Dresden, Leipzig, 1958).

Mecklenburgische Volkskunde, eds Ulrich Bentzien and Siegfried Neumann (Rostock, 1988).

Vollständiges Koch-, Back- und Konfitürenlexikon (Ulm, 1786; new edn, Leipzig, 1986).

Vollständiges Nürnbergisches Koch-Buch (Nuremberg, 1691; new edn, Leipzig, 1979; 2nd edn, 1986).

'Von der Blütezeit Lübbenauer Braukunst im 18. Jahrhundert', *Märkische Rundschau, Ausgabe Cottbus*, 28 (August, 1975), no. 205, p. 6.

'Von Fliesenwurst und schmackhafter Pottsuse', *Liberal-Demokratische Zeitung, Ausgabe Altmark Stendal*, 23 (1977), no. 1, p. 5.

Wähler, Martin, 'Die deutsche Volksnahrung', in Wilhelm Pessler (ed.), *Handbuch der deutschen Volkskunde*, vol. 3 (Potsdam, 1934), pp. 140–55.

Wagner, Annalise, 'Hopfen und Malz', in Annalise Wagner (ed.), *Aus dem alten Neubrandenburg*, vol. 4 (Neubrandenburg, 1973), pp. 32-38.

Wagner, Erich, 'Rudolstädter Wasser und Bier vor 300 Jahren', *Rudolstädter Heimathefte*, (1961), pp. 223-6.

Walter, Hans-Henning, 'Die Entwicklung der Siedesalzgewinnung in Deutschland von 1500–1900 unter besonderer Berücksichtigung chemisch-technologischer Prozesse' (postdoctoral thesis, Freiberg, 1985).

Weber-Kellermann, Ingeborg, 'Fragebogen zu einer Volkskunde des Nahrungswesens', *Deutsches Jahrbuch für Volkskunde*, 4(1958), pp. 190–7.

Weiden, Kurt, 'Wie in der Mark Brot gebacken wurde', *Brandenburgische Neueste Nachrichten*, 33(October/November 1983), nos 229, 253, 288; 34(Januar 1984), no. 21.

Weinhold, Rudolf, *Winzerarbeit an Elbe, Saale und Unstrut* (Berlin, 1973).

Weinhold, Rudolf, '"Gewissermassen ein Bestandteil ihrer Nahrung und Existenz". Frühe Nachrichten über den Kartoffelbranntwein', *Hessische Blätter für Volks- und Kulturforschung*, 20(1986), pp. 75–80.

Weisse, Angelika, '*Der Brau- und Schankbetrieb der ehemaligen Kommun-Brauerei in Bad Klosterlaussnitz*, mimeo (Jena, 1962).

Widera, Bruno, 'Beginn und Umfang der deutschen Getreideausfuhr in die vormongolische Rus', *Jahrbuch für Wirtschaftsgeschichte*, (1963), no. 2, pp. 79ff.

Winter, Renate, 'Pommersche Antworten auf die Frage: Wat gifft to eten', *Korrespondenzblatt des Vereins für niederdeutsche Sprachforschung*, 68(1961), pp. 42–6.

Winter, Renate, '*Die Milch und ihre Verarbeitung im niederdeutschen Wortschatz der ehemaligen Provinz Pommern*' (doctoral thesis, Rostock, 1963).

Wüstefeld, Karl, 'Eichsfelder Schlachtfest im 19. Jahrhundert', *Eichsfelder Heimatstimmen*, 22(1978), pp. 448–52, 496–7, 543–7.

Zahmel, Jutta, 'Vom Brotbacken in Emstal', *Brandenburger Kulturspiegel*, 4(1984), pp. 6–11.

Zeun, K., 'Rund um das Erzgebirgische Butterfass', *Glückauf. Zeitschrift des Erzgebirgs-Vereins*, 12(1965), no. 1, pp. 6–9.

Zirnstein, Gottfried, '*Zur Geschichte der Beziehungen von Pflanzenzüchtung und Biologie von den Anfängen bis in die dreissiger Jahre des 20. Jahrhunderts*' (doctoral thesis, Jena, 1977).

Zur Geschichte von Kultur und Lebensweise der werktätigen Klassen und Schichten des deutschen Volkes, ed. Bernhard Weissel, Hermann Strobach and Wolfgang Jacobeit (Berlin, 1972).

9 Nutrition in Austria in the industrial age

Roman Sandgruber

The growth of interest in Austrian food history

As indispensable as food is, the social relations connected with it are no less manifold, and its effect on all aspects of life is no less fundamental. To put it briefly, we already know precisely, *what* and *how much* people eat or should eat, but we know little about *why* they eat what they eat.

Any scientific investigation on food and its history, however, must not only ask 'what' and 'how much'; it must also include 'where', 'how' and 'with whom'. Apart from the diversity of food and the quantity available, its preparation, the places where it is eaten and the customs attending mealtimes must be considered, that is to say, all the economic, disciplining, socially differentiating and communicative functions of food.

This paper on the state of Austrian food history is designed precisely with these questions in mind. In recent years the study of food history in Austria has gathered considerable pace, for this is a problem in which several different disciplines are interested.

In studies of goods and material culture, much attention has always been given to the food people eat, and in connection with collecting and processing material for the *German and Austrian Ethnological Atlas* (Atlas der deutschen Volkskunde und Österreichischer Volkskundeatlas) many important results have been found. Continuing the long tradition of folklore studies and European ethnology, more and more attention has been paid during the last decade to the question of changes in food brought about by industrialization, urbanization, new ways of preservation and preparation, instant meals and fast food.[1] In addition, the connections with sociology and the history of civilization have become stronger.

In connection with an increasing interest in the history of everyday life, historical research became intensively involved with the question of nutrition. In the field of medieval history the Institut für mittelalterliche Realienkunde (Institute for Studies of Medieval Realities) of the Austrian Academy of Sciences in Krems played a leading role. This was caused by an earlier interest in the history of material culture, and by considering new questions of everyday life and using quantitative and iconographical methods.[2]

For more recent work in economic and social history, food history plays an important role in the history of everyday life. It is also referred to in connection with the classical topics of economic and social history, especially in the interpretation of industrialization, the analysis of agricultural societies, and as an indicator in the discussion on the development of the standard of living.[3] Concerning the question of living standards the complex indicator of body height was added to the classical indicators, – the consumption of meat, various luxuries etc. – in recent times.[4]

Sociologists, with their interest in the process of civilization,[5] have also shown a new interest in food history, no longer confining themselves to examining the eating habits of fringe groups or drug addiction.[6] Agronomy[7] and food studies[8] have also turned to historical questions concerning food. Even linguistics have produced articles on such topics.[9]

The Austrian as a man of pleasure

From the late Middle Ages up to the 19th century, Austria and Vienna enjoyed a reputation as a bastion of good food and hedonism. The Viennese had the reputation of consuming more food than any other European town-dwellers. At the end of the 18th century Vienna was said to be the most hedonistic city in Germany, if not in Europe. Usually, it was ranked right below London and Paris, but far above Rome, Naples, Berlin, Copenhagen or Stockholm.[10] Friedrich Nicolai, one of the sternest critics of Viennese pleasures of the table, summed up his impressions as follows: 'The feasting and luxurious living in Vienna is known to the world and strikes a foreigner all too quickly at the first glance'. Not only the upper class but also the middle and the lower classes seemed to fit into this picture. 'One would imagine that the tables of distinguished and rich people are full of many and special meals', he said: 'But one has no idea how far feasting and gluttony have spread among the lower classes unless one has seen it.'' Not least because of the judgement and prejudice of this supporter of the Enlightenment from Berlin did the feasting of the Viennese and Austrian people become the preferred topos of travel literature.

Nicolai's report was just one among many. Often these were based on personal experiences, but some were also taken from other travel reports that made fun of Viennese eating habits or were simply an excuse to vent their anger. If the reporters told their own experiences at all they did not go into enormous detail. They wrote about the salons and houses of the aristocracy where the traveller usually found hospitality, and finished with a description of restaurants and the trip to the Prater on Sundays or the theatre visit in the evening. Little was said of the everyday life of the lower classes. Therefore one must not understand these superficial impressions as descriptions of the general situation. Certainly only the *haute bourgeoisie*, the upper clergy and the aristocracy could lead a life such as foreign travellers described it.

The impression that some reports gave that urban income in pre-industrial times was much higher than that of the surrounding countryside was correct, however. Indeed, Vienna was a very rich city because it was here, in the centre of the Empire and near the Emperor's residence, that the upper class was concentrated. They possessed a huge amount of money from money transactions, ground rents and trade, in the shadow of which, many servants and deliverymen could also lead a good life. The already great number of officials increased quickly in the late 18th century because the tasks of the municipality grew more complex. Their income was quite high, in spite of their daily complaints. In addition, travelling became more fashionable and the travellers brought with them to Vienna a great deal of money. And, last but not least, more and more trades and businesses came into being that offered good wages and profits.

Vienna was a city of consumption and luxury. Adolf Schmidl, a geographer and author of travel books, expressed it precisely: 'The Viennese eats more than others, because he has got more to eat.' Empirical and quantitative statements prove this: the average per-capita consumption of meat, beer and sugar in Vienna was much higher than that of the surrounding country, and by 1910 it had almost reached the all-Austrian average of today (see Figure 9.1).

Table 9.1 Annual Viennese per-capita food consumption, 1784–1910

Year	1784	1830	1850	1870	1890	1910
Bread/cereals (kg)	220.4	145.1	147.8	136.3	103.9	–
Rice (kg)	–	1.4	1.5	1.0	2.1	–
Legumes (kg)	9.6	6.2	4.4	2.6	1.8	–
Potatoes, etc. (kg)	–	47.3	61.3	–	–	–
Meat (kg)	72.4	85.3	70.3	79.1	74.2	74.9
Poultry/game (kg)	11.7	8.5	5.0	4.5	6.2	7.5
Fish (kg)	2.2	1.8	1.8	1.7	1.6	1.5
Milk (l)	–	39.0	41.3	75.3	103.0	154.5
Butter (kg)	5.8	4.6	4.5	3.5	4.1	–
Cheese (kg)	2.5	1.5	1.8	2.1	2.1	–
Eggs	–	125.5	102.2	75.7	102.7	–
Wine (l)	133.0	63.0	41.2	35.4	45.4	35.1
Beer (l)	128.6	114.2	101.4	117.2	129.5	135.9

Source: Sandgruber (1982), p. 150.

Investigations into consumption and quantifiable data

Nevertheless, the differences in the urban population were manifold. Therefore, the partly undifferentiated data need empirical proof for each class of the population. For pre-industrial times, for which statistics are unavailable this is only possible qualitatively or in isolated cases. One must rely mostly on norms that are given for the resident households in different states of order or which occur in arguments about the wages or the regulations for board between masters and journeymen, employers and employees, peasants and farmhands, etc. These norms mostly show a situation as it should be, not the real situation.

It is amazing how many notes about household budgets we have from as early as the 19th century.[11] But most of the time these statements were only meant to be guidelines. They showed either 'how a worker and his people could get forward legally and reach a good income' (this is the title of a 'trade primer for the Austrian worker'[12] from 1849 which was edited and prefaced by the Austrian ministry of education), how one could get by on normal or even lower wages, or, on the contrary, if published by the workers' committees and journeymen's societies, they demonstrated how high wages should be to guarantee an adequate standard of living. This may well, however, have been for the most part an exercise in calculation more or less divorced from reality.[13]

An exact access to household consumption first became possible with the beginning of modern consumption statistics and with the monographic method developed by the French Frédéric Le Play. Apart from detailed studies on a Viennese joiner's apprentice's household (with an exact listing of the inventory, furniture, bedlinen, and household equipment), he also wrote a remarkable monograph on a Carinthian charcoal burner who led a hard life in his primitive self-made hut covered with leaves. This man was one of the farmhands of a large farm. He still had his place in a patriarchal house community. Every week he received food from the farm. His meals consisted mostly of soup and butter noodles. A small amount of money was used to buy spirits, tobacco, sugar and coffee, and he also bought a lottery ticket.

This case is isolated, and nothing definite can be said as to whether it is representative. Many of the consumption data which were listed by committed private people working during the 1870s and 1880s therefore might lack empirical proof. This applies to the data of Freiherr von Vogelsang's Christian-social group as well as to the information given by the sociopolitical thinker and university professor Eugen Philippovich.[14]

Modern scientific calculation on household budgets began in Austria with Ignaz Gruber and Karl von Inama-Sternegg.[15] Systematic research, however, began with the studies of the k.u.k. Arbeitsstatistisches Amt (Department for Work Statistics) on 'economic calculation and living standards of Viennese workers' families between 1912 and 1914', whose more or less fully evaluated source material became a victim of official document-destroying rampages during the interwar period just like later studies of the Wiener Arbeiterkammer.[16] Only the systematic studies on consumption which were made yearly by the Viennese Chamber for Workers and Employees since 1925 give a more or less representative chronology of changes in consumption habits.[17]

Such studies on household budgets exist on the whole for 12 years (1912 and 1925–1935), though with very small sample sizes during the interwar period. None can be called a statistically representative mass study. The number of households investigated ranges from 40 to 139, mostly from the upper working class.

After 1945 the household studies were continued on an annual basis, and investigations comparable to those of earlier years were carried out by the Chamber for Workers and Employees. Additionally, there were studies on consumption and census by the Statistisches Zentralamt (Central Office for Statistics).

Additional nutritional balances for the most important food stuffs exist in annual studies after 1945. Figures are also reckoned back for the years 1934–8. Aggregated consumption trends can also be developed for special goods that are subject to a particular tax. For sugar, beer and coffee this can even be done back to the beginning of the 19th century.

Eating habits and nutrition in the 19th century

In the pre- and early industrial period most people took it for granted that much more than half of their income would be spent on food. Because of its high financial importance food was a good means to express prestige and to mark the boundaries of status. The amount and kind of food as well as its preparation, eating utensils and the order of meals served to differentiate social classes.

Contemporary reports always emphasize workers' tendency to spend more on food as their income increases and to adapt to needy times by reducing food consumption. Workers differed from the middle class by not saving any extra money either for housing, education or for cases of emergency. They spent it on consumption, expenses that seemed to be pure waste like senseless boozing, opulent meals or nightly card games.[18] They did not have the ability to plan for the future. Long-lasting consumer goods, especially better dwellings, had proved to be too expensive in relation to the income expected. Thus, they bought mainly food and clothes. Manual labour also called for a totally different emphasis on food that was not necessary for classes that no longer did manual work.

The average income in Austria, demonstrated by the example of Viennese industrial workers and shown in present values, increased from 1830 to 1988 more than tenfold (see Table 9.2). The average number of hours worked per week fell by more than half. In 1830, a worker could buy approximately 35 kg of bread for his week's pay; by 1988 he could buy 270 kg. In 1830 two-thirds of the household budget was spent on food and luxury goods; by 1988 this figure had fallen to a quarter (Table 9.3).

Concerning the relationship between industrialization and nutrition, a structural change can be recognized because of a changed size and structure of households, increased income, better availability of goods, better preservation processes and new methods of preparation; it is striking, however, that in the field of industrial food processing the industry merely continued earlier processes to establish new ways of consumption and spread it to all classes of society.

The information about the diet of urban workers in the second half of the 19th century is as copious as the food is monotonous: coffee and bread in the morning, soup, meat and vegetables for lunch, leftovers from lunch, sausage, cheese and bread

Table 9.2 Weekly income earned and hours worked by an unskilled Viennese industrial worker, 1830–1988

Year	Weekly income	Currency	Schilling equivalent 1989 prices	Bread price per kg	Bread bought by one week's pay (kg)	Hours worked per week
1830	2.5	Florin CM	396.5	0.04 fl	35.7	82.5
1870	6.0	Florin ÖW	563.6	0.16 fl	37.5	78.0
1910	18.0	Kronen	770.4	0.31 K	58.1	58.0
1930	56.0	Schilling	1410.6	0.55 S	101.8	44.0
1950	231.0	Schilling	1360.6	2.40 S	96.3	50.3
1970	961.0	Schilling	2354.5	6.10 S	157.5	44.3
1988	4550.0	Schilling	4550.0	16.80 S	270.8	39.5

CM (= Conventionsmünze)
ÖW (= Österreichische Währung)
Sources: Tafeln zur Statistik der Österreichisch-Ungarischen Monarchie; Österreichisches Statistisches Handbuch; Statistisches Handbuch für die Republik Österreich; Wirtschafts- und Sozialstatistisches Handbuch; Wirtschafts- und Sozialstatistisches Taschenbuch; Österreichisches Statistisches Zentralamt.

Table 9.3 Average expenditure on consumption in Viennese workers' households, 1830–1988 (in per cent)

Year	Foodstuffs/ luxury foods	Clothing	Rent	Heating	Furnishing	Others
1830	63.0	8.0	11.0	11.0	7	
1870	60.0	8.0	20.0	5.0	8	
1910	59.2	8.8	14.2	4.5	1.3	12.0
1930	52.6	11.6	4.0	4.3	4.5	23.0
1950	50.7	13.6	4.1	4.9	3.9	22.8
1970	31.9	13.1	6.9	4.3	8.2	35.2
1988	25.5	10.4	10.5	5.5	6.8	41.3

Sources: see Table 9.1. (Figures of 1870 and 1970 are rounded off).

in the evening. The side dishes consisted mostly of potatoes, prepared in various ways. The vegetables, cabbage, endive, herbs, beets and beans were stewed.

Poorer families with many children could not afford much meat. The worse the financial situation of the workers, the more coffee became a main part of their diet. The men often replaced coffee with alcohol. People who had to eke out their resources tended to drink coffee in the morning and at noon, ate mostly one piece of bread and had a watery soup or bread, bacon and sausage in the evening. They could afford meat only at weekends, and then it was mostly horsemeat because this was comparatively cheap.

The average meat consumption of an adult, 49.3 kg per year, in a Viennese worker's family in 1912–13 was, on the one hand, only half the Viennese average, but still well in excess of the level of workers in the countryside. Although meat and sausage were part of the daily diet of most workers, the amounts could hardly compare either qualitatively or quantitatively. In particular, the difference between men and women was very large: while the men usually ate meat for lunch the women's diet consisted for the most part of smaller quantities of meat or was even meatless, which was certainly due to their much lower wages. In the workers' poor world meat was for the men, the economic heads of the family, while the women ate bread which was supplemented with sugar, jam, coffee or tea. 'Bread was always the cheapest. We lived mainly on bread. We were quite happy if we had some lard on the bread ... ', working women said. This was the reason why women and children consumed more sugar than men. In terms of its calorie content, sugar was much cheaper than meat in the late 19th century and was a good substitute. The expression 'sweet girl' has something to do with this.

Average figures, even if they are scaled according to income, hide the difficulties the workers had to cope with. Getting as well as preparing food had become a problem for most of the workers. The poorest had to pay the most for their goods, because they could only afford to buy them in small amounts. Most of the time they lived on credit. Only a small part of the Viennese workers' households which were investigated in 1912–13 could get cheap foodstuffs from relatives. Even the foundation of consumer cooperatives could not completely solve the problem.

Once the food was selected and bought, its preparation was far from ideal. If a woman was working, the family lunch was either warmed up or cold. Most women, indeed, were just too tired to cook. The meal was prepared the evening before or in the morning. Everything had to be done quickly, leaving the choice of meals remarkably limited: lunches that needed long cooking times or that had to be prepared fresh could not be done. Besides, facilities for cooking were rather strained. Because of the narrowness of dwellings the kitchen was used more for sleeping than for cooking. The solution was often to get a portion of food from a restaurant and supplement it with bread so that it would be enough for two or three people. The alternatives were little cold snacks, coffee and a drop of spirits.

If it was possible to go home and prepare lunch there this was the cheapest solution. Married workers usually ate at home if their lunchbreak was long enough and home was not too far away. In a Viennese factory, where 50% of the workers were married, 44.7% ate at home before 1914. In another factory 53.2% took their main meal at home while 29.2% ate in a restaurant, 11.5% in the factory, 1.5% in a grocery shop, 2.3% at private dinner tables and 2.3% in an unknown place.[19]

Käthe Leichter investigated the lunching habits of Viennese working women during the interwar period: 68% took their meal with them to the factory where they usually had a chance to warm it up, 9% went to the factory's cafeteria, 3.3% went to a restaurant. One fifth ate at home.[20] Time budgets and inventory lists could be another source for calculating household expenses.[21]

The First World War

The First World War and the period immediately following brought serious changes in food consumption. The increased needs of the army, blockades, import prohibition and difficulties in transportation caused shortages and hunger. In February 1915 the Kriegs-Getreide-Verkehrsanstalt (War Cereals Office) began to manage food issues at the state level. The longer the war lasted the more the state was involved with food. The most serious problem was lack of fat. The fat card was the most worthless of all food ration cards. Every week hundreds of thousands of cards became invalid. By 1916 the weekly amount of 1200 g per capita could no longer be supplied. Thus, in June 1916 days without fat were introduced. Hungary's supply of meat fell by 97% after Galicia was lost, and in autumn 1916 a third meatless day was introduced. Mutton was still excluded from this rule. From 1917 horsemeat also became popular.

In 1916 oats became human food for the first time in addition to corn and barley. The following year became the year of substitute food. In the first half of 1917 the continuing poor supply of potatoes forced the Viennese community to sell German rutabaga, also called *Wrucken*, as well as Burgundian beets, sugar-beets and the like. In May 1917 young clover, nettles and forest leeks were offered as substitutes for vegetables.

One of the most important events in 1918 was the reduction of the bread ration in January and June. The breakdown in the bread supply in July 1918 was caused by poor harvests and the loss of Hungarian imports. The crisis reached a climax with a decrease in the ration from 1260 g per week to 630 g for the ordinary consumer and from 2240 g to 1120 g for the heavy manual worker. For many Viennese citizens, October 1918 was a fateful month. The announcement on 21 October of a reduction of the fat ration from 40 to 20 g by the Amt für Volksernährung (Office for Public Nutrition), caused an outrage.

According to all reports, the first year of peace, 1919, was the year of the greatest famine and deprivation. Although the blockade was lifted, Vienna, the worst-supplied city of German Austria, was still blockaded. This was not only because all transportation routes were cut as a result of the foundation of national states, but also because of the part-time food embargo on the part of the country surrounding Lower Austria. The food ration card of 1919 guaranteed only 1143 kcal per day: 236 g flour (754 kcal), 164 g potatoes (123 kcal), 18 g meat (18 kcal), 17 g fat (153 kcal) and 25 g sugar (95 kcal).

Between the wars

During the 1920s many changes in workers' food intake occurred. The consumption of meat, eggs, cheese, animal and vegetable fats, potatoes, fruit and sugar increased while that of sausage, milk, legumes and alcoholic drinks decreased. The consumption of flour, bread and butter did not change.[22]

Table 9.4 Average annual food consumption in Viennese workers' households (in kg per NAVE*)

Year	Cereals	Rice	Fat	Meat	Fish	Eggs	Milk	Cheese	Vegetables	Potatoes
1912	157.3	3.4	16.1	49.3	0.8	139	198.3	1.7	–	48.8
1925	169.6	4.8	21.3	57.4	–	160	158.6	2.1	33.4	61.8
1930	138.4	4.9	25.2	60.5	3.4	252	195.7	3.1	47.5	48.2
1935	141.5	5.9	26.4	53.7	2.0	202	168.8	3.4	47.5	53.1
1946	142.9	–	7.0	11.2	6.4	4	32.3	0.5	43.8	143.0
1947	185.0	–	12.4	16.8	5.6	27	43.3	0.4	39.6	81.8
1948	181.1	1.5	15.8	21.2	9.9	45	55.9	0.8	51.1	103.2
1949	155.3	4.8	20.6	29.5	4.7	78	104.9	3.0	43.8	59.9
1950	156.3	6.4	24.2	43.4	2.8	119	176.6	3.7	38.1	68.9
1955	136.8	6.2	27.0	41.0	4.0	151	169.4	4.9	41.6	55.2
1960	119.1	5.1	24.2	49.0	3.7	195	182.6	5.7	54.1	50.4
1965	104.2	5.2	25.0	50.0	4.0	224	177.0	7.0	50.5	46.6
1970	90.9	4.2	22.0	55.4	3.6	207	146.9	7.8	51.8	37.9
1975	75.1	4.1	17.8	57.5	3.5	181	128.1	6.7	47.0	32.8
1980	76.9	3.1	18.3	56.3	3.3	192	102.6	6.6	44.6	29.3
1985	75.4	4.1	15.9	55.6	3.9	172	102.2	6.3	48.4	27.1
1988	84.3	4.7	17.6	63.8	4.3	159	115.3	7.3	54.5	24.8

Year	Legumes	Fruit	Jam	Sugar	Coffee	Tea, cocoa, chocolate	Beer	Wine	Spirits	Salt
1912	3.5	22.2	–	19.4	–	–	69.9	8.5	1.0	–
1925	2.1	29.2	–	23.6	5.2	1.2	11.4	1.7	0.8	–
1930	1.6	47.5	1.0	27.7	6.0	2.4	21.6	3.8	1.3	3.2
1935	2.1	46.0	0.6	25.7	5.7	1.3	10.4	4.9	1.0	3.5
1946	15.6	18.4	0.5	7.0	2.0	0.4	13.1	4.3	0.1	3.8
1947	8.2	17.2	1.9	8.8	1.3	0.1	9.7	5.8	0.2	3.6
1948	6.5	40.0	1.7	19.0	2.6	0.5	12.3	5.1	0.9	3.6
1949	0.9	42.1	1.5	25.3	2.7	1.7	15.4	3.9	1.4	3.4
1950	1.7	48.8	0.8	24.9	2.9	1.8	14.5	4.8	1.2	2.9
1955	1.5	48.0	0.7	28.9	2.7	2.2	13.0	6.5	1.1	2.5
1960	0.9	80.8	1.7	29.1	2.9	4.0	22.4	6.6	1.2	2.2
1965	0.9	69.5	4.4	28.2	3.3	4.5	32.1	9.4	1.0	1.9
1970	0.6	67.1	5.3	21.6	3.1	3.6	34.8	11.0	1.5	2.0
1975	0.3	54.9	5.3	15.9	3.5	4.5	42.1	11.7	2.0	1.7
1980	0.5	56.1	4.7	15.3	3.8	5.4	42.7	16.5	2.7	1.7
1985	0.3	54.3	4.9	13.5	4.0	4.8	43.1	14.9	1.9	1.6
1988	0.3	61.9	5.2	11.4	4.4	5.9	34.2	9.2	1.7	1.4

NAVE = Nutritional equivalent for adult consumers

Sources: *Wirtschafts- und sozialstatistisches Handbuch; Wirtschafts- und sozialstatistisches Taschenbuch*

The difference between the consumption of brown bread and white baked goods reflected a big change in lifestyle. From 1926 till 1930 the ratio of consumption of brown bread to white baked goods was approximately 3:1, increasing to nearly 5:1 in 1933. In the households of unemployed workers the relation was 11:1.

The consumption of alcohol declined. Although it must be admitted that research here is partly wanting, it is known that many families used neither alcohol nor tobacco.[23] The decrease in alcohol consumption during the interwar period is also proved by production data and estimates of average per-capita consumption.

The consumption of luxury items was strongly influenced by the world depression. In 1930 the consumption of alcohol rose, while the consumption of bread and meat continued a downward trend. In the further course of the crisis, the consumption of alcohol and tobacco began to fall. In contrast, the consumption of flour, bread and sugar increased.

The survey on consumption by the Viennese Workers' Chamber proved that food expenditure decreased in percentage terms as income increased. In 1925 the percentage was 72.3 on the lowest income level (less than 2,000 S) and 48.6 on the highest income level (more than 5,000 S).

Over time, the share of expenses taken up by food until 1931 showed a distinct decreasing tendency after it had fallen to less than 50% for the first time in 1928. During the world depression Ernst Engels's principle was also confirmed. It is remarkable that the expenditure on flour, sugar and rent increased not only relatively but also absolutely alongside a marked fall in incomes in 1933. In particular, expenditure on meat decreased during the world depression.

In 1932 the diets of 13 workers' families were investigated separately. The consumption of almost all foodstuffs decreased sharply, except for brown bread, semolina, rice, lard, horsemeat, bones, legumes and potatoes. While the consumption of meat and milk decreased sharply, an extraordinary consumption of horsemeat was evident. The consumption of offal was around the average, while that of lard was above average. The fall in the consumption of eggs, vegetables and fruit was relatively steep, and the consumption of alcohol was far below average.

The total calorie intake of unemployed people was about 500 kcal lower per day than that of average households. Natural produce accounted for 328 kcal, almost an eighth of daily needs. Benefactions had also increased. This showed how much unemployed people depended on private help besides welfare. There was no talk yet of physiological undernourishment, though. But it was agreed that that would happen if the allowance was allowed to fall. Then, only 2000 – 2100 kcal per NAVE (Nutritional equivalent for adult consumers) would be available. The famous Marienthal study by the sociologists Lazarsfeld, Jahoda and Zeisel gives good examples of the unemployed people's diet. They spent most of their money on milk, bread, flour, coal and lard, which already consumed one-third of their budget.[24]

The Viennese Workers' Chamber also studied body height and weight among the unemployed. In 1932, the adult men, 45 years old on average, were approximately 169 cm tall. From 1931 to 1932 their weight decreased from 65.4 to 63.7 kg. The women's weight at an average age of 42 years and height of 156 cm did not change from 59.6 kg.

The Second World War and the postwar period

The common cliché of an intact nourishment system which, in contrast to the First World War, worked in the main for those people who were bound to the state rationing system and were thereby 'accepted' as consumers up to the Second World War needs decisive correction. Most 'ordinary consumers', subjected to a strict quota system, suffered from a lack of regularly available, freely selectable and quantitatively as well as qualitatively sufficient everyday foodstuffs from the beginning of the war. The shortage of unrationed goods and the increased bodily needs brought about by the increased stress situation and additional work caused by wartime economy brought difficulties in addition to the drastic restriction of rationed goods compared to the pre-war standard. The regime succeeded almost perfectly in disciplining the society through nutrition policy.

The long-lasting period of deficient food economy within a society which was subject to the rationing system led to collective misguided eating habits with far-reaching physical consequences. In addition, nutrition was never as closely associated with politics as in the years of National Socialism, which created the term 'political ration' as an expression for deliberately created shortages as a means for the harm and physical destruction of man. The National Socialist state used hunger as a political 'weapon' against enemies, persecuted groups and minorities.

The disastrous food situation did not become clear until after the final collapse. Although a worsening supply during the war years was expected, it was unheard of in 1945 that even basic needs were no longer ensured. Austria had become the worst-supplied country in Europe.

The Allied and neutral states helped. From a modern point of view their campaigns, the Marshall Plan of the USA as well as the May Contribution of the Red Army, might easily be underrated or played down. And, indeed, from today's point of view the amounts involved might seem small. But at that time CARE packages, UNRRA help and the food deliveries of the Marshall Plan guaranteed pure survival.

'I cannot give you anything, no bread, no coal for heating, no glass to cut.' The famous speech of Chancellor Leopold Figl showed the situation in 1945 clearly. The situation at Christmas 1945 seemed hopeless. A slice of bread was a noble gift. Before the end of the war the consumer had the right to 5.9 kg brown bread, 1.5 kg white bread or flour and 1.5 kg white baked goods every four weeks. From the end of fighting until 20 April 1945, one got approximately 0.25 kg of bread, from 20 April to the end of May 0.5 kg–1.0 kg per week! The consumption of bread reached record heights up to 1947, but it decreased again slowly from 1948.

The black market and hoarding blossomed. While the average daily ration for ordinary consumers was around 2,000 kcal per day in 1944 (compared to 3,200 kcal before the war), only 500–800 kcal per day were available in the spring and summer of 1945. From 23 September 1945, 1,549 kcal per day. In 1946 the situation became to some extent worse than in 1945. For a short period only around 950 kcal per day were available, and in the summer only 1,183 kcal.

Table 9.5 Expenditure on food and luxuries in Viennese workers' households (in per cent)

Year	Cereals	Milk, cheese, eggs	Fat	Meat Sausage Fish	Sugar, coffee	Vegetables Fruit	Alcohol	Others	Meals out
1925	20.1	17.0	12.2	26.9	6.5	9.0	2.1	6.2	–
1930	14.6	17.7	10.0	27.2	7.7	10.7	3.7	8.4	–
1935	19.9	17.4	10.3	22.1	9.1	10.9	3.0	6.5	–
1946	21.9	5.1	13.8	9.5	6.4	22.1	5.6	15.6	–
1950	15.6	13.6	11.8	26.1	9.5	10.9	5.0	7.5	–
1955	15.9	18.4	7.1	24.4	11.4	11.5	3.9	7.4	–
1960	13.9	16.2	5.1	25.0	12.1	15.3	4.3	0.9	8.7
1965	13.1	16.2	4.2	24.7	11.3	16.1	5.0	1.2	8.2
1970	12.0	15.1	3.1	26.2	11.5	13.2	5.0	1.7	12.2
1975	10.2	12.9	2.8	24.9	10.8	11.5	5.3	2.1	19.5
1980	10.1	13.2	2.3	21.7	11.8	10.6	5.1	2.3	22.9
1985	11.2	14.2	2.4	19.3	9.1	10.1	4.0	2.9	23.4
1987	11.6	13.9	1.9	19.4	8.2	10.4	3.6	3.7	23.4

Sources: *Wirtschafts- und sozialstatistisches Handbuch; Wirtschafts- und sozialstatistisches Taschenbuch.*

Faced with the drastic situation of 1945–47, it might be surprising that the daily calorie supply for the ordinary consumer increased from 1800 to 2100 in autumn 1947, and that food controls were lifted by 1948. At the end of 1950 only sugar and subsidized edible oil were controlled. Moreover, sugar was allowed on to the free market in autumn 1950. The year 1950–1 was the first since the war with an almost free choice of food.

In 1951, however, fat and meat became scarce again as a result of the Korean crisis and a misguided pricing policy. New controls became necessary. Although the supply with bread grains, milk and milk products was so difficult in 1951 that all imported fat had to be controlled, the production of sausage had to be reduced and a meatless day had to be introduced, the situation became better again in 1952. Thus, at the end of 1952, only imported lard and subsidized vegetable fat were controlled, albeit unnecessarily. In 1953 the food supply improved to such an extent that the last remains of rationing were abolished in the middle of the year. From 1 July 1953, no food ration coupons were needed. Indeed, in 1953, a new concern with agricultural surpluses took over and demanded that precaution should rule the market (see Table 9.5).

Towards a modern consumer society

The structure of economic growth after 1945 was based on mass production and mass consumption. Changes in consumption patterns are revealed by the varying participation of production groups in the increasing consumption. Expenditure on food and clothes decreased as real revenue increased. On the other hand, expenditure on furniture, transportation and leisure increased. From 1950 to 1960 consumption in private households increased by 71%. For housing and maintenance, however, an increase of only 31% was recognizable, for food and luxuries around 50% and for heating and lighting around 53%. The increase in expenditure on clothing was also below average (68%). On the other hand, expenditure on education and entertainment increased by 81%, on means of transport by 169% and on furniture and household equipment by as much as 228%.

The expenditure on consumption of Viennese workers' and employees' households shows the new spending patterns. While during the earliest post-war years goods were in general so scarce that expenditure on unrationed goods, services and luxuries accounted for a large slice of the cake because of high black market prices, the pattern of expenditure changed gradually during the following years. First, expenditure on food increased; then the need for clothing was satisfied. After the mid-1950s expenditure on furniture increased, and in the last third of the decade expenditure on transportation, holidays and entertainment increased.

Although everything had improved since the first post-war years, the pattern of food consumption in the early 1950s, compared to the prewar period, still showed a preference for relatively cheap vegetable products, which was characteristic of an impoverished economy. While the consumption of plant foods was 9% higher in 1952 than in 1937, the consumption of animal products was still 17% lower. Specifically, the supply of grain products, sugar, potatoes and fruit was better while the supply of meat, fat, eggs, milk and vegetables was worse than before the war. This was also due to the fact that most plant products were cheaper than before the war because they were subsidized, in contrast to animal products.

Thus, in 1935 the consumption of bread in Viennese workers' and employees' households amounted to 25% of the daily calorie intake, in 1947 this figure was 44%, falling in 1949 to 30% and in 1950 to around 25%. In addition to the general reduction of bread consumption, a switch from brown bread to white bread appeared: whereas consumption of white bread amounted to 17% before the war, it increased to approximately 34% in 1949. At the same time the percentage of wheat flour in wheat and rye bread had increased by 50%.

In 1960–1 the consumers payed about 52% more for food than in 1950–1. Food consumption was almost 30% higher, but the number of calories increased by only 8%. The population preferred more relatively expensive low-calorie products to cheap high-calorie products. They bought better-quality and more processed or already prepared food.

The high bread consumption during the years 1945–7 was mainly due to the lack of high-grade food. Therefore, the decreasing bread consumption during the normalization of the nutrition situation after 1948 was caused by the developing tendency to prefer high-grade food containing protein rather than carbohydrates.

The consumption of bread grains, processed foodstuffs and potatoes tended to decrease. The need for carbohydrates decreased. The increasing numbers leaving the countryside lowered the bread consumption, which was almost twice as high in rural households as in the city. Shorter working hours and the establishment of factory canteens might have displaced the custom of taking sandwiches to work, even though the price of bread had fallen.

The consumption of milk and milk products in 1950 had reached only 71% of the pre-war period, although it had increased steadily after 1945. During the earliest years after the war the production of butter was furthered at the cost of milk consumption in order to help overcome the lack of fat. By 1949 butter consumption had already reached 102% of 1937 figures. However the fat content of milk had been reduced to 2.5%.

The demands for various kinds of fat developed differently. The annual per-capita consumption of vegetable fat increased from 4.3 kg in 1950–1 to 8.3 kg in 1960–1. Additional demand was mostly for edible oil, margarine and coconut oil. The consumption of olive oil, margarine and synthetic edible fat remained mainly constant. Edible oil and coconut oil had replaced lard, whose consumption decreased from 9 kg to 4.7 kg. The consumption of butter decreased when margarine came on to the market.

In 1946, the average Viennese consumed only 3.8 kg of sugar – 16% of the average before the war. The consumption of sugar increased quickly after 1948 once the supply difficulties of the early pre-war years had been overcome. While in 1950 food consumption on the whole was still far below pre-war levels, people were already consuming more sugar than before the war. The amount per capita was 24.4 kg in 1950–1 compared to 23.3 kg during the last pre-war years. Compared to other western European countries this amount was still rather low, however. Considerable differences by class were evident. The consumption of sugar had increased especially in agricultural households and also in workers' households, while decreasing in civil servants' and employees' households. This increase was caused particularly by the increased consumption of sweets. The domestic sales of the confectionary industry were almost twice as high in 1951 as in 1937. Sugar, sweets and chocolate products accounted for more than 11% of the gross calorie intake (compared to 9% before the war).

In 1949, Viennese workers' and employees' households consumed 25.3 kg of sugar and sweets and 1.2 kg of chocolate per NAVE, – 107% and 150%, respectively, of the pre-war consumption. This is astonishing, because the prices for sweets had sharply increased. And the consumption of sugar increased further.

The year 1956–7 was the first in which the pre-war level of nutrition in terms of calorie intake and protein and fat consumption was reached again. But the average consumption of 2,940 kcal per day during the depression years of 1934–8 hid big differences between the consumption of the hundreds of thousands of unemployed people and their families and that of the rest of the population. Such differences narrowed considerably during the 1950s.

Some products (poultry, citrus fruits) were consumed in quantities almost six times greater in 1960–1 than in 1950–1, others (milk, veal, vegetables) only slightly more, and still others (bread and flour, potatoes, lard) less. This was partly caused by the rise in incomes and partly a result of different rates of price increases. Thus, relatively cheap poultry was substituted for the more expensive veal. Oranges, dates and bananas became popular luxuries.

Table 9.6 Annual food consumption per capita in Austria (nutritional balances) 1934–88 (kg)

	1934/1938	1947/1948	1950/1951	1960/1961	1970/1971	1980/1981	1986/1987
Flour	120.0	126.1	117.1	98.9	85.9	67.3	64.0
Processed food	7.3	11.2	7.0	4.8	2.7	1.9	2.4
Rice	4.3	0.7	3.1	3.4	4.0	3.3	3.7
Potatoes	96.3	113.1	107.1	87.7	67.4	59.9	61.4
Sugar	24.1	11.7	23.6	35.4	32.7	39.9	35.4
Honey	0.2	0.1	0.6	0.9	1.2	1.4	1.5
Legumes	2.2	5.7	0.6	0.8	0.9	0.7	1.0
Beef	13.0	7.8	11.0	14.0	18.7	22.4	20.2
Veal	2.8	1.8	2.9	3.1	2.9	2.7	2.0
Pork	28.1	7.9	20.7	33.4	35.7	45.2	47.8
Poultry	1.2	0.3	0.5	3.0	8.5	11.0	12.6
Sum of meat	48.7	19.7	37.7	56.9	70.9	87.4	89.0
Eggs	6.7	2.3	4.8	11.5	15.0	14.4	14.6
Fresh fish	0.9	1.0	1.5	2.1	2.0	3.1	3.3
Milk	174.7	78.6	151.4	159.0	143.1	127.9	128.8
Cream	–	–	0.7	2.0	2.9	4.2	4.7
Cheese	2.2	0.7	1.6	3.0	4.0	5.6	7.0
Butter	3.6	2.3	3.6	4.5	5.7	5.1	5.3
Plant oils	5.1	3.5	4.3	8.3	12.0	15.3	15.6
Fat	9.2	3.8	9.4	5.0	9.4	11.8	12.2
Vegetables	57.8	39.3	61.0	68.9	66.5	90.4	73.0
Fresh fruit	37.2	21.2	50.3	93.1	71.6	72.0	72.1
Citrus fruit	4.4	1.0	2.1	11.7	16.4	17.5	18.8
Fruit juice	–	–	–	–	7.3	9.3	14.5
Wine	17.3	14.0	15.6	20.4	35.9	35.7	32.1
Beer	37.0	21.3	37.9	75.3	100.8	105.4	114.1
Kilocalories per capita per day	2,936	2,298	2,786	2,995	–	3,086	3,071

Sources: Wirtschafts- und sozialstatistisches Handbuch; Wirtschafts- und Sozialstatistisches Taschenbuch.

Problems 'around the waistline'

As long as hunger was a part of everyday life, an abundance of food signalled high prestige. This was true for country weddings as well as for courtly feasts. There was a connection between food and power: the sovereign had to be several sizes larger than everyone else, as Elias Canetti wrote in *Masse und Macht*. Fatness was a status symbol of the Renaissance sovereign and the monarch and even more of the duodecimo prince, who ate and drank with their companions.[25] If he was not the biggest eater, at least his provisions had to be the greater. As long as there was a lack of food, the waist of the king who ate the most and also the gluttony of the ruling classes showed their superiority. 'The sovereign is the stomach of the country', said the Austrian mercantilist, Wilhelm von Schröder, and he certainly did not mean this only in a figurative sense.

In the 19th century corpulence was a status symbol for the middle classes. Adalbert Stifter and his chronic gluttony might serve as an example: his correspondence shows that he would eat dozens of crayfish or six or more trout just as an *hors d'oeuvre*, followed by a main meal of roast beef, roast venison, chicken, hazel hen, pigeon, roast veal, ham, sour liver, roast pork, sardines, paprika chicken, roast mutton... At teatime he would have tea and hazel hen, tea and ham, etc. In a letter written in 1861 he said: 'Then I work again at the Witiko until 9 o'clock, and then a whole duck is waiting for me. But I am already so hungry that I think I will eat two.' In late summer, when time usually assumes less importance, food was constantly on his mind: 'After breakfast ... At lunch all guests are together again ... After the meal several guests left ... After we had tea ...". People seemed simply to exist from one meal to the next.[26]

In the bourgeois cuisine of the 19th century, an opulent diet signified that 'one had made it': corpulence as a sign of higher status in contrast to the slenderness of those for whom enough to eat was the exception rather than the rule. Embonpoint, the well-filled belly decorated with watch chain and orders, was proudly presented.

At the end of the 19th century a new beau ideal came into being: the full-bosomed woman who stresses her womanly curves by lacing herself up was supplanted by the slender, youthful and sporty woman. Empress Elisabeth might have been the most popular pioneer: wearing tight corsets, raw diet, massage, physical exercise, everything had to serve the preservation of slenderness. Now the trend was reversed: slenderness in the upper classes and corpulence in the lower classes.

Franz Kafka embodied the opposite of Stifter. Throughout his entire adult life he remained vegetarian. When he was employed as an insurance company lawyer he weighed only 61 kg, very little for a man 182 cm tall. He did not eat very much. When he died his weight was less than 50 kg. Suffering from laryngeal tuberculosis, he literally starved to death. His last literary activity was to read the proofs of 'Ein Hungerkünstler' (The Hunger Artist).[27]

During the years of National Socialism and the Second World War the old female beau ideal made a brief comeback. Slenderness could not be connected with the role of the mother. Therefore women were told not to care too much about their waist. The sturdy and well-rounded Brünnhilde type was back in vogue. Hunger prevailed and only the privileged could be corpulent. Corpulence once again conveyed a certain status.

The post-war era has made slender waistlines fashionable again. Wonder drugs and wonder diets have appeared on the market to plaudits from women's magazines. *Nouvelle cuisine* offers small portions on large plates, satisfying the eyes more than the belly. Nevertheless, we grow fatter and fatter.

References

1 Hörandner (1979); Gamerith (1988). For an overview on the older literature on economic history and ethnology, see Sandgruber (1982); Sandgruber (1985); Sandgruber (1988a); Schulz (1982); Valentin (1978); Burgstaller (1982); Burgstaller (1983); Grass and Holzmann (1982); Neuber (1985); Neuber (1988); Woidich (1987); Dollinger-Woidich (1989).
2 *Alltag im Spätmittelalter* (1984); Mülleder (1989); Mülleder (1988); Hundsbichler (1979); Schempf (1978); Stasnik (1988); Mueller (1987).
3 *Wiener Beisln* (1985); *Grazer Gastlichkeit* (1985); Katschnig-Fasch (1984); Kerschbaumer (1983–4); Sinhuber (1980); Ziak (1979); Weigel (1989); Prehsler (1985); *Im Café* (1987); *Das Prager Kaffeehaus* (1988); Sandgruber (1986).
4 *Hunger* (1985); Löwenfeld-Russ (1986); Sandgruber (1982); Sandgruber (1986); *100 Jahre Knorr* (1985); '100 Jahre Maggi Suppen' (1983/84); Wagner and Weishaupt (1971); Komlos (1989–90); Komlos (1985); Komlos (1986); Komlos (1989).
5 Girtler (1985); *Essen und Trinken* (1988); Sandgruber (1988b); Schimatschek (1988); Eisenbach-Stangl (1988a), Pilgram (1988); Girtler (1988); Jansen (1988).
6 Eisenbach-Stangl (1988b); Gehmacher (1987).
7 Hohenecker (1979); Fesl (1980); Sigloch (1985); Schneider (1988).
8 Schultheis (1986); Endler (1988); Floecklmueller (1988); *Probleme um Ernährungserhebungen* (1979); Krajasits (1988); Arnhof (1983); Drumbl (1983).
9 Baran (1988); Abegg-Mengold (1979); Stabéj (1977).
10 See especially Sandgruber (1982).
11 *Der Lebensstandard* (1959); Kautsky (1937); Papp (1980); Kresbach (1953); Rieger (1960); Regler (1932).
12 Müller (1849).
13 Dinklage (1976), pp. 75, 166, 234; Schwarzer (1857), p. 151f.; Witlacil (1847); *Statistischer Bericht* (1889); *Die Arbeits- und Lohnverhältnisse* (1870); Raunig (1892–3); *Bericht* (1894).
14 Philippovich (1894); *Österreichische Monatsschrift für Gesellschafts-Wissenschaft und Volkswirthschaft* (1879ff.).
15 Gruber (1887).
16 *Wirtschaftsrechnungen* (1916).
17 *Löhne und Lebenshaltung* (1928). The others have only been published in an edited form in: *Wirtschaftsstatistisches Jahrbuch* (1924–37); *Wirtschafts- und sozialstatisches Handbuch* (1945–69); Arlt (1925).
18 Braun (1979); Lüdtke (1979), pp.494ff.
19 Sorer (1911).
20 Leichter (1932); *Handbuch der Frauenarbeit* (1930).
21 *Nutzung der Freizeit* (1924); Friedrich (1924).
22 *Löhne und Lebenshaltung* (1928).
23 Langewiesche (1979).
24 Jahoda (1933, 1978); Stiefel (1979).
25 Canetti (1960), pp. 243ff.
26 Augustin (1964), pp. 96ff.; Seebald (1985), pp. 170ff.
27 Demmer (1987); Schlösser (1987).

Literature

Abegg-Mengold, Colette, *Die Bezeichnungsgeschichte von Mais, Kartoffel und Ananas im Italienischen. Probleme der Wortadoption und -adaptation* (Berne, 1979).
Alltag im Spätmittelalter, ed. Harry Kühnel (Graz, Vienna, Cologne, 1984).
Die Arbeits- und Lohnverhältnisse in den Fabriken und Gewerben Niederösterreichs (Vienna, 1870).
Arlt, Ilse, 'Der Einzelhaushalt', in Julius Bunzel (ed.), *Geldentwertung und Stabilisierung in ihren Einflüssen auf die soziale Entwicklung in Österreich* (Munich, 1925), pp. 161–76.
Arnhof, Hans, '*Ernährungsverhalten von Schichtarbeitern*' (doctoral thesis, Vienna, 1983).
Augustin, Hermann, *Adalbert Stifters Krankheit und Tod. Eine biographische Quellenstudie* (Basel, 1964).
Baran, Hanny, 'Die Terminologie der Bierbrauerei im Deutschen und im Tschechischen' (unpublished ms., Vienna, 1988).
Bauer, Josef M., '1900–1934: Politik und Grazer Gaststätten. Eine Betrachtung' in Herwig Ebner and Gerhard Dienes (eds), *Grazer Gastlichkeit. Beiträge zur Geschichte des Beherbergungs- und Gastgewerbes in Graz* (Graz, Vienna, 1985), pp. 113–18.
Bericht über die wirtschaftlichen Verhältnisse des Erzherzogthums Salzburg im Jahre 1893 (Salzburg, 1894).
Braun, Rudolf, 'Einleitende Bemerkungen zum Problem der historischen Lebensstandardforschung' in Werner Conze and Ulrich Engelhardt (eds), *Arbeiter im Industrialisierungsprozess. Herkunft, Lage und Verhalten* (Stuttgart, 1979), pp. 128–35.
Burgstaller, Ernst, *Vom Korn zum Brot. Katalog* (Linz, 1982).
Burgstaller, Ernst, *Österreichisches Festtagsgebäck. Brot und Gebäck im Jahres- und Lebensbrauchtum* (Linz, 1983).
Canetti, Elias, *Masse und Macht* (Hamburg, 1960).
Celedin, Gertrude, 'Das Gasthaus als Ausflugsziel – eine Sonderform des Gastgewerbes' in Herwig Ebner and Gerhard Dienes (eds), *Grazer Gastlichkeit. Beiträge zur Geschichte des Beherbergungs- und Gastgewerbes in Graz* (Graz, Vienna, 1985), pp. 206–42.
Cerwinka, Günter, 'Student und Gasthaus in Graz' in Herwig Ebner and Gerhard Dienes (eds), *Grazer Gastlichkeit. Beiträge zur Geschichte des Beherbergungs- und Gastgewerbes in Graz* (Graz, Vienna, 1985), pp. 75–88.
Demmer, Erich, 'Franz! Essen bei Kafka', *Lesezirkel. Literaturmagazin der Wiener Zeitung*, 4(1987), no. 29, p. 12.
Dienes, Gerhard M., 'Gastwirte – Bemerkungen über einen Berufsstand', in Herwig Ebner and Gerhard Dienes (eds), *Grazer Gastlichkeit. Beiträge zur Geschichte des Beherbergungs- und Gastgewerbes in Graz* (Graz, Vienna, 1985), pp. 46–54.
Dinklage, Karl, *Geschichte der Kärntner Arbeiterschaft* (Klagenfurt, 1976).
Dollinger-Woidich, Angelika, *Fertignahrung in Österreich. Ernährung und Gesellschaft im Wandel* (Graz, 1989).
Drumbl, Peter, '*Studien zur Entwicklung des Ernährungsverhaltens an der Bevölkerungsgruppe der 60–70jährigen in Wien*' (doctoral thesis, Vienna, 1983).
Eisenbach-Stangl, Irmgard, 'Der Bier-, Wein- und Spirituosenkonsum in der Republik Österreich' in Hubert Christian Ehalt, Manfred Chobot and Rolf Schwendter (eds), *Essen und Trinken* (Vienna, 1988a), pp. 21–9.
Eisenbach-Stangl, Irmgard, 'Zum Bedeutungswandel eines Konsumgutes. Die Geschichte des Alkohols in der Republik Österreich 1918–1984' mimeo (Vienna, 1988b).
Endler, Peter Christian, '*Ernährungsgewohnheiten älterer Menschen. Eine Untersuchung an 153 ausgewählten Grazern und Grazerinnen zwischen 60 und 103 Jahren und einer Vergleichsgruppe*

von 30–40jährigen' (doctoral thesis, Graz 1988).
Essen und Trinken, eds Hubert Christian Ehalt, Manfred Chobot and Rolf Schwendter (Vienna, 1988).
Fesl, Johann, *Die Milchwirtschaft in Österreich. The Austrian Dairy Sector* (Vienna, 1980).
Floecklmueller, Sabine, 'Alternative Getreidearten in der menschlichen Ernährung mit besonderer Berücksichtigung des Dinkels' (unpublished ms., Vienna, 1988).
Friedrich, Rager, 'Das Problem der Freizeit der Arbeiter in Österreich', *Arbeit und Wirtschaft*, 2 (1924), pp. 23–6, 57–62.
Gamerith, Anni, *Speise und Trank im südoststeirischen Bauernland* (Graz, 1988).
Gehmacher, Johanna, *'Die "Alkoholfrage" als "Frauenfrage"*. Zur Behandlung des Alkohols in der Theorie der österreichischen Sozialdemokraten mit besonderer Berücksichtigung sozialdemokratischer Frauenzeitschriften in Österreich 1918–1934'* (unpublished ms., Vienna, 1987).
Girtler, Roland, 'Das Beisl: Seine sonderbare und freundliche Tradition', in Hubert Christian Ehalt (ed.), *Wiener Beisln. Bilder & Geschichten* (Vienna, Munich, 1985), pp. 103ff.
Girtler, Roland, 'Vaganten, Studenten und die Kultur des Alkohols. Eine kultursoziologische Betrachtung', in Hubert Christian Ehalt, Manfred Chobot and Rolf Schwendter (eds), *Essen und Trinken* (Vienna, 1988), pp. 67–85.
Grass, Nikolaus und Hermann Holzmann, *Geschichte des Tiroler Metzgerhandwerks und der Fleischversorgung des Landes* (Innsbruck, 1982).
Grazer Gastlichkeit. Beiträge zur Geschichte des Beherbergungs- und Gastgewerbes in Graz, eds Herwig Ebner and Gerhard M. Dienes (Graz, Vienna, 1985).
Gruber, Ignaz, *Die Haushaltung der arbeitenden Klassen* (Jena, 1887).
Handbuch der Frauenarbeit in Österreich, ed. by Kammer für Arbeiter und Angestellte in Wien (Vienna, 1930).
Hohenecker, Josef, *Analyse der mengenmässigen Nachfrage nach Milch und Milchprodukten in Österreich und Voraussschätzung des Verbrauchs bis zum Jahre 1985* (Vienna, 1979).
Hörandner, Edith, 'Morgenmahlzeiten werktags im Sommer vor dem Ersten Weltkrieg' in *Österreichischer Volkskundeatlas*, 6th edn, part 2 (Vienna, Cologne, Graz, 1979), pp. 105–6.
Hundsbichler, Helmut, *'Reise, Gastlichkeit und Nahrung im Spiegel der Reisebücher des Paolo Santonino'* (doctoral thesis, Vienna, 1979).
Hunger. Special issue of the *Beiträge zur Historischen Sozialkunde*, 15 (Vienna, 1985), no. 2.
Im Café. Vom Wiener Charme zum Münchner Neon, ed. René Zey (Dortmund, 1987).
Jahoda, Marie, Paul Lazarsfeld and Hans Zeisel, *Die Arbeitslosen von Marienthal. Ein soziographischer Versuch* (Leipzig, 1933; new edn, Frankfurt am Main, 1978).
100 Jahre Knorr Österreich (Wels, 1985).
'100 Jahre Maggi Suppen', *Maggi Revue*, special issue, 2 parts (Vienna, 1983/84).
Jansen, Isolde, 'Nüchterne Idealisten und rote Spiesser. Zur Geschichte des Arbeiter-Abstinentenbundes in Österreich' in Hubert Christian Ehalt, Manfred Chobot and Rolf Schwendter (eds), *Essen und Trinken* (Vienna, 1988), pp. 86–97.
Jontes, Günter, 'Gasthaus, Wirte und Gäste in Alt-Graz vom 16. bis zum 18. Jahrhundert' in Herwig Ebner and Gerhard M. Dienes (eds), *Grazer Gastlichkeit. Beiträge zur Geschichte des Beherbergungs- und Gastgewerbes in Graz* (Graz, Vienna, 1985), pp. 21–54.
Katschnig-Fasch, Elisabeth, *Im Wirtshaus bin i wia z'haus. Zur kulturellen Bedeutung des Gasthauses für eine städtische Region. Eine volkskundliche Gegenwartsuntersuchung* (Graz, 1984).
Kautsky, Benedikt, 'Die Haushaltsstatistik der Wiener Arbeiterkammer 1925 bis 1934', *International Review of Social History*, (1937), pp. 177–232.
Kerschbaumer, Gert, 'Gausuppe und tausendjähriger Juchezer. Gasthauskultur im Dritten

Reich – am Beispiel Salzburg', *Zeitgeschichte*, 11 (1983–4), pp. 213–34.

Komlos, John, 'Stature and nutrition in the Habsburg monarchy: the standard of living and economic development in the eighteenth century' *American Historical Review*, 90 (1985), pp. 1149–61.

Komlos, John, 'Patterns of children's growth in east-central Europe in the eighteenth century' *Annals of Human Biology*, 13 (1986), pp. 33–48.

Komlos, John, *Nutrition and Economic Development in the Habsburg Monarchy. An Anthropometric History* (Princeton, N. J., 1989).

Komlos, John, 'Height and social status in eighteenth-century Germany' *Journal of Interdisciplinary History*, 20 (1989–90), pp. 607–21.

Krajasits, Eveline, 'Der Wandel der Ernährungsgewohnheiten unter besonderer Berücksichtigung von Getreide und Fleisch und die Entwicklung der Tischsitten und einer Esskultur' (unpublished ms., Vienna, 1988).

Kresbach, Robert, *'Die Stellung des Arbeiters als Konsument. Eine statistische Untersuchung für die Jahre 1925–1935'* (unpublished doctoral thesis, Vienna, 1953)

Kropac, H., 'Das Gast- und Schankgewerbe vom Beginn des 19. bis ins 20. Jahrhundert', in Herwig Ebner and Gerhard M. Dienes (eds), *Grazer Gastlichkeit. Beiträge zur Geschichte des Beherbergungs- und Gastgewerbes in Graz* (Graz, Vienna, 1985), pp. 33–45.

Langewiesche, Dieter, *Zur Freizeit des Arbeiters. Bildungsbestrebungen und Freizeitgestaltung österreichischer Arbeiter im Kaiserreich und in der Ersten Republik* (Stuttgart, 1979).

'Der Lebensstandard von Wiener Arbeiterfamilien im Lichte langfristiger Familienbudgetuntersuchungen', *Arbeit und Wirtschaft*, 13 (1959), no. 12, pp. 1–16.

Leichter, Käthe, *Wie leben die Wiener Heimarbeiter? Eine Erhebung über die Arbeits- und Lebensverhältnisse von tausend Wiener Heimarbeitern* (Vienna, 1928).

Leichter, Käthe, *So leben wir... 1320 Industriearbeiterinnen berichten über ihr Leben. Eine Erhebung* (Vienna, 1932).

Löhne und Lebenshaltung der Wiener Arbeiterschaft im Jahre 1925 (Vienna, 1928).

Löwenfeld-Russ, Hans, *Im Kampf gegen den Hunger. Aus den Erinnerungen des Staatssekretärs für Volksernährung 1918–1920*, ed. Isabella Ackerl (Vienna, 1986).

Lüdtke, Alf, 'Erfahrung von Industriearbeitern', in Werner Conze and Ulrich Engelhardt (eds), *Arbeiter im Industrialisierungsprozess. Herkunft, Lage und Verhalten* (Stuttgart, 1979), pp. 494–512.

Österreichische Monatsschrift für Gesellschafts-Wissenschaft und Volkswirthschaft (1879ff.).

Mülleder, Gerhard, *'Beiträge zur Geschichte des Alkohols und der Gastlichkeit in Ostösterreich vom Spätmittelalter bis Ende des 17. Jahrhunderts'* (unpublished ms., Vienna, 1988).

Mülleder, Gerhard, 'Alkoholkonsum im 15., 16. und 17. Jahrhundert', *Unsere Heimat. Monatsblatt des Vereins für Landeskunde von Niederösterreich und Wien*, 60 (1989), pp. 198–213.

Müller, Karl, *Der Haushalt des Arbeiters oder: Wie soll es der Arbeiter anfangen, um sich und den Seinigen ein rechtliches Fortkommen und ein reichliches Auskommen zu sichern? Eine allgmeine Gewerbslehre mit besonderer Berücksichtigung des österreichischen Arbeiters* (Vienna, 1849).

Mueller, Sylvia, *'Die Fastengebote der Römisch-Katholischen Kirche und ihre Auswirkung auf die Ernährung und Kochkunst in Österreich'* (unpublished ms., Vienna, 1987).

Naschenwerg, Hannes P., 'Grazer Gast- und Kaffeehäuser und ihre Bedeutung für das Kulturleben', in Herwig Ebner and Gerhard M. Dienes (eds), *Grazer Gastlichkeit. Beiträge zur Geschichte des Beherbergungs- und Gastgewerbes in Graz* (Graz, Vienna, 1985), pp. 62–74.

Neuber, Berta, *'Die Ernährungslage in Wien während des Ersten Weltkrieges und in den ersten Nachkriegsjahren'* (unpublished ms., Vienna, 1985).

Neuber, Berta, *Die Ernährungssituation in Wien in der Zwischenkriegszeit, während des Zweiten Weltkriegs und in den ersten Nachkriegsjahren* ((doctoral thesis) Vienna, 1988).
'Nutzung der Freizeit in Österreich', *Internationale Rundschau der Arbeit*, 2 (1924), pp. 458ff.
Papp, Magdalene, *Wiener Arbeiterhaushalte um 1900. Studien zur Kultur und Lebensweise im privaten Reproduktionsbereich* (unpublished doctoral thesis, Vienna, 1980).
Philippovich, Eugen von, 'Wiener Wohnungsverhältnisse', *Archiv für soziale Gesetzgebung und Statistik*, 7 (1894), pp. 215–77.
Pilgram, Arno, 'Von der agrarischen zur industriellen Alkoholproduktion. Alkoholwirtschaft im 19. Jahrhundert' in Hubert Christian Ehalt, Manfred Chobot and Rolf Schwendter (eds), *Essen und Trinken* (Vienna, 1988), pp. 30–45.
Das Prager Kaffeehaus. Literarische Tischgesellschaften, ed. Karl-Heinz Jähn (Berlin, 1988).
Prehsler, Ilse, *'Das Kaffeehaus als kulturelle Einrichtung im Europa des 18. und 19. Jahrhunderts'* (unpublished ms., Vienna, 1985).
Probleme um Ernährungserhebungen. Berichte, vorgelegt auf dem Symposium der Österreichischen Gesellschaft für Ernährungsforschung am 4. und 5. April 1979 in Wien, ed. Wilhelm Auerswald, Berta Brandstetter and S. Gergely (Vienna, Munich, Berne, 1979).
Raunig, G., 'Ein Wiener Haushalt in Beziehung zu den indirekten Steuerlasten', *Deutsche Worte. Wöchentliche Rundschau über Politik und Gesellschaft, geistiges und wirtschaftliches Leben*, 3 (1892–3), p. 134.
Regler, Melanie, *'Ernährungsverschiebungen. Dargestellt auf Grund ganzjähriger Haushaltsrechnungen minderbemittelter Familien vor und nach dem Weltkrieg'* (doctoral thesis, Vienna, 1932).
Rieger, Philipp, *'Änderungen in den Lebensverhältnissen und den Verbrauchsgewohnheiten von Wiener Arbeitnehmerhaushalten 1952/57'* (unpublished doctoral thesis, Vienna, 1960).
Sandgruber, Roman, *Die Anfänge der Konsumgesellschaft. Konsumgüterverbrauch, Lebensstandard und Alltagskultur in Österreich im 18. und 19. Jahrhundert* (Vienna, 1982).
Sandgruber, Roman, 'Knödel, Nudel, Topfenstrudel. Österreichische Ernährungsgewohnheiten und regionale Unterschiede in Mitteleuropa' in Günter Wiegelmann (ed.), *Nord-Süd-Unterschiede in der städtischen und ländlichen Kultur Mitteleuropas* (Münster, 1985), pp. 265–87.
Sandgruber, Roman, *Bittersüsse Genüsse. Kulturgeschichte der Genussmittel* (Vienna, Cologne, Graz, 1986).
Sandgruber, Roman, 'Arme Leute, arme Küche. Vom früheren Essen und Trinken im Mühlviertel' in *Das Mühlviertel. Katalog der oberösterreichischen Landesausstellung 1988* (Linz, 1988a), pp. 339–46.
Sandgruber, Roman, 'Träume vom Schlaraffenland' in Hubert Christian Ehalt, Manfred Chobot and Rolf Schwendter (eds), *Essen und Trinken* (Vienna, 1988b), pp. 7–11.
Schempf, Herbert, 'Kleine Fische. Ein Kapitel Rechtsarchäologie besonders nach österreichischen Quellen', *Forschungen zur Rechtsarchäologie und rechtlichen Volkskunde*, 1 (1978), pp. 63–80.
Schimatschek, Erna, 'Die Dicken und die Dünnen' in Hubert Christian Ehalt, Manfred Chobot and Rolf Schwendter (eds), *Essen und Trinken* (Vienna, 1988), pp. 12–15.
Schlösser, Hermann, 'Franz Kafkas "ein Hungerkünstler"' *Lesezirkel. Literaturmagazin der Wiener Zeitung*, 4 (1987), no. 29, pp. 11ff.
Schneider, Matthias and Michael Wüger, *Nachfrage nach Nahrungsmitteln und Getränken. Analyse und Vorschau bis 1995/96*, 2 vols (Vienna, 1988).
Schultheis, Martina, *Die Ernährung älterer Menschen* (unpublished ms., Vienna, 1986).
Schulz, Friedrich, *Brot in Volksmedizin und Aberglaube* (Vienna, 1982).

Schwarzer, Ernst von, *Geld und Gut in Neu-Österreich* (Vienna, 1857).
Sebald, W. G., *Die Beschreibung des Unglücks. Zur österreichischen Literatur von Stifter bis Handke* (Salzburg, 1985).
Sigloch, Georg, '*Die räumliche Organisation der Milchwirtschaft in Österreich nach 1945*' (unpublished ms., Vienna, 1985).
Sinhuber, Bartel F., *Das grosse Buch vom Wiener Heurigen* (Vienna, Stuttgart, 1980).
Sorer, Richard, *Auslese und Anpassung der Arbeiterschaft in der Automobilindustrie und in einer Wiener Maschinenfabrik* (Munich, 1911).
Stabéj, Joze, *Kruk ubogik. Kulturnozgodovinski in jezikovni zacrt zgadovine krompirja na Slovenkskem* [The Bread of the Poor. A Brief Account of the Cultural and Linguistic History of the Potato in Slovenia] (Ljubljana, 1977).
Stastnik, Brigitte, '*Wien und der Alkohol im Spätmittelalter*' (unpublished ms., Vienna, 1988).
Statistischer Bericht über Industrie und Gewerbe des Erzherzogthums Österreich unter der Enns im Jahre 1885 (Vienna, 1889), pp. 88–112.
Staudinger, Eduard, 'Gasthaus und frühe Arbeiterbewegung. Grazer Gasthäuser als Versammlungs- und Vereinslokale', in Herwig Ebner and Gerhard M. Dienes (eds), *Grazer Gastlichkeit. Beiträge zur Geschichte des Beherbergungs- und Gastgewerbes in Graz* (Graz, Vienna, 1985).
Stiefel, Dieter, *Arbeitslosigkeit. Soziale, politische und wirtschaftliche Auswirkungen am Beispiel Österreichs 1918–1938* (Berlin, 1979).
Valentin, Hans E., *Brezen, Kletzen, Dampedei. Brot im süddeutschen und österreichischen Volksbrauchtum* (Regensburg, 1978).
Wagner, Johann and Rudolf Weishäupl, *Ein Jahrhundert österreichischer Spirituswirtschaft* (Vienna, 1971).
Weigel, Hans, *Wiener Kaffeehausführer* (Vienna, 1989).
Wiener Beisln. Bilder & Geschichten, ed. Hubert Christian Ehalt (Vienna, Munich, 1985).
Wirtschaftsrechnungen und Lebensverhältnisse von Wiener Arbeiterfamilien in den Jahren 1912 bis 1914 (Vienna, 1916).
Wirtschafts- und sozialstatistisches Handbuch 1945–1969, ed. Kammer für Arbeiter und Angestellte in Wien (Vienna, 1970).
Wirtschaftsstatistisches Jahrbuch, ed. Kammer für Arbeiter und Angestellte in Wien, Vol. 1–12 (Vienna, 1924–1937).
Witlacil, Andreas, 'Verhältnisse der handarbeitenden Bevölkerung in Wien', *Zeitschrift des Vereins für deutsche Statistik*, 1 (1847), part 2, pp. 177–87.
Woidich, Angelika, 'Convenience Food. Entwicklung und Funktion der Fertignahrung in Österreich' (unpublished ms., Vienna, 1987).
Ziak, Karl, *Des Heiligen Römischen Reiches grösstes Wirtshaus. Der Wiener Vorort Neulerchenfeld* (Vienna, Munich, 1979).

10 Food history in Switzerland: a survey of the literature

Martin R. Schärer

Introduction

There can be no such thing as a history of Swiss food because the subject does not exist. There simply is no such entity as 'Swiss cooking' – this patchwork quilt of a country, a nation by act of will, straddles too many of the great European cultures to have a single characteristic cuisine of its own. Neither is there as yet a history of food in Switzerland, which would be more relevant; unfortunately, the subject seems likely to remain a gap in our bookshelves for the foreseeable future. As a result we are obliged to make do with individual pieces of the mosaic which, substantial as some of them may be, can hardly make up for the lack of a complete picture. It is amazing how much work is currently being done on food history and food ethnology; hardly a term goes by without some lecture being devoted to the subject somewhere or other, generally with the 18th to 20th centuries in the foreground. Before taking a closer look at the various parts of the mosaic – and this, let us not forget, is an annotated bibliography, not an outline of food history – a few preliminary remarks are in order.

A great many studies large and small – and this seems typical of all food history – are not the outcome of historical research and, strictly speaking, therefore do not really belong here. This is partly because many of them are the work of amateurs with a bent for history (but they are none the less valuable here because of the dearth of other research) and partly because many are theses authored by people from other disciplines such as law, economics, medicine and ethnology, all of which address different aspects of food industry, farming, public health and lifestyles, trade and professional associations, co-operatives and food supply systems. These studies are interesting less for the often rudimentary nature of their historical basis than for their depiction of a state of affairs, for instance, that of the processed cheese industry between the wars. Thus, such reports do have a certain legitimate source value for the modern historian. It is for this reason that this survey deliberately includes publications which are not the work of professional historians.

As an exhaustive bibliography of this kind would have to deal with more than

1,000 titles, further limits must be set – not to mention the often all too subjective nature of decisions on the importance and representative nature of many works. Reports drawn up for political reasons of the time, commemorative volumes published by companies, professional associations, guilds, consumer co-operatives, etc., and academic works existing only in typescript are not included. Also omitted are general histories of Switzerland and listings of statistical source material.[1] The only statistical surveys quoted concern agriculture and nutrition; some useful economic compendia are also mentioned.[2]

We are taking food history in a very broad sense of the term here,[3] including all phases of the 'food chain' from production through processing, preservation, transport, trade and preparation to consumption. These stages, which obviously do not always fit into watertight compartments, form the bones of this text and bibliography in its three main sections devoted to food production, processing and consumption. Breaking down the subject matter into these thematic subdivisions seems to us a more convenient way of dealing with the mass of material than attempting what would be a very difficult chronological approach. Time and place, particulary important in the case of Switzerland with its numerous regional studies, only come into play if the subject-matter is subdivided even further. Some classification problems arise in connection with the food trade, which comes into the food chain at several points. The different publications are slotted in at the point where there is a link from the product – for example, the trade in wheat and cattle is dealt with under 'Production', the trade in cheese under 'Processing', and the food trade in general together with meat and salt under 'Consumption' (Food Supplies).

General surveys

Until very recently, the history of everyday life, and hence also of food, was hardly touched upon in general Swiss history books. Only the latest 'holistic' publication[4] which attempts to give an overall view of the matter stands apart from the matrix of political history, placing considerable weight on economic and socio-historical developments. However, because of its extremely piecemeal approach to the food situation it is just as far from conveying a concise overview as are the economic and social histories of Switzerland[5] which touch upon numerous aspects of food history, with farming and industry taking pride of place over living standards and eating habits in the topics dealt with. It goes without saying that this also applies to the many regional accounts of economic history.

This category of publications also includes general surveys of agricultural history[6] which, like the history of food consumption, has in general received better treatment than processing and preservation. Christian Pfister describes the development of agriculture and food with new methods and a considerably broader interdisciplinary approach.[7] Starting with an account of climatic changes in modern times and an examination of land systems and their productivity, he develops elements of an ecological theory of demography via quality and quantity, taking into account the buffering strategies which are easier to apply in cereal-growing areas. This new context makes it possible to explain the frequent subsistence crises and their various effects in the different economic areas as well as the interlinking of the various factors of agricultural modernization in the 18th and early 19th centuries. Three key innovations – new cultivated plants (potatoes, green fodder); summer stall-feeding, and hence an increase in the useful amount of stall manure; and changes in land-use patterns, above all the abandonment of fallow – combined to bring about a decisive improvement in food, especially carbohydrates, animal proteins and vitamin C, and enabled two important gaps of the traditional system to be filled: the lack of protein in spring and of carbohydrates in early summer.

Of the sociological and demographic studies[8] the comprehensive history of Swiss demography by Markus Mattmüller is of major interest. It is based on a whole series of regional theses and, approaching the subject from the viewpoints of traditional economic and social history, comes to similar conclusions. In a section on growth-inhibiting forces, Mattmüller also deals in detail with the economic background and demographic effects of famines. The final analysis of the growth process describes the demography of early modern times (1500–1700) as a demography of scarcity with regard to the food margin and labour supply in non-farming sectors, as mortality-regulated growth: a substantial increase in the early 16th century due to expansion of the means of subsistence was followed by a period of resource scarcity and hence slower growth interrupted by another rise in the food ceiling, above all in regions which had been industrialized at any early date (home industry). The 18th century saw a substantial decline in mortality thanks to better food (dairy products, cereals, potatoes). Thus, economic factors come to the fore which are examined for the various food zones which have evolved since the late Middle Ages (and which should be regarded as rough points of reference only): cereal-growing country (the three-field system), mixed subsistence zones (rotational system of tilling and pasturing), Alpine autarkical subsistence zones without rotation, and cattle-breeding country (an export economy based on cattle and cheese). New research concerning these areas allows a better understanding of their geographical extension and specific agricultural problems.[9] The cattle-breeding area, which is probably perceived as being the most 'Swiss' of economic areas, was described by Ralph Bircher in the 1930s.[10]

Besides these analyses contained in major comprehensive works, there exist a number of general surveys of food history.[11] Even though these rough sketches of mostly a few pages cannot be classified as to the character of their research, as with one exception (Bergier) they are not the work of historians and are marked by huge oversimplifications or idealized pictures of food in earlier times (Bircher), they can still be quite useful when approaching the subject for the first time.

Food production

As is already clear from the general surveys mentioned above, farming was not only the first area of the production–processing–consumption chain to be investigated (think of the economic societies of the 18th century) but also for a long time the best researched.[11] In the following, the available material has therefore been screened particularly strictly, inevitably leaving technical aspects of agriculture and legal matters, for example, out of the picture.

Many of the general works not specially devoted to individual food items place the transition to modern farming in the foreground.[12] What Pfister did for Switzerland, Anne-Marie Piuz [13] has done for the region at the western end of Lake Geneva in form of a contribution to ecological history which attempts to link the consequences of climate and agricultural developments to daily life. Samuel Huggel[14] gives a detailed account of land enclosure as part of the general process of the individualization of agriculture as an important new factor in raising production. Of the agricultural 'pioneers' of the 18th century who practised these and other innovations, the peasant-philosopher Jacob Guyer,[15] also known as 'Kleinjogg', became known far beyond the confines of Switzerland. Not only does he provide a wealth of detailed information of all new aspects of agricultural modernization, he also discusses his progressive farming methods in the *Bauerngespräche* [Farmers' Talks] of the Zurich Natural Science Society. Guyer is a typical representative of an enlightened peasantry within the larger context of the debate on farming issues in the Economic-Patriotic Society of the second half of the century. The decisive role played by these advocates of modern farming methods was described by Georg Schmidt in the framework of agricultural modernization.[16]

The Lucerne study by Max Lemmenmeier deserves special mention as an important contribution to research in economic, social, legal and political developments in agriculture.[17] It attempts to point out the long-term trends in a limited zone between cattle-raising and cereal-growing areas within the general framework. It is an exemplary study of the transition from cereal growing to livestock raising and dairy farming and its effects on farmers' living standards.

As far as contemporary history is concerned, agricultural research has done no more than touch upon the particular problems of neutral Switzerland in the Second World War[18] when the country was forced, in order to feed its people, to restrict consumption, to double the national acreage under cultivation, to bring in compulsory land service and in general to modernize its agriculture.

Research on the production of specific food items is dominated by cereals, livestock/dairy products and viniculture. It relies heavily on traditional research methods, except for cereals – often virtually synonymous with food – where quantitative analysis is widely applied. Such analysis, in conjunction with climate research findings, can provide a highly informative picture of the state of modern agriculture and hence of the food situation and demographic developments:[19] the most important growth phase is revealed as being the 1666–1742 period, which is also marked by an increase in population. Works dealing with cereal trading and policies can be assigned to a second group covering various periods and regions through to the 20th-century debate on the cereal monopoly and cereal laws.[20] In a study centred on Calvin's city of Geneva, Jean-François Bergier of the Swiss Federal Institute of Technology (ETH) in Zurich[21] shows the important transition after the end of the

Middle Ages to the capitalistic organization of the cereal trade, powered by a small group of dynamic entrepreneurs acting on a new set of basic principles and deriving from a new economic outlook. Finally, there are a number of works which deal in fair detail with millet and oats, cereals which are otherwise largely ignored, chestnuts and onions, also generally bypassed by the literature, and oilseeds.[22]

Cattle[23] is another subject of extensive research, such that we are once again forced to set ourselves limits and concentrate above all on the trade in cattle – extremely important for Switzerland – and dairy products. The historical, cultural-anthropological work of Rudolf Ramseyer examines in detail the world of the cowherd[24] and the rise, 18th-century zenith and decline (due mainly to the spread of cheese dairies in the valleys during the 19th century) of these rich and respected entrepreneurs. Paul Hugger[25] depicts the living tradition of present-day Alpine herdsmen in his ethnological study. The economic rise of the cattle-breeding economy in early modern times was influenced by the cattle trade, above all with Italy.[26] Alain Dubois[27] shows that this transalpine trade and hence cattle-breeding were particularly strong in the 16th century, during the Thirty Years War, and again in the second half of the 18th century, mainly because of hefty price rises and growing demand for cheese and, in the last half of the 19th century, also a burgeoning demand for fresh milk for direct sale and industrial use.

Dairy products research concentrates mainly on processing. Thomas Steiger[28] shows the production-oriented side in a detailed presentation of 19th century statistical material which he interprets in relation to farmers' decision-making (reactions to changes in price relations) and places it in an overall economic context. Whereas the world market had a very great impact on cereal prices, it had hardly any effect at all on meat and milk prices. However, there were few opportunities for farmers to adapt their production structure to price developments, mainly because of a lack of sources of information and biological, organizational and technical limitations. Mention may be made in passing of a few works, some rather old and most ethnologically oriented, on pigs, goats, fish, snails and bees – subjects which are otherwise rarely dealt with.[29]

Wine-making plays such a dominant role in some parts of Switzerland, above all on many of the lakes, that Pfister has suggested adding to the 'cattle-raising' and 'cereal-growing' areas another region called 'wine country' with very specific production conditions and lifestyles. As part of his ecologically oriented historical studies Pfister also looked at the fluctuations in earnings and their economic effects.[30] Two further studies are worth mentioning because they provide a historical overview and a representative picture of a wine-growing area.[31]

Unlike the trade in cattle and cereals, which is nearer to the production than to the consumption end of the chain, we shall leave the third area – salt and the trade in salt – on which an extensive literature is available, to the section on consumption which also deals with supply problems. This is justified by the fact that prior to the 19th century Switzerland had only insignificant sources of salt of its own.

Food processing

The first products to be manufactured on an industrial scale in Switzerland were chocolate (1819), pasta (1839), condensed milk (1866), baby food (1867), canned food (1868), powdered soup (1883), margarine (1889), biscuits (1899), beet sugar (1911) and canned cheese (1913). As late as 1895 the nascent food industry occupied a modest place in the country's economy, employing only about 7 per cent of industrial workers.

There are several large research gaps in everything to do with food processing. And, at the same time, in neither the area of food production nor of food consumption have non-historians made such a major contribution as here. Mention should be made of most company histories and of the commemorative brochures published by various associations, but there is no room for them here, nor for the biographies of individual entrepreneurs.[32] This is also an area in which juridical and political-science dissertations on specific areas of industry abound; they are of special value because there is hardly anything else available on the subject. The striking absence of professional historical studies is obviously related to the desolate source situation, that is, the lack of or difficulty of access to company archives. The pickings are very meagre.

Apart from a few small general surveys[33] which also touch upon the question of geographical location, works devoted to the food sector in general are concerned with two principal aspects: food law,[34] in which the Swiss law of 1905/1909 marks a major milestone, and food science.[35]

Monographs dealing with individual foodstuffs or areas of industry are, as might be expected, concerned mainly with cereal and dairy products, chocolate and beer. Milling[36] is placed in its socio-economic and legal context in a work by Anne-Marie Dubler[37] relating to Lucerne. The work reveals that millers ranked alongside large farmers as the most influential occupational group. In particular, the strong rise in prices due to the Thirty Years War filled their coffers, and thanks to a broad-based economic underpinning they came through the postwar crisis without losses, though also without growth throughout the entire 18th century – a situation which was to remain unchanged until the production rises of the 19th century.

Studies both large and small of bread and bakeries abound.[38] Emigration had always been a major factor in little Switzerland. It has been studied in relation to confectioners,[39] with – in a purely economic light – a positive verdict: the money which the expatriate confectioners earned abroad was invested in the burgeoning tourist industry at home. This sector of activity also includes milk cure centres run by Swiss in other countries.[40] Economic, business-management and legal problems of the interwar period are dealt with in non-historical theses relating to the biscuit, pasta and soup industries.[41]

The dairy industry[42] is a favourite area of research in food processing, especially cheese-making and trading. A good, thoroughly historically oriented introduction was provided by the now rather dated study by Karl Gutzwiller,[43] who traces the development of upland and valley cheese dairies. Two compilations[44] provide extensive cross-sections of production fundamentals, mainly about milk processing, thereby outlining the situation in the 1930s and 1940s. Special wartime problems (reduced cattle holdings, pricing, organizational structures in a wartime economy) have been examined.[45]

While there is no lack of publications dealing with cheese[46] we unfortunately are still missing a broad, truly historical work on the subject. Authors from the cheese industry, journalists, ethnologists, jurists, economists, philologists, and, rarely, historians have turned their attentions to regionally or thematically limited topics and individual cheeses: the shift from upland to valley cheese dairies in the 19th century,[47] the cheese trade,[48] processed cheese,[49] the Jura,[50] Emmental[51] (not forgetting the novels of the Berne pastor and writer Jeremias Gotthelf, with their realistic depictions of everyday life written during the period of turmoil in the dairy sector 150 years ago;[52] and studies also of Appenzell,[53] Tête de Moine[54] and Gruyère[55] cheeses. This last study by Roland Ruffieux and Walter Bodmer provides an exemplary picture of the importance of cheesemaking and the cheese trade against a historico-economic background (the fact that in pre-industrial times Gruyère cheese was, along with mercenaries, the canton of Fribourg's chief 'foreign currency earner' underlines the economic importance of this foodstuff). The 19th century then saw the completion of the important shift to cheese manufacture in the valleys and the rise of marketing co-operatives.

Chocolate as another successful Swiss product[56] has also attracted a lot of attention. What the confectioners were to Grisons, the *cioccolatieri* were to the valleys of the Upper Ticino. They, too, sought and often found their fortune abroad.[57] The chocolate industry has attracted the attentions of numerous jurists, economists and political scientists as a subject for their theses but not, surprisingly, so far of any historians. These works[58] already convey some useful insights, especially into the first half of the 20th century.

The same applies to works on the sugar industry[59] and studies on the mineral water industry[60] and breweries.[61] The last of these areas is dominated by the critical period during and immediately after the First World War and the difficulties in raw-materials procurement, among other things. Brewing is the subject of innumerable commemorative brochures produced by the breweries, and of publications of local interest, which are beyond the scope of this survey. Works on distilled alcoholic liquors focus on the development of the state alcohol monopoly and the relevant federal law of 1886.[62] We would like to round out this menu of the food industry – a copious one but one in which real historical meat is unfortunately rather lacking – with a true 'green fairy' story. Absinthe[63] had long been an important industry, above all in the Neuchâtel Jura, until its prohibition was enshrined in 1908–10 in the Swiss constitution. This aperitif may act as a bridge to the third main section of this survey.

Food consumption

This final link in the food chain, telescoped by many into the history of food as a whole, is in contrast covered in copious detail, though without much attention being paid to food preparation. Researchers tend to concentrate all their energies on food consumption and budgetary matters, and to neglect cooking! We shall not attempt to list here all the cookery-books that have been published and so have nothing more to say on this matter except that there is scope for a scientific treatment of it. As there is much more general literature available on food consumption in the broadest sense of the term, and less in the way of monographs, than in the areas of food production and processing, we must adopt a different approach to sub-dividing the subject in order to do justice to aspects of consumption which have evolved since the 19th century. We will deal, first, with the question of food supplies, then with living standards and consumption.

Food supplies

General food supply policy breaks down naturally into two parts: the *ancien régime*, quite clearly the preserve of the historians; and the 20th century, a period for economists and jurists to get their teeth into; the 19th century lies like a fallow field between them.

All studies of food policy up to the 18th century[64] are regional studies which exemplify specific problems. They are concerned with Brugg and Baden,[65] the former a Bernese country town, the latter part of an area under common sovereignty, that is, a territory administered jointly by bailiffs of the confederation of the original cantons with a complicated customs and excise system; Glarus,[66] a rural area without an urban focus, with a typical Alpine peasant economy and significant imports of cereals; Basel[67] and Geneva,[68] the latter, with a population of some 25,000, being the largest city in the confederation's 18th-century networks of alliances (Geneva was only an ally and did not become a full member of the confederation until 1815), with large town markets and a considerable hinterland, necessary for its food supplies; Lausanne,[69] a centre of the Bernese subject territory of the Vaud; and finally, Neuchâtel,[70] a Prussian principality allied with the confederation, with lakeside vineyards and extensive dairy-farming in the Jura mountains, which faced particularly severe supply problems during the revolutionary period in neighbouring France.

Little neutral Switzerland, so often surrounded by warring nations, has always faced enormous problems in keeping itself supplied with food in times of crisis. The numerous studies of legal, economic and administrative provenance devoted to these problems[71] have a certain source value for the modern historian. They deal with the Franco-Prussian War,[72] the First World War[73] and, above all, the Second World War.[74]

With only a few exceptions, often concerning salt, studies dealing with the supply of individual foodstuffs are dominated largely by discussions of problems of the first half of the 20th century; thus, theses on food are also highly popular in the field of food supply – above all among non-historians. As might be expected, they are concerned mainly with cereal and bread supplies[75] but also with fruit,[76] vegetables,[77] milk[78] and eggs,[79] not forgetting several studies devoted to meat.[80] Though water supplies are important for more than just food, they nevertheless have to play a vital role in this sector, as documented in an extensive monograph.[81]

Salt is a subject which is enormously popular with historians. It is one of the best researched of foodstuffs in monographs and studies cover all parts of the country. The only thing that is lacking at the present time is a synthesis covering the whole country. The reason why salt is such a popular subject of research may reside in the fact that – from a Swiss point of view – there is almost no need to go into the production aspect (apart from the salt mines of Aigle/Bex in the canton of Vaud, which were of regional significance only), Switzerland had no sources of salt of its own until major deposits were discovered near Rothaus/Schweizerhalle (Canton Basel Land) in 1835–36; as a result, trade and supply are in the foreground, forging very close links with traditional political and economic history. Of the twenty or so leading publications, we can mention here only a few supraregional studies[82] and the most comprehensive regional one,[83] by way of example.

Food supply also embraces the wholesale[84] and retail food trade,[85] yet another area for economists and legal experts. Also of interest, because of the wealth of statistical material they contain, are the studies of the cumulative and steadily growing price differentials in the food trade from producer to consumer, including all stages in between.[86] Of particular interest, in view of our discussion below of living standards and household budgets, is the development of the consumer co-operative movement[87] which is the subject of a wealth of studies and reports including numerous jubilee publications by individual co-operatives which we cannot go into here and studies arising from political issues of topical interest.

The hotel and restaurant business[88] is part of the supply situation in the broadest sense of the term, and it is an area which has so far almost entirely escaped the attention of historical research.

Living standards

Living standards are a prime focus of research among social and economic historians, so it is not surprising to find a rich crop of studies dealing with this topic. Research covers the entire period from the late Middle Ages to the present day, especially the 18th century and the period since 1850. A wealth of source material is available for the latter period thanks to the development of statistics, interest in the 'worker question' and several periods of high prices.

Two hundred years ago, to dabble in social history was to risk one's neck – literally. Let us merely recall the Zurich pastor, Johann Heinrich Waser,[89] who was executed as a subversive on 27 May 1780 for, among other things, unauthorized publication of certain economic reports, including demographic data, which he seems to have drawn up also on the basis of stolen official documents. For most research historians, times have certainly changed for the better.

Ulf Dirlmeier's detailed study on German living standards,[90] which is also of key interest to Switzerland, examines the transition from the Middle Ages to early modern times. He comes to the conclusion that the cost of living was very high in comparison with the level of people's incomes. Living standards, already relatively modest, deteriorated even further in the 16th century – a finding which, among other things, leads him to revise our notions of a very high meat consumption in the late Middle Ages onwards. Hugo Wermelinger[91] examines the links between rising food prices and politics in the same period, giving a detailed account of price movements. He shows how the anger of the people, impotent in the face of the massive price rises of the first half of the 16th century, was directed against 'speculators' as scapegoats and exploded in peasant revolts. Plenty of examples of odd prices are given, either in the form of simple lists, in an interpretative context[92] or as a part of larger studies.

A whole series of regional theses directed by Markus Mattmüller in Basel,[93] mentioned earlier in connection with his demographic history, deals with various aspects of food history. They more or less specifically describe food aspects in a historical context, thus above all putting the nutritional situation in perspective. These studies, together with a similar Zurich work,[94] therefore form part of the category concerned with 'living conditions'. They mainly deal with the 18th century, the time of early industrialization with its multiple transitional forms such as homeworkers and day labourers with a small agricultural activity.[95]

Rudolf Braun traces similar developments but from a more socio-historical angle, with regard to changes in lifestyles, for a rural industrial area in the 18th to 20th centuries.[96] The study devotes considerable attention to food and indicates the evolution of the traditional stew standards under the influence of the town and, above all, the totally new way of life in the factories. The 'regimentation' characteristic of the industrialization process was depicted against the backcloth of tensions subsisting between the peasantry, out- workers and factory workers with their different eating patterns – cyclical nourishment as dictated by the seasons, as against linear food patterns organized for the short term, based on variety (chocolate, biscuits, snacks and schnapps to pass the time) and conditioned by rigorously enforced working hours – which also, when there was no work, for example, made hard times harder and thus made people more receptive to new foodstuffs such as the potato.

Erich Gruner[97] focuses mainly on the working population in the factories of the century of the 19th. He examines living standards as part of the 'social question'. The workers' basket of goods, with food in particular, is put in the context of wage and price movements, not forgetting the consumer co-operatives and the food industry touched upon in the previous section.

We owe a lot of important information to Hansjörg Siegenthaler's wide-ranging research project at Zurich University on the real wages of Swiss industrial workers between 1890 and 1920, which is part of a planned historical-statistical survey of Switzerland. The work provides a wealth of data of relevance to food history:[98] wages, prices and the pattern of expenditure of private households derived from a wide variety of source material such as official price lists, consumer association price lists and family budgets, drawn up in a manner which allows valid comparisons to be made.

As these new studies contain all the material concerning the period up to 1920 and published since the second half of the 19th century, especially the numerous individual studies of living standards, and above all housekeeping accounts (mainly of blue-collar workers rather than clerical staff), there is no need to go into theme at length here – and we could not in any case list them all. We will therefore concentrate on a few of the more outstanding publications on living standards in the years after the First World War.[99] Since 1943, annual accounts of the housekeeping expenditure of non-independent employees have been published in Switzerland.[100]

Other consumption-related topics with a bearing on living standards and food are problems of domestic management, especially orderliness and cleanliness – new watchwords in the second half of the 19th century. Geneviève Heller[101] and Beatrix Mesmer[102] show the means which were used to get the ideals across – chief amongst them cookery courses and popular cookbooks.

Food

While agriculture, as the first phase of food's journey from farmer to consumer, has been well researched, receiving substantial new impulses in recent years, and processing has been neglected, food itself – including mainly consumption and eating habits as well as living standards – is the preserve of the food historian. Looking at preindustrial Switzerland, the very different patterns of nourishment in cattle-raising and cereal-growing areas have been established: in the Alpine regions the staple diet consisted of milk foods, cheese, game, wild nuts, berries and mushrooms, together with a little fruit and vegetables. Bread was rather scarce, cattle were mostly exported. For people living on the plateau, the diet included stew and soups, bread, and toward the end of the 18th century potatoes, as well as vegetables (mainly chard, cabbage, root crops, onions and legumes) and occasionally sausage, dried and stewed fruit, as well as water, light wine, milk and, from the end of the 18th century, coffee. Fresh meat was mainly reserved for the urban upper classes. Much of the food (including cereals) had to be imported and large sectors of the population suffered from malnutrition. Between these two zones there existed many transitional areas with mixed diets. Industrialization then ushered in a levelling and balancing process, marked since the beginning of the 20th century by the ever-increasing presence of industrially manufactured products.

The period we are interested in is heralded by the Reformation, an event which was also of key importance to food history. Zwingli's 1522 sermon on the choice and freedom of food[103] in which the Zurich pastor proved by reference to the Scriptures that church bans on certain foodstuffs were incompatible with Christian freedom, pointed the way to new eating habits marked since the 16th century by an increasing range and choice of foodstuffs – though it was a very slow process and, prior to industrialization, hardly of relevance to the lower layers of society.

Various studies are concerned with food in both the Middle Ages and modern times, making it possible to observe long-term changes. Whereas Dietrich Schwarz[104] provides a very condensed survey of everyday life as a whole, focusing on material aspects of the history of civilization, Andreas Morel[105] presents two highly important sources from the 16th century: the diary of the Basel doctor, Felix Plattner, and the first German-language cookery-book by a woman, Anna Wecker, a doctor's wife also from Basel; it was reprinted ten times by the end of the 17th century.

The study of food and drink in old Zurich by Albert Hauser, which also incorporates elements of cultural anthropology, is a pioneering work of its kind.[106] The author describes food and drink in both town and country in great detail and also gives a vivid rendering of urban and rural eating and drinking habits. This attention to detail throws up some intriguing comparisons, especially in view of the work's large timespan of several centuries. Food (though less the way it is prepared) is surprisingly similar in both town and country, especially in the 18th century, this being partly explained by the keen interest which townsfolk then showed in farming. Hauser's recently published major history of daily life in the 15th to 19th centuries[107] again deals with food, living standards, eating and drinking habits in great detail, placing them in the setting of the environment, where and how ordinary people lived, their dress, religion, etc. The work also addresses the thorny problem of quantifying consumption, and an attempt is made, as in his Zurich study, to compare standards of living then and now through an examination of purchasing power.

Other works focus more directly on the gastronomical aspect, be it in almost all old town halls,[108] the meals served in the guildhalls and patricians' houses such as François de Capitain (Berne Historical Museum) describes for Berne,[109] or in the Swiss heartland.[110] Besides Zurich, Berne, and Uri, Geneva is represented by a few special studies on wine and meat consumption and hospital food.[111]

Undernourishment as well as the countless supply shortages and famines feature prominently in modern history before the French Revolution. Despite the extraordinary difficulty of drawing up a qualitative record of each period, we do have some essays on the subject.[112] Otherwise, apart from larger works (Mattmüller, Pfister) which approach the topic from the demographic and agricultural angles, there is as yet no comprehensive study of this subject. Like gastronomic history, only more so, supply shortages in particular, affecting as they do all aspects of food and nutrition, are characterized by the broad range of literature typical of the history of everyday life, as exemplified by the famine of 1816-17.[113] In addition to archive material, a large number of printed sources are available: contemporary accounts in magazines and calendars, travel reports,[114] official writings, sermons, price surveys, accounts of the weather and practical food hints. Numerous useful accounts, rich in detail, are to be found in jubilee articles, most of them published in journals to mark an anniversary. Finally, modern historical scholarship has now addressed the subject in three unpublished degree theses and an important overall study in theoretical economics.[115]

Literature also provides a key to the question of nourishment in the age of transition from an agricultural to an industrial society. The works of two major Swiss writers, Jeremias Gotthelf (1797-1854) and Gottfried Keller (1819-90) have been thoroughly combed for all references to food and drink.[116] The studies on living standards in this age of transition mentioned in the previous section which also deal in detail with food consumption,[117] with primary reference to factory workers,[118] relate to a period which was marked by the development of statistics and hence benefit from a much improved situation as regards sources. The result is a much broader base for establishing reasonably accurate nutritional balances, even if these attempts, the first since the 1870s, are inevitably punctuated with several large question marks. There was at the same time an enormous surge of scientific interest in the nutrition of workers. Contemporary reports on this subject are a further important source: it was the economist and statistician, Victor Böhmert,[119] and the doctor and factory inspector, Fridolin Schuler,[120] who exposed the malnutrition among the working population. Whereas Böhmert concentrates more on food prices, inflation and steps to improve the situation, Schuler presents a list of elements and causes: price rises, adulteration, the inadequate fare offered by soup kitchens and insufficient time for preparing meals at home. He proposes numerous measures to ameliorate the situation, in particular arguing for the leguminous meal developed by Julius Maggi and propagated by the Swiss Public Benefit Society (Schweizerische Gemeinnützige Gesellschaft').[121] He was also vigorously involved with that typically 19th-century phenomenon,[122] the temperance movement.[123]

From the first Swiss nutritional balance for the year 1870 to the latest nutritional report there has been a whole series of attempts to draw up a statistical record of food consumption.[124] The early accounts, however crude and incomplete they may be, represent an essential source of information and would provide an admirable starting-point for a still non-existent general survey of Swiss food consumption. From the beginnings of the 'age of statistics' (we will not go into sporadic earlier attempts to capture food consumption in figures) to the Second World War, nutritional balances are available for the years 1870,[125] 1908–12,[126] 1917[127] (Comparisons with soldiers' wartime rations are also revealing;[128] they surprisingly seem to be smaller than in the armies of the surrounding countries), 1920–22,[129] 1934–6.[130] From 1923 onwards, annual surveys are also available. Only a few individual foodstuffs have special statistics: frozen meat,[131] fats and oils[132] and dairy products.[133]

The physician, Alfred Fleisch,[134] has authored a comprehensive study for the period of the Second World War. It takes as its point of departure the wartime feed-the-people plan, presents details of farm production and rationing and their nutritional fundamentals, discusses wartime food and social problems, and comes to the following conclusion: even when rations were below the approved minimum, there was no general deterioration in public health.

The postwar years do not seem to interest food historians. All studies, surveys and food reports are the work of doctors, trophologists and food chemists. However, a note on the most important publications[135] would appear justified not only because the subjects they deal with are tomorrow's history but also because we historians cannot complain about nutrition scientists ignoring history if we ourselves fail to take account of contemporary developments!

In addition to the works of historians, statisticians, economists and nutrition experts, there is another group of studies by cultural anthropologists (often also interested in history) for whom food and drink has always been an important field of research. The regional diversity which is of such particular interest in Switzerland is illuminated by historico-cultural and ethnological studies.[136]

Conclusion

This annotated bibliography of food history inevitably leaves out a great deal, not least because we have chosen to cast our net very wide, taking in everything from the farmer to the consumer. As a result, we have obviously had to include many works which do not stem from the pens of professional historians.

Our stroll through the literature of food history reveals certain focal points which, however, are outnumbered by the gaps it contains. It can be seen that the historian is interested principally in agricultural production and consumption, while most of the contributions on processing are the work of lawyers and economists. In terms of time, the accent is mainly on the period from the 18th to the early 20th century, with the interplay between the shifting factors of farming, eating patterns and demography clearly of great importance.

Against this background the gaps are plain to see. The most obvious deficiency is the lack of a work which pulls together all the various strands of our knowledge. In the light of the present state of research, it would inevitably be a very provisional work, not yet capable of presenting an overall picture, but still an extremely important one. Studies are also needed which dig deeper into individual aspects of the huge area represented by processing, preservation and preparation, again with special reference to the period of transition from the agrarian to the industrial age. Furthermore, early modern times and the 20th century urgently require attention. However, these vast, still fallow fields should not be allowed to divert our attention from fields which are still being turned over by older means, and above all the many which are being worked with the help of the most advanced methods and excellent seeds. In Switzerland at any rate, as elsewhere, the history of food is an increasingly exciting field of research.

References

1 Bundesamt für Statistik (1985).
2 *Statistische Erhebungen* (1923–59); *Statistische Erhebungen* (1960ff); Brugger (1968); Franscini (1848–51); Furrer (1887–92); Reichesberg (1901–11); Handbuch (1939,1955).
3 See Teuteberg (1987).
4 *Geschichte* (1986).
5 Hauser (1961); Bergier (1983); Braun (1984); *Ein Jahrhundert* (1964); Bairoch (1984).
6 Brugger (1956–87).
7 Pfister (1975); Pfister (1984); Pfister (1978–9).
8 Walter (1966); Bickel (1947); Mattmüller (1987).

9 *Die Agrarzonen* (1989).
10 Bircher (1938).
11 Aebi (1963); Aebi (1974); Ziegler (1975); Bircher (1981); Bergier (1984a).
12 Howald (1951); Piuz (1985a); Chevallaz (1949); Brühwiler (1975); Huggel (1979); Guyer (1972); *Lob der Tüchtigkeit* (1985); Schmidt (1932); Dürst (1951); Lemmenmeier (1983); Hauser (1972); Hauser (1974); Wahlen (1946); Maurer (1985).
13 Piuz (1985a).
14 Huggel (1979).
15 Guyer (1972); *Lob der Tüchtigkeit* (1985).
16 Schmidt (1932).
17 Lemmenmeier (1983).
18 Wahlen (1946); Maurer (1985).
19 Pfister (1940); Pfister (1978); Pfister (1982); Pfister (1986); Head-König (1970); Head-König (1979); Head-König (1972); Head-König (1987).
20 Rundstedt (1930); Bosch (1913); Dubler (1968); Bergier (1984b); Blanc (1941); Zumkeller (1985); Piuz and Zumkeller (1981); Mottu-Weber (1983); Buscher (1942); Mesmer (1972); Fleischmann (1921); Quinche (1960).
21 Bergier (1984b).
22 Brandstetter (1917); Hilber (1935); Kaeser (1932); Woessner (1945); Rebmann (1943).
23 Wirth (1942); Ramseyer-Hugi (1961); Radeff (1974); Hugger (1972); Marty (1951).
24 Ramseyer-Hugi (1961).
25 Hugger (1972).
26 Marty (1951); Dubois (1979); Bodmer (1981); Kaufmann (1988).
27 Dubois (1979).
28 Steiger (1982).
29 Sturzenegger (1917); Fankhauser (1887); Liebenau (1897); Wildhaber (1949–50); Sooder (1952).
30 Pfister (1981).
31 Schlegel (1973); Altwegg (1980).
32 Mention should be made of *Schweizer Pioniere der Wirtschaft und Technik* (Zürich 1955ff.), which introduces also some personalities from the food sector in biographies: Suchard (1), Nestlé (2), Cailler (6), Peter (7), Wander (8), Bühler (12), Dietschy (15), Sprüngli und Lindt (22), Müller-Thurgau (29), Aebi (38), Duttweiler (42).
33 Strahlmann (1970); Oetiker (1915); Neumann (1945).
34 Strahlmann (1969); Schwab (1912); Meyer (1929); Strahlmann (1983); Robert (1989).
35 Numerous essays by Berend Strahlmann on the history of food science can be found in *Mitteilungen aus dem Gebiete der Lebensmitteluntersuchung und Hygiene* (1962ff).
36 Keller (1912); Dubler (1978); Geiser (1946).
37 Dubler (1978).
38 Meier (1939); Währen (1971); Dorschner (1936); *Das Buch vom Schweizer Brot* (1952).
39 Kaiser (1985); Hirn (1974).
40 Neff (1961).
41 Frater (1948); Wildeisen (1929); Stoffel (1957).
42 Gutzwiller (1923); *50 Jahre Schweizerische Milchwirtschaft* (1938) (includes a useful survey of official rules from the period 1869–1937); *Die schweizerische Milchwirtschaft* (1948); Fuchs (1946); Wahlen (1979).
43 Gutzwiller (1923).
44 *50 Jahre Schweizerische Milchwirtschaft* (1938); *Die schweizerische Milchwirtschaft* (1948).

45 Fuchs (1946).
46 Montandon (1980); Roth (1970); Roth (1977); Sommer (1965); Glauser (1971); Reichen (1989); Lustenberger (1926); Gallati (1943); Hugger (1971); Schneider (1916); Roth (1966); Littell (1977); Koller (1964); Burkhalter (1979); Ruffieux (1972).
47 Roth (1977).
48 Glauser (1971); Reichen (1989); Lustenberger (1926).
49 Gallati (1943).
50 Hugger (1971). Further relevant titles of the same series (1963ff): *Le boucher ambulant* (11), *Der Tirggelbäcker* (14), *Une huilerie vaudoise* (23), *Le Moulin de Vaulion* (29).
51 Schneider (1916); Roth (1966).
52 Littel (1977).
53 Koller (1964).
54 Burkhalter (1979).
55 Ruffieux (1972).
56 Bruni (1946); Schiess (1913); Hartmann (1919); Mulhaupt (1932); Gutzwiller (1932); Hout (1933); Frei (1951); Senn (1939).
57 Bruni (1946).
58 Schiess (1913); Hartmann (1919); Mulhaupt (1932); Gutzwiller (1932); Hout (1933); Frei (1951); Senn (1939).
59 Kientsch (1929); Luy (1945); Moser (1987).
60 Kottelat (1953).
61 Wick (1914); Weber (1920); Schmidt-Bellod (1919); Schoellhorn (1929).
62 Hauck (1899).
63 Berthoud (1969).
64 Siebert (1911); Kundert (1936); Vettiger (1941); Piuz (1985b); Piuz (1985c); Radeff (1980); Gern (1976).
65 Siebert (1911).
66 Kundert (1936).
67 Vettiger (1941).
68 Piuz (1985b); Piuz (1985c).
69 Radeff (1980).
70 Gern (1976).
71 Jöhr (1912); Käppeli (1926); Schmid (1942); Rosen (1946); Rosen (1947) (useful survey in English); Schneebeli (1948). An important source with much organizational, legal and statistical information is: *Die Schweizerische Kriegswirtschaft* (1950).
72 Jöhr (1912).
73 Käppeli (1926).
74 Schmid (1942); Rosen (1946); Rosen (1947); Schneebeli (1948); *Die Schweizerische Kriegswirtschaft* (1950).
75 Reichlin (1912); Rufer (1931); Wirz (1902, 1917); Egli (1919); Kaufmann (1923); Stisser (1953).
76 Schellenberg and Gosselke (1938); Anliker (1945) (also concerned with the trade in fruit).
77 Anliker (1945); Bertschi (1945); Meyer (1945).
78 Scheuermann (1923); Deitmer (1930).
79 Kraft (1945).
80 Bühler (1906) (includes a useful survey on regulations, arranged by canton); Frey (1922); Jacky (1927); Schäublin (1960); Bloch (1949); Stübi (1946); Vogt (1947).
81 Suter (1981).

82 Hauser-Kündig (1927); Livet (1981); Gern (1984); Ribeaud (1895); Waldmeyer (1928).
83 Dubois (1965).
84 Felber (1939); Wegst (1947).
85 Faes (1943).
86 Howald (1923); Petricevic (1948); Angehrn (1966).
87 Mühlemann (1939); Wyss (1949); Wunderle (1957); Boson (1965).
88 Liebenau (1891); Egger (1940) (also gives a useful survey of legal history since 1848).
89 Anderegg (1933); Stückelberger (1933).
90 Dirlmeier (1978).
91 Wermelinger (1971).
92 Bodmer (1984); Mühlemann (1882).
93 Wicki (1979); Bucher (1974); Bielmann (1972); Menolfi (1980); Schürmann (1974); Ruesch (1979).
94 Tanner (1982).
95 Mattmüller (1985); Mattmüller (1980).
96 Braun (1960); Braun (1965).
97 Gruner (1968); Gruner (1987).
98 The material is not printed, but can be examined in Swiss university libraries: '*Reallöhne*' (1981). A presentation of this project can be found at Beck (1987).
99 Ackermann (1963), Vilímovská (1952); Jenny (1923); *Haushaltungsrechnungen* (1942); Wartenweiler (1946); Freudiger (1946).
100 *Haushaltungsrechnungen* (1987ff).
101 Heller (1979).
102 Mesmer (1982).
103 Zwingli (1904).
104 Schwarz (1970).
105 Morel (1985). No. 3 of the 8th year (pp. 117–228 of the *Magazin Archäologie der Schweiz* is dedicated to food, especially in prehistory and the Middle Ages.
106 Hauser (1973).
107 Hauser (1987); Hauser (1989).
108 Kopp (1978).
109 Capitani (1982).
110 Iten (1972).
111 Bergier (1984c); Piuz (1985d).
112 Piuz (1985e); Piuz (1985f); Mattmüller (1982); Pfister (1990).
113 Schärer (1981).
114 See the two main descriptions in Scheitlin (1820); Zollikofer (1818/19).
115 Stolz (1977).
116 Riedhauser (1985); Karthaus (1987).
117 Braun (1960); Braun (1965).
118 Gruner (1968); Gruner (1987).
119 Böhmert (1873).
120 Schuler (1882); Schuler (1889).
121 Schuler (1885).
122 Schuler (1884).
123 Mattmüller (1979); Wunderlin (1986).
124 Strahlmann (1975); Mesmer (1989).
125 Simler (1873/1874/1875).

126 Schneider (1917).
127 Schneider (1919).
128 Morin (1917); Hürlimann (1880).
129 Howald (1924).
130 Brugger (1947).
131 Jacky (1928).
132 Sturzenegger (1932).
133 Sturzenegger (1935).
134 Fleisch (1947).
135 *Vergleichende Untersuchungen* (1962–4); Verzár (1962); *Zur Ernährungssituation* (1975); *Zweiter Schweizer Ernährungsbericht* (1984); Müller (1987).
136 Weiss (1978–82); Geiger (1951–3); Caduff (1986); Lurati (1971); Schlup (1984); Hugger (1984); Preiswerk (1982–3).

Literature

Ackermann, Ernst, *Sechs Jahrzehnte. Wandlungen der Lebenshaltung und der Lebenskosten seit der Jahrhundertwende* (Wetzikon, 1963).

Aebi, Hugo, 'Unsere Ernährungsgewohnheiten im Wandel der Zeit', *Mitteilungen aus dem Gebiet der Lebensmitteluntersuchung und Hygiene*, 54 (1963), pp. 230-58.

Aebi, Hugo, *Unsere Ernährung im Spiegel des gesellschaftlichen Wandels* (Berne, 1974).

Die Agrarzonen der Alten Schweiz. Referate gehalten an der Tagung der Arbeitsgemeinschaft zur Sozialgeschichte vom 23. Januar 1988 in Basel, ed. André Schluchter (Basel, 1989).

Altwegg, Andreas Manuel, *Vom Weinbau am Zürichsee. Struktur und Wandlungen eines Rebgebietes seit 1850* (doctoral thesis, Zurich 1979, Zurich, 1980).

Anderegg, Emil, *Johann Heinrich Waser, sein Leben und Werk. Ein Beitrag zur Geschichte der Volkswirtschaft der Stadt Zürich in der zweiten Hälfte des 18. Jahrhunderts* (doctoral thesis, Zurich 1933).

Angehrn, Otto, *Der Nahrungsmittelverbrauch in der Schweiz 1950–1964. Entwicklung der Verbrauchswerte, der Marktspanne und der landwirtschaftlichen Produzentenerlöse bei Nahrungsmitteln* (Zürich, 1966).

Anliker, Fritz, *Die Marktverhältnisse der Stadt Bern, mit spezieller Berücksichtigung der Entwicklung und des Einzugsgebietes ihres Gemüsemarktes* (doctoral thesis, Berne, 1945).

Bairoch, Paul, 'L'économie suisse dans le contexte européen: 1913–1939', *Revue suisse d'histoire*, 34 (1984), pp. 468–97.

Beck, Bernehard *et al.*, 'Die Entwicklung der Reallöhne Schweizerischer Arbeiter 1890 bis 1920. Zielsetzungen eines Forschungsprojektes', in Werner Conze and Ulrich Engelhardt, (eds), *Arbeiterexistenz im 19. Jahrhundert. Lebensstandard und Lebensgestaltung deutscher Arbeiter und Handwerker* (Stuttgart, 1987), pp. 46–56.

Bergier, Jean-François, *Die Wirtschaftsgeschichte der Schweiz* (Zurich, Cologne, 1983).

Bergier, Jean-François, 'Manger en Suisse, jadis. Quelques notes sur l'histoire de l'alimentation', in Jean-François Bergier, *Hermès et Clio. Essais d'histoire économique* (Lausanne, 1984a), pp. 173–84.

Bergier, Jean-Francois, 'Commerce et politique du blé à Genève aux XVe et XVIe siècles', in Jean-François Bergier, *Hermès et Clio. Essais d'histoire économique*, (Lausanne, 1984b), pp. 185–206.

Bergier, Jean-François 'Le Vin des Genevois. Consommation et politique du vin à Genève vers 1500' in Jean François Bergier, *Hermès et Clio. Essais d'histoire économique* (Lausanne, 1984c), pp. 207–21.

Berthoud, Dorette, 'La "Fée verte". Pour une histoire de l'absinthe', *Revue suisse d'histoire*, 19 (1969), pp. 638–61.

Bertschi, Fred, *Die Gemüsebelieferung der Stadt Zürich aus den schweizerischen Produktionsgebieten. Eine wirtschaftsgeographische Untersuchung* (doctoral thesis, Zurich, 1945).

Bickel, Wilhelm, *Bevölkerungsgeschichte und Bevölkerungspolitik der Schweiz seit dem Ausgang des Mittelalters* (Zurich, 1947).

Bielmann, Jürg, *Die Lebensverhältnisse im Urnerland während des 18. und zu Beginn des 19. Jahrhunderts* (doctoral thesis Basel, Basel/Stuttgart, 1972).

Bircher, Ralph, *Wirtschaft und Lebenshaltung im schweizerischen 'Hirtenland' am Ende des 18. Jahrhunderts* (doctoral thesis Zurich, Lachen 1938).

Bircher, Ralph, *Ursprünge der Tatkraft. Beiträge zur Ernährungsgeschichte der Schweiz* (Erlenbach, 1981).

Blanc, Herman, *La chambre des blés à Genève 1628–1798* (Geneva, 1941).

Bloch, René, *Die Organisationsformen des Schlachtviehmarktes in der Schweiz* (doctoral thesis, Basel, 1949).

Bodmer, Walter, 'Der Zuger und Zürcher Welschlandhandel mit Vieh und die von Zürich beeinflusste Entwicklung der Zuger Textilgewerbe', *Schweizerische Zeitschrift für Geschichte*, 31 (1981), pp. 403–44.

Bodmer, Walter, 'Die Bewegungen einiger Lebensmittelpreise in Zug zwischen 1610 und 1821 verglichen mit denjenigen in Luzern und Zürich', *Schweizerische Zeitschrift für Geschichte*, 34 (1984), pp. 449–467.

Böhmert, Victor, *Arbeiterverhältnisse und Fabrikeinrichtungen in der Schweiz. Bericht ... für die Wiener Weltausstellung* (Zurich, 1873).

Bosch, Reinhold, *Der Kornhandel der Nord-, Ost-, Innerschweiz und der ennentbirgischen Vogteien im 15. und 16. Jahrhundert* (doctoral thesis, Zurich, 1913).

Boson, Marcel, *Co-op in der Schweiz. Betrachtungen zu den Anfängen und zur Entwicklung der Co-op Genossenschaften* (Basel, 1965).

Brandstetter, Renward, 'Die Hirse im Kanton Luzern', *Der Geschichtsfreund*, 72 (1917), pp. 71–109.

Braun, Rudolf, *Industrialisierung und Volksleben. Veränderungen der Lebensformen unter Einwirkung der verlagsindustriellen Heimarbeit in einem ländlichen Industriegebiet (Zürcher Oberland) vor 1800* (doctoral thesis, Zurich, Winterthur, 1960).

Braun, Rudolf, *Sozialer und kultureller Wandel in einem ländlichen Industriegebiet (Zürcher Oberland) unter Einwirkung des Maschinen- und Fabrikwesens im 19. und 20. Jahrhundert* (Erlenbach, Stuttgart, 1965).

Braun, Rudolf, *Das ausgehende Ancien Régime in der Schweiz. Aufriss einer Sozial- und Wirtschaftsgeschichte des 18. Jahrhunderts* (Göttingen, Zurich, 1984).

Brühwiler, Jürg, *Der Zerfall der Dreizelgenwirtschaft im schweizerischen Mittelland. Ein Beitrag zur Geschichte des Individualeigentums* (doctoral thesis, Berne, Zurich 1975).

Brugger, Hans, 'Produktion und Verbrauch von Nahrungsmitteln in der Schweiz 1934–36, 1943–45', *Schweizerische Zeitschrift für Volkswirtschaft und Statistik*, 83 (1947), pp. 243–70.

Brugger, Hans, *Statistisches Handbuch der schweizerischen Landwirtschaft* (Berne, 1968).

Brugger, Hans, *Geschichte der schweizerischen Landwirtschaft*, vol.I: *Die schweizerische Landwirtschaft in der ersten Hälfte des 19. Jahrhunderts*, (Frauenfeld, 1956), vol.II: *Die schweizerische Landwirtschaft 1850–1914* (Frauenfeld, 1978), vol.III: *Die schweizerische Landwirtschaft 1914–1980. Agrarverfassung, Pflanzenbau, Tierhaltung, Aussenhandel.*

(Frauenfeld, 1985), vol.IV: *Die Ertragslage der schweizerischen Landwirtschaft 1914 bis 1980* (Frauenfeld, 1987).

Bruni, Frederico, *I cioccolatier, dall'artigianato all'industria* [The Chocolatier, from the artist to the industry] (Bellinzona, Lugano, 1946).

Das Buch vom Schweizer Brot. Vom Samenkorn zum Brot. Eine Würdigung der am Werdegang des Brotes beteiligten Gewerbe und Industrien. Die Bedeutung des Brotes als Volksnahrungsmittel, ed. Hans W. Daetwyler (Zurich, 1952).

Bucher, Silvio, *Bevölkerung und Wirtschaft des Amtes Entlebuch im 18. Jahrhundert. Eine Regionalstudie als Beitrag zur Sozial- und Wirtschaftsgeschichte der Schweiz im Ancien Régime* (doctoral thesis, Basel, Lucerne, 1974).

Bühler, Robert, *Die Fleischschau der Schweiz, mit besonderer Berücksichtigung ihrer geschichtlichen Entwicklung* (doctoral thesis, Zurich, Teufen, 1906).

Bundesamt für Statistik (ed.), *Verzeichnis der Veröffentlichungen 1860–1985* (Berne, 1985).

Burkhalter, Guido, *Der Bellelay Käse (Tête de moine) und sein Ursprungsgebiet* (Schaffhausen, 1979).

Buscher, Josef, *Getreidebau und Getreidehandel der Schweiz von 1914–1939* (doctoral thesis, Basel, 1942).

Caduff, Moritz, 'Essen und Trinken im Lugnez', *Schweizerisches Archiv für Volkskunde*, 82 (1986), pp. 223–6.

Capitani, François de, *Festliches Essen und Trinken im alten Bern. Menüs und Rezepte vergangener Jahrhunderte* (Berne, 1982).

Chevallaz, Georges André, *Aspects de l'agriculture vaudoise à la fin de l'ancien régime. La terre, le blé, les charges* (doctoral thesis Lausanne, 1949).

Deitmer, Wilhelm, *Die städtische Milchversorgung in der Schweiz und die Tätigkeit der milchwirtschaftlichen Organisationen* (doctoral thesis, Bonn, 1930).

Dirlmeier, Ulf, *Untersuchungen zu Einkommensverhältnissen und Lebenshaltungskosten in oberdeutschen Städten des Spätmittelalters (Mitte 14. bis Anfang 16. Jahrhundert)* (Heidelberg, 1978).

Dorschner, Fritz, *Das Brot und seine Herstellung in Graubünden und Tessin. Ein Beitrag zur Wort- und Sachforschung der romanischen Süd- und Ostschweiz* (doctoral thesis, Zurich, Winterthur 1936).

Dubler, Anne-Marie, 'Das Fruchtwesen der Stadt Basel von der Reformation bis 1700', *Jahresbericht des Staatsarchives Basel-Stadt* (1968).

Dubler, Anne-Marie, *Müller und Mühlen im alten Staat Luzern. Rechts-, Wirtschafts- und Sozialgeschichte des luzernischen Landmüllergewerbes 14. bis 18. Jahrhundert* (Lucerne, Münich, 1978).

Dubois, Alain, *Die Salzversorgung des Wallis 1500–1610. Wirtschaft und Politik* (doctoral thesis Zurich, Winterthur, 1965).

Dubois, Alain, 'L'exportation de bétail suisse vers l'Italie du XVIe au XVIIIe siècle: esquisse d'un bilan', in Ekkehard Westermann (ed.), *Internationaler Ochsenhandel (1350–1750). Akten des 7th International Economic History Congress Edinburgh 1978* (Stuttgart, 1979), pp. 11–38.

Dürst, Elisabeth, *Die wirtschaftlichen und sozialen Verhältnisse des Glarnerlandes an der Wende vom 18. Jahrhundert* (doctoral thesis, Zurich, 1951).

Egger, Victor and Georg Egger, *Das schweizerische Gastgewerbe im Rahmen von Wirtschaft und Staat* (Zurich, 1940).

Egli, Albert, *'Die Getreideversorgung der Schweiz, unter besonderer Berücksichtigung des Mannheimer Umschlagplatzes'* (doctoral thesis, Heidelberg, 1918; Zurich, 1919).

Eidgenössische Volkswirtschafts-Departementes (ed.), *Die Schweizerische Kriegswirtschaft 1939–48* (Berne, 1950).

Escher, Walter, 'Stand der Nahrungsforschung in der Schweiz', *Ethnologia Europaea*, 5 (1971), pp. 78–83.

Faes, Maurice, *Le Commerce de détail en Suisse. Son évolution, sa structure, l'aide de petit commerce de détail* (doctoral thesis, Lausanne, 1943).

Fankhauser, Frank, 'Die Bedeutung der Ziegenwirtschaft für die schweizerischen Gebirgsgegenden in forstlicher und statistisch-volkswirtschaftlicher Hinsicht', *Zeitschrift für schweizerische Statistik*, 23 (1887), pp. 50–134.

Felber, Karl Ernst, *Die Strukturwandlungen im schweizerischen Kolonialwarengrosshandel* (doctoral thesis, Basel, 1939).

Fleisch, Alfred, *Ernährungsprobleme in Mangelzeiten. Die schweizerische Kriegsernährung 1939–1946* (Basel, 1947).

Fleischmann, Edgar, *Das Getreidemonopol in der Schweiz. Seine rechtlichen, wirtschaftlichen und geschichtlichen Grundlagen* (doctoral thesis, Leipzig, Zurich, 1921).

Franscini, Stefano, *Neue Statistik der Schweiz*, 3 vols (Berne, 1848–51).

Frater, Charles, *Die Biscuit-Industrie und ihre wirtschaftliche Bedeutung, mit besonderer Berücksichtigung der schweizerischen Verhältnisse* (doctoral thesis, Berne, 1948).

Frei, René, *Über die Schokolade im allgemeinen und die Entwicklung der Berne,ischen Schokoladeindustrie* (doctoral thesis, Berne, Lucerne, 1951).

Freudiger, Hans, *Die Kosten der Lebenshaltung in den Städten Zürich, Basel, Bern, Biel und Neuenburg und in den Kantonen Zürich und Tessin im Jahre 1943. Haushaltrechnungen von 104 Familien öffentlicher Funktionäre* (Berne, 1946).

Frey, Arthur, *Die schweizerische Fleischpreispolitik während des Weltkrieges 1914/18* (doctoral thesis, Zurich, 1922).

Fuchs, Hans, *Die schweizerische Milchwirtschaft während des Krieges 1939/45* (doctoral thesis, Fribourg, Mörschwil, 1946).

50 Jahre Schweizerische Milchwirtschaft. Festschrift Schweizerischer milchwirtschaftlicher Verein 1887–1937 (Schaffhausen, 1937).

Furrer, Alfred, *Volkswirtschafts-Lexikon der Schweiz*, 3 vols (Berne, 1887–92).

Gallati, Werner, *Die schweizerische Schachtelkäse-Industrie und der Verband Schweizerischer Emmentaler Schachtelkäsefabrikanten* (doctoral thesis, Berne, 1943).

Geiger, Paul and Richard Weiss, *Atlas der schweizerischen Volkskunde*, part 1 (Basel, 1951–5).

Geiser, Ernst, *Die schweizerische Müllerei im Zweiten Weltkrieg* (doctoral thesis, Berne, 1946).

Gern, Phillipe, 'L'Helvétique et le sel français, ou la loi du plus fort', *Revue suisse d'histoire*, 34 (1984), pp. 206–19.

Gern, Phillipe, 'L'approvisionnement de Neuchâtel pendant la Révolution française', *Musée neuchâtelois*, 3, 13 (1976), pp. 57–86.

Geschichte der Schweiz und der Schweizer, 3 vols (Basel, Frankfurt, 1986).

Glauser, Fritz, 'Handel mit Entlebucher Käse und Butter vom 16.–19. Jahrhundert', *Schweizerische Zeitschrift für Geschichte*, 21 (1971), pp. 1–63.

Gruner, Erich, *Die Arbeiter in der Schweiz im 19. Jahrhundert. Soziale Lage, Organisation, Verhältnis zu Arbeitgeber und Staat* (Berne, 1968).

Gruner, Erich and Hans-Rudolf Wiedmer, *Arbeiterschaft und Wirtschaft in der Schweiz 1880–1914. Soziale Lage, Organisation und Kämpfe von Arbeitern und Unternehmern, politische Organisation und Sozialpolitik*, vol. I: *Demographische, wirtschaftliche und soziale Basis und Arbeitsbedingungen* (Zurich, 1987).

Gutzwiller, Karl, *Die Milchverarbeitung in der Schweiz und der Handel mit Milcherzeugnissen.*

Geschichte, Betriebsformen, Marktverhältnisse und volkswirtschaftliche Bedeutung (Schaffhausen, 1923).
Gutzwiller, Alfred, *Die schweizerische Schokoladenindustrie und die Weltkakaowirtschaft* (doctoral thesis, Basel, Liestal, 1932).
Guyer, Walter, *Kleinjogg, der Zürcher Bauer 1716–1785* (Erlenbach, Stuttgart, 1972).
Handbuch der schweizerischen Volkswirtschaft, 2 vols (Berne, 1939, 2nd edn, Berne, 1955).
Hartmann, Hans, *Zur ökonomischen Theorie der schweizerischen Schokoladenindustrie mit besonderer Berücksichtigung der Standortfrage* (doctoral thesis, Berne, 1919).
Hauck, Franz F., *Beiträge zur Entwicklungsgeschichte des schweizerischen Alkoholmonopols* (doctoral thesis, Basel, Berne, 1899).
Hauser, Albert, *Schweizerische Wirtschafts- und Sozialgeschichte* (Erlenbach, Stuttgart, 1961).
Hauser, Albert, 'Produktivität und Lebenshaltung in der schweizerischen Landwirtschaft', in Albert Hauser, *Wald und Feld in der alten Schweiz. Beiträge zu schweizerischen Agrar- und Forstgeschichte* (Zurich, Munich, 1972), pp. 162–93.
Hauser, Albert, *Vom Essen und Trinken im alten Zürich. Tafelsitten, Kochkunst und Lebenshaltung vom Mittelalter bis in die Neuzeit* (3rd. edn, Zurich 1973).
Hauser, Albert, 'Zur Produktivität der schweizerischen Landwirtschaft im 19. Jahrhundert', in *Wirtschaftliche und soziale Struktur im säkularen Wandel. Festschrift für Wilhelm Abel*, vol. 3 (Hanover, 1974), pp. 597–616.
Hauser, Albert, *Was für ein Leben. Schweizer Alltag vom 15. bis 18. Jahrhundert* (Zürich, 1987).
Hauser, Albert, *Das Neue kommt. Schweizer Alltag im 19. Jahrhundert* (Zürich, 1989).
Hauser-Kündig, Margrit, *Das Salzwesen der Innerschweiz bis 1798* (doctoral thesis, Zurich, Zug 1927).
'Haushaltungsrechnungen von Familien unselbständig Erwerbender. Berne, 1943–1986', in *Die Volkswirtschaft. Haushaltsrechnungen von unselbständig Erwerbenden und Rentnern* (Berne, 1987ff.).
Haushaltungsrechnungen von Familien unselbständig Erwerbender. 1936/37 und 1937/38 (Berne, 1942).
Head-König, Anne-Lise and Béatrice Veyrassat-Herren, 'La production agricole du plateau suisse aux XVIIe et XVIIIe siècles', *Revue suisse d'histoire*, 20 (1970), pp. 562–600.
Head-König, Anne-Lise, and Béatrice Veyrassat-Herren, 'Les revenus décimaux à Genève de 1540 à 1783', in *Les fluctuations du produit de la dîme. Conjuncture décimale de la fin du Moyen-Age au XVIIIe siècle* (Paris, The Hague 1972), pp. 165–79.
Head-König, Anne-Lise, 'Les fluctuations des rendements et du produit décimal céréaliers dans quelques régions du plateau suisse (1500–1800)', *Revue suisse d'histoire*, 29 (1979), pp. 575–604.
Head-König, Anne-Lise, Lucienne Hubler and Christian Pfister, 'Evolution agraire et démographie en Suisse (XVIIe-XIXe siècles)', in Antoinette Fauve-Chamous (ed.), *Evolution agraire et croissance démographique* (Liège, 1987), pp. 233–61.
Heller, Geneviève, *'Propre et en ordre'. Habitation et vie domestique 1850–1930: l'exemple vaudois* (doctoral thesis, Lausanne; Lausanne, 1979).
Hilber, Paul, *Hafer in der Schweiz* (Lützelflüh, 1935).
Hirn, Sven, 'Sockerbagaren från Graubünden [Confectioners from Girsons]', *Historika och Litteraturhistorika Studier*, 49 (1974), pp. 171–232.
Hout, Theodor van, *Entwicklung und volkswirtschaftliche Bedeutung der schweizerischen Schokoladenindustrie* (doctoral thesis, Freiburg, Herzogenbuchsee, 1933).
Howald, Oskar, 'Die Verarbeitungs-, Veredelungs- und Verteilungskosten im Lebensmittelverkehr der Schweiz', *Zeitschrift für schweizerische Statistik und Volkswirt-*

schaft, 59 (1923), pp. 315–43.

Howald, Oskar, 'Die Ernährung der schweizerischen Bevölkerung in den Jahren 1920/22', *Zeitschrift für schweizerische Statistik und Volkswirtschaft*, 60 (1924), pp. 237–51.

Howald, Oskar, 'Entwicklung und Stand der Forschung auf dem Gebiete der Wirtschaftslehre des Landbaus in der Schweiz', in *Stand der Forschung auf dem Gebiete der Wirtschaftslehre des Landbaus. Festschrift für Ernst Laur* (Brugg, 1951), pp. 125–50.

Hürlimann, Josef, 'Ueber die Ergebnisse der Sanitarischen Rekruten-Musterung in der Schweiz während den Jahren 1875 bis 1879. Eine populäre militärärztliche Skizze', *Schweizerische Zeitschrift für Gemeinnützigkeit*, 19 (1880), pp. 417–69.

Huggel, Samuel, *Die Einschlagsbewegung in der Basler Landschaft. Gründe und Folgen der wichtigsten agrarischen Neuerung im Ancien Régime*, 2 vols. (doctoral thesis, Basel, Liestal, 1979).

Hugger, Paul, *Die Alpkäserei im Waadtländer Jura* (Basel, 1971).

Hugger, Paul, *Hirtenleben und Hirtenkultur im Waadtländer Jura* (Basel, 1972).

Hugger, Paul, 'Les Cafés. Les nourritures traditionnelles', in *Encyclopédie vaudoise*, vol. XI, *La Vie quotidienne*, part 2: *Maisons, Fêtes, Sport, Langage* (Lausanne, 1984), pp. 126–60.

Iten, Karl, *Vom Essen und Trinken im alten Uri*, 2 vols (Altdorf, 1972).

Jacky, Wilhelm, *Fleischversorgung der Schweiz mit besonderer Berücksichtigung der Stadt Zürich* (doctoral thesis, Zurich, 1927).

Jacky, Wilhelm, 'Der Konsum von Gefrierfleisch in der Schweiz', *Zeitschrift für schweizerische Statistik und Volkswirtschaft*, 64 (1928), pp.387–96.

'Ein Jahrhundert Schweizerischer Wirtschaftsentwicklung', *Schweizerische Zeitschrift für Volkswirtschaft und Statistik*, 100 (1964), pp. 1–368.

Jenny, Oscar Hugo, 'Diagramme zur Veränderung der Kosten der Lebenshaltung 1911–1922', *Zeitschrift für schweizerische Statistik und Volkswirtschaft*, 59 (1923), pp. 68–74.

Jöhr, Adolf, *Die Volkswirtschaft der Schweiz im Kriegsfall* (2nd edn, Zürich, 1912).

Käppeli, Joseph and Max Riesen, 'Die Lebensmittelversorgung der Schweiz unter dem Einfluss des Weltkrieges von 1914–22', *Landwirtschaftliches Jahrbuch der Schweiz*, 40 (1926), pp. 1–134.

Kaeser, Hans, *Die Kastanienkultur und ihre Terminologie in Oberitalien und in der Südschweiz* (doctoral thesis, Zurich, Aarau, 1932).

Kaiser, Dolf, *Fast ein Volk von Zuckerbäckern? Bündner Konditoren, Cafétiers und Hoteliers in europäischen Ländern bis zum Ersten Weltkrieg. Ein wirtschaftsgeschichtlicher Beitrag* (Zurich, 1985).

Karthaus, Ulrich, 'Kulinarisches bei Gottfried Keller', in Irmgard Bitsch *et al.* (eds), *Essen und Trinken in Mittelalter und Neuzeit. Symposium Giessen* (Sigmaringen, 1987), pp. 85–93.

Kaufmann, Robert Uri, *Jüdische und christliche Viehhändler in der Schweiz 1780–1930* (doctoral thesis, Zurich, 1988).

Kaufmann, Rudolf, *Die Weizenvorräte der Schweiz und die Sicherung der Landesversorgung mit Brotgetreiden im Kriegsfalle* (doctoral thesis, Berne, 1923).

Keller, Robert, *Die wirtschaftliche Entwicklung des schweizerischen Mühlengewerbes aus ältester Zeit bis zirka 1830* (doctoral thesis, Berne, 1912), (=Beiträge zur schweizerischen Wirtschaftskunde, 2).

Kientsch, Erwin, *Die Rübenzuckerfabrikation in der Schweiz unter besonderer Berücksichtigung des Standortes* (doctoral thesis, Berne, 1929).

Koller, Franz, 'Appenzeller Käse', in *Die appenzellische Land-, Milch- und Alpwirtschaft im Wandel der Zeiten* (Appenzell, 1964), pp. 11–52.

Kopp, Peter, 'Vom Essen und Trinken in alten Rathäusern', *Schweizerisches Archiv für*

Volkskunde, 74 (1978), pp. 46–69.
Kottelat, Marcel, *Die schweizerische Mineralwasserindustrie und ihre Organisationsfragen* (doctoral thesis, Berne, 1953).
Kraft, Jörg, *Die Bewirtschaftung der Eier in der Schweiz während der vier Kriegsjahre Sept. 1939 – Sept. 1943* (doctoral thesis, Berne, 1945).
Kundert, Fridolin, *Die Lebensmittelversorgung des Landes Glarus, bis 1798. Eine volkswirtschaftliche Studie* (doctoral thesis, Berne, Glarus, 1936).
Lemmenmeier, Max, *Luzerns Landwirtschaft im Umbruch. Wirtschaftlicher, sozialer und politischer Wandel in der Agrargesellschaft des 19. Jahrhunderts* (doctoral thesis, Zurich, Lucerne, Stuttgart, 1983).
Liebenau, Theodor von, *Das Gasthof- und Wirtshauswesen der Schweiz in ältester Zeit* (Zurich, 1891).
Liebenau, Theodor von, *Geschichte der Fischerei in der Schweiz* (Berne, 1897).
Littel, Katherine M., *Jeremias Gotthelf's 'Die Käserei in der Vehfreude'. A didactic satire* (doctoral thesis, Berne, Frankfurt, Las Vegas, 1977).
Livet, Georges, 'La Suisse, carrefour diplomatique des sels européens. Pressions politiques et tension sociales dans la Confédération Helvétique sous l'ancien régime', in Guy Cabourdin (ed.), *Le Sel et son histoire. Actes du colloque de l'Association interuniversitaire de l'Est* (Nancy, 1981), pp. 405–33.
Lob der Tüchtigkeit. Kleinjogg und die Zürcher Landwirtschaft am Vorabend des Industriezeitalters. Zum zweihundertsten Todesjahr Kleinjogg Guyers (1716–1785 (Zurich, 1985).
Lurati, Ottavio, 'Alltags- und Festtagsspeisen im Tessin. Stand der Forschung und Wandel der Speisen', *Ethnologa Europaea*, 5 (1971), pp. 84–90.
Lustenberger, Maurice, *Organisation des schweizerischen Käsehandels seit 1914, die Genossenschaft schweizerischer Käseexportfirmen und die schweizerische Käseunion* (doctoral thesis, Berne, 1926).
Luy, Marcel, *Le Marché mondial du sucre et le problème de l'économie sucrière suisse* (doctoral thesis, Fribourg; Paris, Lucerne, 1945).
Marty, Albin, *Die Viehwirtschaft in der Urschweiz und Luzerns, insbesondere der Welschlandhandel 1500–1798* (doctoral thesis, Zurich, 1951).
Mattmüller, Markus, *Der Kampf gegen den Alkoholismus in der Schweiz. Ein unbekanntes Kapitel der Sozialgeschichte im 19. Jahrhundert* (Berne, 1979).
Mattmüller, Markus, 'Bauer und Tauner im schweizerischen Kornland um 1700', *Schweizer Volkskunde*, 70 (1980), pp. 49–62.
Mattmüller, Markus, 'Die Hungersnot der Jahre 1770/71 in der Basler Landschaft', in *Gesellschaft und Gesellschaften. Festschrift für Ulrich Im Hof* (Berne, 1982), pp. 271–91.
Mattmüller, Markus, 'Die Landwirtschaft der schweizerischen Heimarbeiter im 18. Jahrhundert', in Paul Bairoch and Anne-Marie Piuz (eds), *Les passages des économies traditionelles européennes aux Sociétés industrielles. Quatrième rencontre franco-suisse d'histoire économique et sociale* (Geneva, 1985), pp. 317–41.
Mattmüller, Markus, *Bevölkerungsgeschichte der Schweiz*, 2 vols (Basel, Frankfurt am Main, 1987).
Maurer, Peter, *Anbauschlacht. Landwirtschaftspolitik, Plan, Wahlen, Anbauwerk 1937–1945* (doctoral thesis, Berne, Zurich, 1985). Summary: Peter Maurer, 'Landwirtschaft und Landwirtschaftspolitik der Schweiz im Zweiten Weltkrieg', in Bernd, Martin and Alan S. Milward (eds), *Landwirtschaft und Versorgung im Zweiten Weltkrieg* (Ostfildern, 1985), pp. 103–16.

Meier, Albert, *Das Bäckerhandwerk im alten Bern*, (14.–18. Jahrhundert), (doctoral thesis, Berne, 1939).

Menolfi, Ernest, *Sanktgallische Untertanen im Thurgau. Eine sozialgeschichtliche Untersuchung über die Herrschaft Bürglen (TG) im 17. und 18. Jahrhundert* (doctoral thesis, Basel, St Gallen, 1980).

Mesmer, Beatrix, 'Reinheit und Reinlichkeit. Bemerkungen zur Durchsetzung der häuslichen Hygiene in der Schweiz', in *Gesellschaft und Gesellschaften. Festschrift für Ulrich Im Hof* (Berne, 1982), pp. 470–94.

Mesmer, Beatrix, 'Rationelle Ernährung. Sozialmedizinische Reaktionen auf den Wandel der Ess- und Trinkgewohnheiten', in P. Saladin, H. J. Schaufelberger and P. Schläppi (eds), *'Medizin' für die Medizin. Arzt und Ärztin zwischen Wissenschaft und Praxis. Festschrift für Hannes G. Pauli* (Basel, Frankfurt am Main, 1989), pp. 329–43.

Mesmer, Heinz, 'Die Errichtung einer definitiven Getreideordnung in der Schweiz (1919–29)', in Roland Ruffieux (ed.), *La Démocratie référendaire en Suisse au XXe siècle*, vol. 1 (Fribourg, 1972), pp. 183–257.

Meyer, Konrad, *Die Gemüseversorgung der Stadt Zürich. Eine wirtschaftsgeographische Betrachtung mit besonderer Berücksichtigung des örtlichen Gemüsegürtels* (doctoral thesis, Zurich, 1945).

Meyer, Wilhelm, *Die Lebensmittelpolizei der Stadt Basel von ihren Anfängen bis zum eidgenössischen Lebensmittelgesetz von 1905* (doctoral thesis, Basel, 1929).

Die schweizerische Milchwirtschaft (Thun, 1948).

Montandon, Jacques, *Les Fromages de Suisse. Origines, histoire, traditions et folklore, la cuisine au fromage* (Lausanne, 1980).

Morel, Andreas, 'Zu Quellen für Speise und Trank um die Wende des Mittelalters', *Archäologie der Schweiz*, 8 (1985), pp. 204–22.

Morin, Jean, *Contribution à l'étude de la ration alimentaire du soldat suisse* (doctoral thesis, Lausanne, 1917).

Moser, Werner and Rolf Haeberli, *Zucker. Geschichte und Bedeutung für die Schweiz* (Aarberg, Frauenfeld, 1987).

Mottu-Weber, Liliane, 'Contrats de voiture et comptes des blés et du sel. Contribution à l'étude des couts de transports (1550–1630)', *Revue suisse d'histoire*, 33 (1983), pp. 269–296.

Mulhaupt, Armand, *L'Industrie chocolatière suisse avant, pendant et après la guerre* (doctoral thesis, Lausanne, 1932).

Mühlemann, Carl, 'Einfluss der wichtigsten Nahrungsmittelpreise auf die Bewegung der Bevölkerung im Kanton Berne, während des 100jährigen Zeitraumes 1782–1881', *Zeitschrift für Schweizerische Statistik*, 18 (1882), pp. 59–70.

Mühlemann, Hans E., *Anfänge der schweizerischen Konsumgenossenschaftsbewegung* (doctoral thesis, Berne, 1939).

Müller, Elisabeth *et al.*, *Ernährung der Einwohner ländlicher Gebiete. Eine Erhebung in der Schweiz* (Berne, Stuttgart, Toronto, 1987).

Neff, Karl, 'Innerrhoder Schöttler, Milchkuranstalten und Broderieshändler im Ausland', *Innerrhoder Geschichtsfreund*, 8 (1961), pp. 3–30.

Neumann, Hans and Eduard Weckerle, *Industrien der Nahrungs- und Genussmittel: Brot, Bier, Tabak, Zucker, Schokolade u.a.* (Olten, 1945).

Oetiker, Karl, 'Die Standorte der schweizerischen Industrien der Lebens- und Genussmittel' (doctoral thesis, Basel), *Zeitschrift für schweizerische Statistik*, 51 (1915), pp. 143–76.

Petricevic, Jure, 'Die Verschleissspanne im Nahrungsmittelverkehr der Schweiz', *Mitteilungen des schweizerischen Bauernsekretariates*, 141 (1948), pp. 14–64.

Pfister, Christian, *Agrarkonjunktur und Witterungsverlauf im westlichen Schweizer Mittelland zur Zeit der Ökonomischen Patrioten 1755–1797* (doctoral thesis, Berne, 1975).

Pfister, Christian, 'Climate and economy in 18th century Switzerland', *Journal of Interdisciplinary History*, 9 (1978–9), pp. 223–43.

Pfister, Christian, 'Die Fluktuationen der Weinmosterträge im schweizerischen Weinland vom 16. bis ins frühe 19. Jahrhundert. Klimatische Ursachen und soziöokonomische Bedeutung', *Schweizerische Zeitschrift für Geschichte*, 31 (1981), pp. 445–91.

Pfister, Christian, 'Lang- und kurzfristige Fluktuationen der Getreideproduktion im schweizerischen Mittelland vom 16.–19. Jahrhundert in ihrer Abhängigkeit von Natur- und Humanfaktoren', in Joseph Goy and Emmanuel le Roy Ladurie (eds), *Prestations paysannes, dîmes, rente foncière et mouvement de la production agricole à l'époque préindustrielle. Actes du Colloque préparatoire (1977) au VIIe Congrès international d'histoire économique à Edinbourg 1978* (Paris, The Hague, New York 1982), pp. 283–92.

Pfister, Christian, *Das Klima der Schweiz von 1525–1860 und seine Bedeutung in der Geschichte von Bevölkerung und Landwirtschaft*, vol. 1: *Klimageschichte der Schweiz 1525–1860*, vol. 2: *Bevölkerung, Klima und Agrarmodernisierung 1525–1860* (Berne, Stuttgart, 1984).

Pfister, Christian, 'Bevölkerung, Wirtschaft und Ernährung in den Berg- und Talgebieten des Kantons Bern, 1760–1860', in Markus Mattmüller (ed.), *Wirtschaft und Gesellschaft in Berggebieten. Kolloquium Graz 1985* (Basel, 1986), pp. 361–91.

Pfister, Christian, 'Food supply in the Swiss canton of Berne, 1850', in L. Newman (ed.), *Hunger in History* (London, 1990), pp. 281–303.

Pfister, Willy, 'Getreide- und Weinzehnten 1505–1798 und Getreidepreise 1565–1770 im berneischen Aargau', *Argovia*, 52 (1940), pp. 237–64.

Piuz, Anne-Marie, 'L'alimentation hospitalière à Genève au XVIIIe siècle', in *Lyon et Europe. Hommes et sociétés. Mélanges d'histoire offerts à Richard Gascon*, vol. II (Lyon, 1980), pp. 167–85.

Piuz, Anne-Marie and Dominique Zumkeller, 'Stoccagio de grani e sistema annoario a Ginevra nel secolo XVIII', *Quaderni storici*, 16 (1981), pp. 168–91.

Piuz, Anne-Marie, 'La Disette de 1693/1694 et ses conséquences démographiques', in Anne-Marie Piuz, *Genève et autour de Genève aux XVIIe et XVIIIe siècles. Etudes d'histoire économique* (Lausanne, 1985), pp. 82–90.

Piuz, Anne-Marie, 'Climat, récoltes et vie des hommes à Genève, XVIe-XVIIIe siècles', in Anne-Marie Piuz, *Genève et autour de Genève aux XVIIe et XVIIIe siècles. Etudes d'histoire économique* (Lausanne, 1985a), pp. 61–81.

Piuz, Anne-Marie, 'Le marché urbain', in Anne-Marie Piuz, *Genève et autour de Genève aux XVIIe et XVIIIe siècles. Etudes d'histoire économique* (Lausanne, 1985b), pp. 45–58.

Piuz, Anne-Marie, 'Les Politiques de subsistances (vers 1650–1760)', in Anne-Marie Piuz, *Genève et autour de Genève aux XVIIe et XVIIIe siècles. Etudes d'histoire économique* (Lausanne, 1985c), pp. 139–51.

Piuz, Anne-Marie, 'Le marché du bétail et la consommation de la viande au XVIIIe siècle', in Anne-Marie Piuz, *Genève et autour de Genève aux XVIIe et XVIIIe siècles. Etudes d'histoire économique* (Lausanne, 1985d), pp. 112–23.

Piuz, Anne-Marie, 'Alimentation populaire et sous-alimentation au XVIIe siècle', in Anne-Marie Piuz, *Genève et autour de Genève aux XVIIe et XVIIIe siècles. Etudes d'histoire économique* (Lausanne, 1985e), pp. 93–111.

Preiswerk, Yvonne, *Le repas des morts. Catholiques et protestants aux enterrements. Visage de la culture populaire en Anniviers et aux Ormonts* (doctoral thesis, Lyon 1982; Sierre, 1983).

Quinche, Jean, *Le Régime du blé en Suisse* (doctoral thesis, Lausanne, Neuchâtel, 1960).

Radeff, Anne, 'Aspects de l'exploitation laitière à Genève et au Pays de Vaud au XVIIe siècle', *Revue historique vaudoise*, 82 (1974), pp. 65–76.

Radeff, Anne, *Lausanne et ses campagnes au XVIIe siècle* (doctoral thesis, Lausanne, 1980).

Ramseyer-Hugi, Rudolf, *Das altberneische Küherwesen* (doctoral thesis, Berne, 1961).

'Reallöhne schweizerischer Industriearbeiter von 1890–1921', ed. Hansjörg Siegenthaler, 5 vols (Zurich, 1981).

Rebmann, Hans, *Die kriegsbedingte Ölproduktion durch vermehrten Ölpflanzenanbau in der Schweiz* (doctoral thesis, Berne, 1943).

Reichen, Quirinus, *Auf den Spuren des Käses nach dem Süden: Vom frühen Sbrinz-Export über die Alpenpässe Grimsel und Gries* (2nd edn, Berne, 1989).

Reichesberg, Naum, *Handwörterbuch der Schweizerischen Volkswirtschaft, Sozialpolitik und Verwaltung*, 4 vols (Berne, 1901–11).

Reichlin, August, *Die Brotversorgung der Stadt Basel mit besonderer Berücksichtigung des Bäckergewerbes*, (doctoral thesis, Basel; Aarau, 1912).

Ribeaud, Emile, *Zur Geschichte des Salzhandels und der Salzwerke in der Schweiz* (Lucerne, 1895).

Riedhauser, Hans, *Essen und Trinken bei Jeremias Gotthelf. Darstellung und Motivation des Rekreativen in Alltag und Fest* (doctoral thesis, Zurich; Berne, Stuttgart, 1985).

Robert, Olivier, 'Les vins falsifiés du XIXe siècle: image d'un certain quotidien vaudois?', *Revue historique vaudoise*, 97 (1989), pp. 69–105.

Rosen, John Rosenwasser, Josef) 'Der Inlandsanteil der schweizerischen Lebensmittelversorgung im Kriege nach dem Nährwert', *Schweizerische Zeitschrift für Volkswirtschaft und Statistik*, 82 (1946), pp. 151–68.

Rosen, John (Rosenwasser, Josef), *Wartime Food Developments in Switzerland* (Stanford, California, 1947).

Roth, Alfred, *Aus der Geschichte des Emmentaler Käses* (Burgdorf, 1966).

Roth, Alfred G., *Aus der Geschichte des Schweizerkäses. Neue Quellen und Forschungen zu seiner Geschichte* (Burgdorf, 1970).

Roth, Alfred G., *Talkäsereien. Zur Aufnahme ihres Betriebes in der Schweiz* (Burgdorf, 1977).

Ruesch, Hanspeter, *Lebensverhältnisse in einem frühen schweizerischen Industriegebiet. Sozialgeschichtliche Studie über die Gemeinden Trogen, Rehetobel, Wald, Gais, Speicher und Wolfhalden des Kantons Appenzell Ausserrhoden im 18. und frühen 19. Jahrhundert* (doctoral thesis, Basel; Basel, Stuttgart, 1979).

Rufer, Alfred, 'Das Problem der Brotversorgung während der Helvetik', *Politische Rundschau*, 10 (1931), pp. 30–8, 71–84.

Ruffieux, Roland and Walter Bodmer, *Histoire du Gruyère en Gruyère du XVIe au XXe siècles* (Fribourg, 1972).

Rundstedt, Hans Gerd von, *Die Regelung des Getreidehandels in den Städten Südwest-Deutschlands und der deutschen Schweiz im späten Mittelalter und im Beginn der Neuzeit* (doctoral thesis, Freiburg i. Br., Stuttgart, 1930). .

Schärer, Martin R., '*Herausforderung der Gesellschaft: Wie reagierte sie auf die Hungerkrise von 1816/17 in der Schweiz?*', (paper presented to the Famine in History Symposium, Vevey, 1981).

Schäublin, Rolf, *Der schweizerische Schlachtvieh- und Fleischmarkt 1935–55* (doctoral thesis, Zurich, 1960).

Scheitlin, Peter, *Meine Armenreisen in den Kanton Glarus und in die Umgebungen der Stadt St. Gallen in den Jahren 1816 und 1817, nebst einer Darstellung, wie es den Armen des gesamten Vaterlandes im Jahre 1817 erging* (St. Gallen, 1820).

Schellenberg, Alfred and Rudolf Friedrich Gosselke, 'Schweizerische Obstbauwirtschaft und Import von Trauben und Südfrüchten 1885–1937', *Landwirtschaftliches Jahrbuch der Schweiz*, 52 (1938), pp. 421–56.

Scheuermann, Eduard, *Die Milchversorgung der Schweiz während des Krieges und der Nachkriegszeit* (doctoral thesis, Zurich, Stuttgart, 1923).

Schiess, Edouard, *L'Industrie chocolatière suisse. Étude économique précédée d'un aperçu général sur le cacao et le chocolat* (doctoral thesis, Zurich, Lausanne, 1913).

Schlegel, Walter, *Der Weinbau in der Schweiz. Seine regionale Differenzierung unter dem Einfluss von Landesnatur, wirtschaftlichen und sozialen Entwicklungen* (Wiesbaden, 1973).

Schlup, Michel, *Scènes gourmandes et croquis culinaires d'autrefois (Neuchâtel)* (Hauterive, 1984).

Schmid, Ernst, *Die Ernährungswirtschaft der Schweiz als Problem der wirtschaftlichen Kriegsvorsorge* (doctoral thesis, Berne, 1942).

Schmidt, Georg C. L., *Der Schweizer Bauer im Zeitalter des Frühkapitalismus. Die Wandlung der schweizerischen Bauernwirtschaft im 18. Jahrhundert und die Politik der ökonomischen Patrioten*, 2 vols (doctoral thesis, Basel, Berne, 1932).

Schmidt-Bellod, Gustav, *Die schweizerische Brauereiindustrie insbesondere seit Kriegsausbruch* (doctoral thesis, Zurich, 1919).

Schneebeli, Paul, *Die Lebensmittelversorgung der Schweiz während des Krieges 1939–45* (doctoral thesis, Neuenburg, 1948).

Schneider, Ida, *Die schweizerische Milchwirtschaft unter besonderer Berücksichtigung der Emmentaler Käserei* (doctoral thesis, Zurich, 1916).

Schneider, Salome, 'Die Erzeugung und der Verbrauch von Nährwerten in der Schweiz', *Zeitschrift für schweizerische Statistik und Volkswirtschaft*, 53 (1917), pp. 275–335.

Schneider, Salome, 'Die schweizerische Volksernährung vor und während dem Kriege', *Zeitschrift für schweizerische Statistik und Volkswirtschaft*, 55 (1919), pp. 7–20.

Schoellhorn, Fritz, *Das schweizerische Braugewerbe, seine Krise infolge des Weltkrieges und ihre Überwindung* (Winterthur, 1929).

Schürmann, Markus, *Bevölkerung, Wirtschaft und Gesellschaft in Appenzell Innerrhoden im 18. und frühen 19. Jahrhundert* (doctoral thesis, Basel, Appenzell, 1974).

Schuler, Fridolin, *Über die Ernährung der Fabrikbevölkerung und ihre Mängel* (Zurich, 1882).

Schuler, Fridolin, *Zur Alkoholfrage. Die Ernährungsweise der arbeitenden Klassen in der Schweiz und ihr Einfluss auf die Ausbreitung des Alkoholismus* (Berne, 1884).

Schuler, Fridolin, *Die Leguminosen als Volksnahrung. Gutachten* (Zurich, 1885).

Schuler, Fridolin and Albrecht Eduard Burckhardt, *Untersuchungen über die Gesundheitsverhältnisse der Fabrikbevölkerung in der Schweiz mit besonderer Berücksichtigung des Krankenwesens* (Aarau, 1889).

Schwab, Rudolf, 'Zur Geschichte des eidgenössischen Lebensmittelgesetzes', *Schweizerische Blätter für Wirtschafts- und Sozialpolitik*, 20 (1912), pp. 225–44.

Schwarz, Dietrich W. H., *Sachgüter und Lebensformen. Einführung in die materielle Kulturgeschichte des Mittelalters und der Neuzeit* (Berlin, 1970).

Senn, Christian, *Soziale Betriebspolitik in der schweizerischen Schokolade-Industrie* (doctoral thesis, Zurich, Affoltern a.A., 1939).

Siebert, Ludwig, *Die Lebensmittel-Politik der Städte Baden und Brugg im Aargau bis zum Ende des 17. Jahrhunderts* (doctoral thesis, Freiburg i.Br.; Berne, 1911).

Simler, Theodor, 'Versuch einer Ernährungsbilanz der Schweizer Bevölkerung', *Zeitschrift für schweizerische Statistik*, 9 (1873) pp. 158–69; 10 (1874), pp. 15–26; 11 (1875), pp. 1–22.

Sommer, Peter, *Caseus, Kess, Schweizer Käse macht Schweizer Geschichte* (Berne, 1965).

Sooder, Melchior, *Bienen und Bienenhalten in der Schweiz* (Basel, 1952).
Statistische Erhebungen und Schätzungen auf dem Gebiete der Landwirtschaft (Brugg, 1923–59).
Statistische Erhebungen und Schätzungen über Landwirtschaft und Ernährung (Brugg, 1960ff).
Steiger, Thomas, *Die Produktion von Milch und Fleisch in der schweizerischen Landwirtschaft des 19. Jahrhunderts als Gegenstand bäuerlicher Entscheidungen. Das statistische Bild der Entwicklung der Rindviehhaltung und ihre ökonomische Interpretation* (doctoral thesis, Zurich, Berne, Frankfurt, 1982).
Stisser, Reinhold, *Grundgedanken, Methoden und Ergebnisse der schweizerischen Agrarmarkt- und Ernährungspolitik unter besonderer Berücksichtigung des Getreidemarktes* (Kiel, 1953).
Stoffel, Alexander Erik, *Die Absatzprobleme der schweizerischen Suppenindustrie* (doctoral thesis, St Gallen, 1957).
Stolz, Peter, *Basler Wirtschaft in vor- und frühindustrieller Zeit. Ökonomische Theorie und Wirtschaftsgeschichte im Dialog* (Zurich, 1977).
Strahlmann, Berend, 'Die Entwicklung des Lebensmittelrechtes in der Schweiz', *Mitteilungen aus dem Gebiete der Lebensmitteluntersuchung und Hygiene*, 60 (1969), pp. 343–70.
Strahlmann, Berend, 'Die Entwicklung der Konservierungsmethoden in der Schweiz', *Mitteilungen aus dem Gebiete der Lebensmitteluntersuchung und Hygiene*, 61 (1970), pp. 348–64.
Strahlmann, Berend, 'Erhebungen über den Lebensmittelverbrauch der schweizerischen Bevölkerung in historischer Sicht', in Georg Brubacher and Günther Ritzel (eds), *Zur Ernährungssituation der schweizerischen Bevölkerung. Erster schweizerischer Ernährungsbericht* (Berne, Stuttgart, Vienna, 1975), pp. 42–56.
Strahlmann, Berend, '100 Jahre amtliche Lebensmittelkontrolle im Kanton Bern,', *Mitteilungen aus dem Gebiete der Lebensmitteluntersuchung und Hygiene*, 74 (1983), pp. 383–413; 76 (1985), pp. 277–303.
Stübi, Robert, *Das schweizerische Metzgereigewerbe und die Rückwirkung der Kriegswirtschaft von 1939 bis zum Ende des europäischen Krieges* (doctoral thesis, Geneva, 1946).
Stückelberger, Hans Martin, *Johann Heinrich Waser von Zürich. Geboren am 1. April 1742. Enthauptet am 27. Mai 1780* (doctoral thesis, Zurich, 1933).
Sturzenegger, Otto, *Über den Verbrauch von Kochfett, Margarine und Speiseölen in der Schweiz* (Lausanne, 1932).
Sturzenegger, Otto, *Verbrauch von Milch und Milchprodukten in der Stadt Zürich. Ergebnisse einer Umfrage bei 8309 Haushaltungen im Februar 1935* (Zurich, 1935).
Sturzenegger, Robert, *Die Schweinezucht in der Schweiz. Ein Versuch der Darstellung ihrer Entwicklung von den ersten Anfängen bis zur Gegenwart* (doctoral thesis, Berne, Trogen, 1917).
Suter, Elisabeth, *Wasser und Brunnen im alten Zürich* (doctoral thesis, Zurich, 1981).
Tanner, Albert, *Spulen-Weben-Sticken. Die Industrialisierung in Appenzell Ausserrhoden* (doctoral thesis, Zurich, 1982).
Teuteberg, Hans Jürgen, 'Zum Problemfeld Urbanisierung und Ernährung im 19. Jahrhundert' in Hans Jürgen Teuteberg (ed.), *Durchbruch zum modernen Massenkonsum. Lebensmittelmärkte und Lebensmittelqualität im Städtewachstum des Industriezeitalters* (Münster, 1987), pp. 1–36.
'Vergleichende Untersuchungen über die Ernährung in verschiedenen Gebieten der Schweiz', ed. Fritz Verzár, *Mitteilungen aus dem Gebiet der Lebensmitteluntersuchung und Hygiene*, 53 (1962), pp. 93–148, 55 (1964), pp. 1–43.
Verzár, Fritz and Daniela Gsell, *Ernährung und Gesundheitszustand der Bevölkerung der Schweiz* (Berne, 1962).
Vettiger, Margarete, *Die agrare Preispolitik des Kantons Basel im 18. Jahrhundert* (doctoral

thesis, Basel, 1939, Weinfelden, 1941).
Vilímovská, Libuse, *Die Verschiebungen in der Verbrauchsstruktur in der Schweiz seit 1912* (doctoral thesis, Berne, 1952).
Vogt, Herbert, *Die Fleischversorgung in der Schweiz im Zweiten Weltkrieg 1939–45 mit besonderer Berücksichtigung der Rationierungstechnik und der Statistik* (doctoral thesis, Berne, 1947).
Währen, Max, *Zur Entwicklung der ländlichen Bäckerei* (Berne, 1971).
Wahlen, Friedrich Traugott, *Das schweizerische Anbauwerk 1940–45* (Zurich, 1946).
Wahlen, Hermann, *Rudolf Schatzmann, 1822–1886. Ein Bahnbrecher der schweizerischen Land-, Alp- und Milchwirtschaft und ihres Bildungswesens* (Münsingen, 1979).
Waldmeyer, Ernst, *Die Schweizerische Salz- und Sodaindustrie unter spezieller Berücksichtigung ihrer Beziehungen zur chemischen Grossindustrie im Hochrheingebiet* (doctoral thesis, Berne, Weinfelden, 1928).
Walter, Emil J., *Soziologie der Alten Eidgenossenschaft, eine Analyse ihrer Sozial- und Berufsstrukturen von der Reformation bis zur Französischen Revolution* (Berne, 1966).
Wartenweiler, Oskar, *Haushaltsrechnungen aus Zürcher Landgemeinden und der Stadt Winterthur 1943* (doctoral thesis, Zurich, 1946).
Weber, Walter, *Die Neuorientierung der schweizerischen Brauereiindustrie seit den achtziger Jahren* (doctoral thesis, Berne, Weinfelden, 1920).
Wegst, Oscar, *Der selbständige schweizerische Lebensmittelgrosshandel und die Einkaufsgenossenschaften des Lebensmittel-Detailhandels* (doctoral thesis, Berne, 1947).
Weiss, Richard, *Volkskunde in der Schweiz. Grundriss* (Erlenbach, Zurich, 1978, 2nd edn, Erlenbach, Zurich, 1982).
Wermelinger, Hugo, *Lebensmittelteuerungen, ihre Bekämpfung und ihre politischen Rückwirkungen in Bern, vom ausgehenden 15. Jahrhundert bis in die Zeit der Kappelerkriege* (doctoral thesis, Zurich; Berne, 1971).
Wick, Wilhelm, *Beiträge zur Entwicklungsgeschichte des schweizerischen Baugewerbes 1870–1912* (Zurich, 1914).
Wicki, Hans, *Bevölkerung und Wirtschaft des Kantons Luzern im 18. Jahrhundert* (doctoral thesis, Basel; Munich, Lucerne, 1979).
Wildeisen, Ernst, *Die Teigwarenindustrie in der Schweiz* (doctoral thesis, Berne, 1929).
Wildhaber, Robert, 'Schneckenzucht und Schneckenspeisen', *Schweizerisches Archiv für Volkskunde*, 46 (1949–50), pp. 119–84.
Wirth, Paul, *Die geographische Verbreitung der schweizerischen Viehwirtschaft* (doctoral thesis, Berne, 1942).
Wirz, Jakob, *Die Getreideproduktion und Brotversorgung der Schweiz* (doctoral thesis, Fribourg, 1902; 2nd edn, Fribourg, 1917).
Woessner, Dietrich, 'Geschichtliches über die Zwiebel und ihre Bedeutung als Kulturpflanze im Kanton Schaffhausen', *Mitteilungen der Naturforschenden Gesellschaft Schaffhausen*, 20 (1945), pp. 25–67.
Wunderle, Karl, *Konsumgenossenschaften und privater Detailhandel. Historische Darstellung und kritische Würdigung der schweizerischen Entwicklung* (doctoral thesis, Basel; Zurich, 1957).
Wunderlin, Dominik, 'Die Antialkoholbewegung in der Schweiz', *Hessische Blätter für Volks- und Kulturforschung*, new series, 20 (1986), pp. 113–128.
Wyss, Annemarie, *Die konsumgenossenschaftlichen Grundsätze in der Schweiz von den Anfängen bis zur Gegenwart* (doctoral thesis, Zurich, 1949).
Ziegler, Eugen, *Betrachtungen über den säkularen Wandel der Ernährung in der Schweiz* (2nd edn, Berne, 1975).
Zollikofer, Ruprecht, *Der Osten meines Vaterlandes oder die Kantone St. Gallen und Appenzell*

im Hungerjahre 1817. Ein Denkmal jener Schreckens-Epoche, 2 vols (St. Gallen, 1818–19).

Zumkeller, Dominique, 'Géographie des achats de la Chambre des Blés de Genève 1628–1798' in Paul Bairoch and Anne-Marie Piuz (eds), *Les Passages des économies traditionelles européennes aux Sociétés industrielles. Quatrième recontre franco-suisse d'histoire économique et sociale Genève 1982* (Geneva, 1985), pp. 145–68.

Zweiter Schweizerischer Ernährungsbericht, ed. Hugo Aebi *et al.* (Berne, Stuttgart, Vienna, 1984).

Zur Ernährungssituation der Schweizerischen Bevölkerung. Erster Schweizerischer Ernährungsbericht, ed. Georg Brubacher and Günther Ritzel, (Berne, Stuttgart, Vienna, 1975).

Zwingli, Huldreich, 'Von Erkiesen und Freiheit der Speisen. 16. April 1522' in Emil Egli and Georg Finsler (eds), *Huldreich Zwinglis sämtliche Werke*, vol. I: *Corpus reformatorum*, 88 (Berlin, 1904), pp. 74–136.

11 Food and foodways as the subject of historical analyses in Hungary

Eszter Kisbán

To understand the main aspects of historical food research in Hungary, it must be remembered that the country has in the main always subsisted on its own resources. There was a lively export of cattle to western Europe between the 15th and 18th centuries, though demand fluctuated from time to time; this was backed up by a fairly sophisticated cattle-ranching system in the Hungarian Plain. Improvements in agriculture began slowly in the late 18th century, and large-scale industrialization really did not start until the 1880s. The mid-19th-century boom in agrarian products had a marked effect on Hungarian agriculture: the acreage under wheat doubled between 1847 and 1868, while wheat exports increased by a factor of six during the same period. In spite of this it was not the industrial workers but the landless agricultural labourers – nearly 25% of the population in 1910 and 20% in 1930 – who between 1890 and 1945 constituted the poor (in 1910, when the population was 18 million, they totalled 4.3 million, and in 1930, when the population was 8.6 million, they totalled 1.6 million). In 1930 the agricultural population of farmers, cottagers and labourers amounted to just over 50% of the total population, while industrial workers amounted only to 23%.

Statistical data for the history of Hungarian agriculture have to be reconstructed from different kinds of historical statistics, even for a period as late as 1767–1867.[1] Between 1850 and 1867, Austrian statistical surveys covered Hungary as well.[2] A full-time Central Office of Statistics in Hungary was set up after the Austro-Hungarian Settlement of 1867.

Food and foodways as a subject for historical analysis began fairly late in Hungarian research. Economic historians began taking food consumption into account in the 1960s, and the historical dimension also appeared in ethnological food research. The physiological study of diet has produced contemporary descriptions from time to time, but no historical analyses have as yet been attempted here.

History

In historical scholarship, the question of diet arose in connection with agricultural production and the national economy. Grain production in Hungary was stable up to the 18th century. In view of this, historians concentrated on the diet of the commonalty in the early modern period, the 17th century providing the best sources.

The early modern period

The subject was stimulated by a thesis on army management in the period 1650–1715, published in 1963, in which the strategic role of provisioning the armies was put into focus. To see what the food supplies were like in the area where the army was in service, the author examined the civilian diet. A model of consumption was set up to include only the food that was sufficient for physiological purposes. The starting-point for the model was not the scattered Hungarian sources, but a French hypothesis developed in the 1940s. The author thought the level of 1,800 kcal per capita per day, used by Labrousse and Fourastié, too little and boosted the figure to 2,800 (which means 4,000 kcal a day for an adult male), but accepted the French view that 80% of the calorie intake of the 17th-century French peasant came from grain. These levels would have meant an average annual per-capita consumption of 350 kg of grain in Hungary, this being divided by the author into 250 kg grain for bread (wheat, rye) and 100 kg of other cereal-based foodstuffs.[3]

A lively discussion involving economic historians and historical statisticians developed from this thesis. The volume of agricultural production in Hungary (grain cultivation, animal husbandry) was examined as well as the minimum physiological calorie requirement, and the conclusion was reached and stressed that the use of animal products including meat did not decline in the way it did in western Europe in the early modern period.[4]

The outcome was the publication of the results of current historical research into the production and productivity of grain- and vine-growing at both peasant and estate levels in Hungary,[5] along with revised views of the export-orientated ranching of cattle[6] and an investigation of the scale of animal husbandry in areas beyond the Plain. Beef consumption levels in cities and provincial towns were examined, as well as army meat rations.[7] Comprehensive examination of the tithe collection registers, a source of great importance for grain and vine production, depends on computer analysis, and because of the scale involved this has not yet been completed.[8] Also assembled were data on the yearly wages of farm workers, always received partly in kind to feed themselves and their families in the 16th to 19th centuries, and several studies of the economy of estates sought to establish the daily food rations for workers and officials.[9] Lack of adequate sources prevents the examination of the dietary norms in asylums, hospitals and colleges in Hungary. In international research, Polish studies have brought new light to the history of food consumption, since they give a picture of east central Europe.[10] The dominant belief of Hungarian historians is that in early modern Hungary, with its low population density (averaging 15 persons per square kilometre in the 17th century), animal food products were much more plentiful on the tables of the common people than in western Europe or even Poland.

In 1974, and later in 1979, Makkai drew a provisional balance.[11] He calculated the average food consumption of the 17th century, but buried the point in his original publication, which was printed in French in Poland. When republished in Hungarian at home, he called the article 'Agricultural production and the structure of consumption in Hungary in the mid-17th century'. His main intention was to establish the volume of grain production, using such factors as the extent of cultivated land, grain yields, the annual harvest returns of the average peasant farm and the level of its animal husbandry. The establishment of the average grain consumption at the time and the comparison of this with the peasant harvest were used by him as a check to verify the production calculated. This exercise was felt to be necessary because waste lands were left uncultivated during this period and the main regulator of tillage seemed to be the domestic (national) level of food consumption. Postulating an average family of 4.5 members, he calculated the consumption of the family as well as of the head of the family. For this, following Wyczański for 16th-century Poland, he assessed an average of 3,500 kcal a day. Makkai assigned about a third of the whole family's consumption to the male head, so the average for the family as a whole worked out to about 2,333 kcal a day. In examining the structure of consumption, he took bread grain as his basic starting point. His estimate of bread rations was based on the norms set by contemporaries for the agricultural labourer in the 17th century, that is, the amount allocated daily for the labourer and the amount of grain given in kind for the whole family for the year. The allocation allowed *c.* 1,750 kcal a day (700 g wheat bread) for the head, plus a small amount of other cereal, the two elements totalling nearly 1,800 kcal. A further check took into account the grain harvest of a random regional sample, in which exactly the same net yearly grain supply for the peasant farm emerged. He also figured out where the other essential nutritives might have come from. In some instances he was necessarily on shaky ground. As the second supplier of calories after grain, he named wine (1 litre or 700 kcal per man per day). Third was meat (246 g or 418 kcal per man per day, equivalent to 89 kg a year for the head and an overall average of 60 kg). The latter figures were deduced from the calculated number of animals bred on the peasant farm, and the turnover of butchers' shops in country towns. The food of animal origin totalled 946 kcal per day, that is, 27% of the diet (meat, pig fat and milk products were included, but not fish, the amount of which could not even be guessed). Cereals comprised 51% of the diet. Makkai postulated this dietary pattern for 60% of the population, the middle stratum covering farmers, cottagers and agricultural labourers. One-fifth of the population ate more modestly, and the other fifth more abundantly.

A shortcoming of Makkai's work in both versions is that his conversion techniques and calculations are not easy to follow. Furthermore, neither was published in a readily accessible volume and no wider discussion followed.

Table 11.1 Estimated average daily consumption of an adult man, mid-17th-century Hungary

	Daily ration (g)	Energy value (kcal)	Protein (g)	Fat (g)	Carbohydrate (g)
Bread (wheat)	700	1750	67.7	10.4	347.2
Other cereals (millet, barley, buckwheat)	10	34	0.8	0.1	7.3
Peas	18	63	4.8	0.2	10.8
Wine	1000	700	5.0		60.0
Meat	246	418	38.4	8.2	0.7
Fish	?	?			
Pig's fat	23	122	1.7	12.9	
Lard, Oil	23	195	1.7	15.3	
Milk	639	211	42.1	15.1	30.6
Others		7			
Total		3500	162.2	62.2	456.6
Total (%)			23.8	9.1	67.1

Source: Makkai (1979), p. 269

The 18th to 20th centuries

From the 18th century onwards, demographic conditions, on the one hand, and agricultural production and exports, on the other, entered a period of considerable change in Hungary.[12] The consumption of meat dropped and that of grain increased accordingly. Social stratification also became more complicated. So far historians have not embarked on any comprehensive quantitative analysis of food consumption in the 18th to 20th centuries. Comments were made on the volume of food consumption produced by the Central Office of Statistics in 1887,[13] but long-term continuous data on food have not been collected and analysed, as has been done by Teuteberg for the German evidence.[14]

Some new sources can be tapped in the 18th to 20th centuries, but none occur in large numbers. From the late 18th century, improved farming at higher social levels produced more detailed plans for the feeding of workers and of the family on a daily basis. The instructions included the yearly and weekly sequence and gave the daily allocations of foodstuffs for named dishes.[15]

In mid-19th century, the French social scientist, Frédéric Le Play, introduced the method of household accounting into the country when he constructed such an account himself on a peasant farm in an agro-town on the Plain.[16] The next known household account was made by a Hungarian social politician for industrial workers in the capital in 1888.[17] The classical account for the landless agricultural day-labourer, who was the real problem for social policy, was not completed until the eve of the First World War.[18] The families of clerks did not escape observation either;[19] historians came upon and then discussed a request from the 1830s in which civil servants had asked for a revision of their salaries and specified their demands for food and other household items.[20]

Since 1900, the Hungarian National Health Service has been concerned with the physiological value of overall food consumption, especially for underprivileged groups. A comprehensive survey of agricultural labourers all over the country was based on a special collection of data,[21] while later overall nation-wide analyses used both statistical data and their own collected information.[22] By the Second World War about a dozen case studies had been published in health journals.

In the capital, the cost of living rose by 35–40% during the period 1898 to 1909. Price rises affected cost of food and lodging alike, with the exception of bread. The unions took stock of the situation, and food rations and prices were calculated for the industrial worker as well as for the small burgher. These interesting sources have already been touched on briefly by historians.[23]

Except for the sugar-beet industry,[24] there is no comprehensive monograph on branches of the modern food industry which have had to supply the growing urban population as the transition from agrarian to industrial society took place.

In the late 1940s there occurred a radically new stratification of Hungarian society. There are a few case studies by sociologists who tried to see how people carried the dietary values of former times into their new lifestyles.[25] In historical scholarship, foodways have not as yet received much consideration as a characteristic part of the lifestyles of the different social strata. This did happen, however, in an examination of the meals of the middle classes around 1900 in the new comprehensive history of Hungary.[26]

Statistical records

Only in the final years of traditional agrarian Hungary did the Central Office of Statistics embark on the compilation of the country's first comprehensive food consumption statistics. After data were collected in 1881–3, publication in German and Hungarian followed in 1887.[27] Keleti, head of the Office and author of the volume, studied contemporary methods and gave a precise description of his approach. The net volume of the agricultural product was only used to check the results of data collection and processing. The basis for the work were the oral accounts given by thousands of families all over the country; they itemized meals and menus as well as the kinds of foodstuffs used. Amounts of foodstuffs were not provided. Data processing was based on the physiologically essential nutrients, starting with protein.

The 733 regional research units were divided into three qualitative categories. Thirty-five kinds of staple food were considered, plus luxury items for urban dwellers only. The published results were split up according to the 63 administrative units of the country, and urban settlements were entered separately. The statistics still showed a fairly favourable outcome, though the suggested 17th-century average meat intake of 60 kg a year had fallen to 34.5 kg for the early 1880s. More modern

Table 11.2 Average annual per-capita food consumption in Hungary, 1881–3 (in kg)

Foodstuff	Hungary	Urban	Rural
Meat and eggs	36.75	67.79	30.79
Pig's fat and lard	26.66	33.13	28.37
Milk and milk products	38.83	55.93	35.63
Wheat bread	43.91	60.92	40.74
Rye bread	49.07	52.73	48.39
Barley and oatmeal bread	17.45	3.76	20.00
Maize bread	32.50	11.69	36.39
Bread total	142.93	129.10	145.52
Other flour	58.53	59.24	58.38
Other cereals	10.52	10.41	10.54
Potatoes	112.25	81.48	117.99
Vegetables	112.87	118.50	111.82
Fruit	35.56	33.13	36.02
Wine (litres)	26.15		
Spirits (litres)	23.09		
Beer (litres)	4.06		

Source: Calculated after Keleti (1887) in *Magyarország története* (1979), pp. 1133.

Table 11.3 Average annual per-capita food consumption in Hungary, 1934–85 (main products in kilogram)

Foodstuff	1934/38	1950	1960	1970	1980	1985
Meat and meat products	32.2	34.3	47.6	58.1	71.7	76.9
Fish	0.7	0.6	1.5	2.3	2.1	2.2
Milk and milk products	101.9	99.0	114.0	109.6	166.1	182.0
Eggs	5.2	4.7	8.9	13.7	17.7	18.0
Edible fat	17.0	18.7	23.5	27.7	30.5	34.0
Cereals	147.0	142.1	136.2	128.2	115.1	110.0
Potatoes	130.0	108.7	97.6	75.1	61.2	54.1
Sugar	10.5	16.3	26.6	33.5	37.9	35.3
Fruits and vegetables	95.0	–	139.4	155.7	154.5	146.6
Cocoa	–	0.05	0.3	0.8	1.3	1.1
Coffee beans	–	0.1	0.1	1.6	2.9	2.9
Tea	–	0.01	0.03	0.07	0.1	0.1
Wine (litres)	34.8	33.0	29.9	37.7	34.8	24.8
Beer (litres)	3.1	8.3	36.8	59.4	96.0	92.4
Spirits (litres)	–	1.5	2.8	5.4	9.3	10.9

Source: Statistical Yearbook (1964), p. 288; (1985), p.246.

ideas of physiology have not yet been tested against the Keleti statistics. In Hungarian history, however, Keleti's work has been used as a standard both for the period it deals with and for the decades on either side.

The first continuous annual sequence of statistical data on food consumption was begun for sugar in 1867. Until 1893, the figures were processed outside the Central Office of Statistics. The Office itself did not venture to publish facts on food consumption after the Keleti volume until a new director was appointed. From 1893 onwards, data for per-capita consumption are available in the *Statistical Yearbook* for wheat, rye, sugar, wine, beer, coffee, and tea. For the potato, only the net national product and the supply for the distilleries were given. No meat consumption was specified, though the kinds and numbers of animals slaughtered for public consumption were given. For the period 1934–8 the data were later processed into per-capita figures to provide at least one point of comparison with the new system of publication, which is available from 1950. It gives per-capita figures for different kinds of meat, fish, milk and milk products, eggs, edible fats, grain, rice, potatoes, sugar, cocoa, vegetables, domestic and tropical fruit, coffee, tea, wine, beer and spirits. The daily allocation of nutrients is set out in calories, later in kilojoules, and specified as total protein, animal protein, fat and carbohydrates.

Ethnological food research

Ethnology was established in Hungary as a discipline in 1890. It started as folklife research and concentrated on contemporary rural culture. Today it is more concerned with the whole social complex, past and present, with emphasis on the broad social strata. The descriptions of rural life and of peasant farmers, agricultural labourers and rural craftsmen produced by ethnologists up to the 1950s included food and eating habits in their scope, and have themselves now become an object of historical research.

Sources

Earlier historical evidence for eating habits that have been analysed by modern ethnological research begins to increase in abundance from the 16th century. The sources include documents on practical subjects and lay and learned writing. I shall indicate the most important items in chronological sequence. A bibliography is not provided since it would require a knowledge of Hungarian to be able to use the original documents.

Registers of payments to the feudal landlord, a typical group of sources covering a long period, became numerous in the 16th century. They included food items such as ordinary bread and bread for special occasions, sauerkraut and milk products. Household accounts of burghers and gentlefolk and the daily sequence of meals and side dishes for the landlords' soldiers have survived from the 16th century, though not in great numbers. Regulations by artisans' corporations for the composition of their ceremonial meals are available up to the mid-18th century. Monthly sequences of actual meals with their menus have been recorded for aristocratic households and for the tables of the different officials, either in the presence or absence of their lord. The first large manuscript cookery-book was prepared for professional cooks in the household of the reigning prince during the same period. The first printed cookery-book was addressed to the middle class in the 17th century. Several *mémoires* mark great changes in the eating habits of the literate ranks at this time. In the law courts, briefs of cases began to be recorded in the vernacular, especially concerning female witnesses who provided evidence about the cuisine of lower ranks.

A continuous sequence of descriptions of popular eating habits began in political science in the early 18th century. In keeping with standard army practice, local authorities gave instructions about how the peasant should feed the soldiers billeted on him. Restrictive regulations about the use of luxuries, especially in relation to the number of courses and dishes for meals in cities and in country towns, were numerous at this time.

In the late 18th century, *belles lettres*, the accounts of foreign travellers and studies of dietetics report both peasant and middle-class food in authentic detail. During the same period, chapbooks began to be printed for the use of the master of ceremonies at peasant weddings, at which each course for the main meals was announced in verse as it arrived at the table. Such texts are available spanning long periods and provide evidence for the development of ceremonial meals. The so-called medical topography, which appeared in the early 19th century, described food and foodways for town and village alike. At the same time the period of romanticism brought into fashion the discovery of rural areas and rural lifestyles. In the late 1800s, the Ministry of Agriculture kept yearly accounts of agricultural wages, and since the provision of food was part of the wages on peasant farms, they recorded meals and dishes all over the country, thus supplying an excellent prop for folklife studies and a means of checking ethnological data.

Historical research

Among new foodstuffs and taste stimulants examined by ethnologists were maize (17th century),[28] potatoes (second half of the 18th century),[29] and paprika (early 18th century),[30] introduced both into cultivation and the kitchen. All started as popular foods, and maize never rose to the tables of the privileged. Paprika was to become the leading spice throughout the whole social complex. There were three phases in the introduction of sugar among the peasantry, each with a characteristic form of use. Beet-sugar production started at home in 1831 and by the 1860s was already an export industry. Even so, the average per-capita consumption was 1 kg in 1867. Only around 1900 did sugared pastry and drinks become widely established at peasant feasts, and per-capita consumption reached 8 kg in 1914.[31] Ethnologists also examined the introduction of coffee among the different social classes in Hungary in the 17th to the 19th centuries.[32]

As far as food and meals were concerned, the appearance of leavened bread in the common household and diet was first to be examined. Its adoption in place of flat, unleavened bread seems to have taken place during the 14th century.[33]

The next innovation in cereal foods was the introduction of noodles. Of Italian provenance, they were first served in south central Europe in the 16th century on upper-class tables. By the early 18th century they had become a staple food of the Hungarian peasantry, eaten two or three times a week.[34]

The most important edible fat in the diet of Hungary has been pig fat, which was more costly than any kind of meat until about 1900, since people in the past valued foodstuffs above all for their energy content. Every payment of wages between the 17th and 19th centuries included it in conserved form, salted, and dried or smoked. Up to the 18th century, lard was not melted down for conservation but was conserved and stored as large pieces. It was used for cooking at every social level and was the most desirable cold food for those who undertook hard, physical labour either in agriculture or later in industry.[35]

Goulash is probably the most widely known Hungarian dish, with an interesting domestic history. It was created in the historical cattle-ranching area of the Plain as a herdsman's dish; and the peasants added their new spice, paprika, to it in the mid-18th century. It was to become the most frequent way of cooking meat in the region. In the course of a political conflict with the Habsburg emperor and king of Hungary, the Hungarian nobility became involved in an early case of the invention of tradition in the late 1700s. They elected goulash, at that time only a peasant dish, as a means of characterizing one of the ways in which Hungarians were different from other Habsburg subjects. It became a national dish. This development prepared the way for the passage of goulash to the tables of the higher social strata, whence it later proceeded to the peasantry beyond the Plain.[36]

The modern concept of soup emerged only around 1700 among the upper classes; it was to become an introductory course at every meal. The model also influenced the sequence of peasant dishes. The frequent use of roux, a characteristic feature of Hungarian cooking, is also not earlier than the 18th century.

International ethnological food researchers are convinced that the ethnological analysis of food and foodways should start from the actual meals eaten. This allows historical and regional comparison to be carried out precisely, and diet can also be seen as part of the whole lifestyle.[37]

In this context the basic question is the daily sequence of meals, with two different main systems coming in chronological sequence. The medieval two-meal system with warm meals of equivalent status at about 9–10 a.m. and 4–5 p.m. was once the norm all over Europe at all social levels. The modern three-meal system emerged among the upper classes in the second half of the 17th century and was first recorded in Hungary in the 1690s. The two former meals moved forward in time during the day so that the first came to be eaten at midday, and the new element, breakfast, had a menu that differed from that of the midday and evening meals and became organized around the new warm drinks, tea and coffee. For a time the old and new systems ran parallel, even among the upper classes, and for a much longer time among the

Hungarian peasantry. The agricultural population ate according to the medieval two-meal system during the winter months up to the 20th century, while adopting the three-meal system in summer, although for a long time without tea or coffee. The subject of snacks in-between meals has also been investigated from the 16th century onwards, but shall not be examined here.[38]

The question of the weekly and yearly rhythm of eating has also been followed up historically in ethnological food research, taking into account not only seasonal supply but also the effects of central direction and of the implementation of periods of abstinence and fasting. Regulations regarding abstinence differed regionally already in the 16th century even within the Roman Catholic church. The course of events in Hungary did not mean that the easing of regulations was necessarily followed at once in everyday practice. Friday (formerly a day of fasting) and Wednesday (abstinence) became the noodle days for the people of Hungary, fish being neither universally available nor cheap. Lent and Advent were the only periods when butter was used for cooking instead of pig fat.[39]

As regarding eating customs, people were already eating at high tables in Hungary in the 16th century. The habit of eating out of individual plates instead of out of a common dish is known for peasants only in the Netherlands at this time. We do not yet know how the use of such plates spread among the upper classes in Hungary, nor whether the flat plate proceeded more quickly than the deep one, as was the case in France. The lack of soup might point to a comparable sequence. But at this social level, the use of plates and cutlery had been fully implemented by the late 17th century. The last item to be introduced was the regular use of the fork. Nevertheless, 250 years later, eating out of the common dish and neglecting the fork were still accepted manners among the agricultural population, although plates and forks had been present in their households for a long time.[40]

Following a request from Germany, a comparative survey was tried out on the chronological sequence of innovations in popular foodways in north-west Germany and in Hungary, that is to say, in two diametrically opposite areas in the north-west and south-east of central Europe. Close to the economic centres, the north-west became an area of innovation in the early modern period; the south-east, however, maintained forms of traditional behaviour where innovations penetrated slowly, later, and only in part.[41]

Future tasks

In this third decade of historical ethnological food research, the main task of the discipline in Hungary is to summarize what has already been done. Hungarian historians are not fully aware of the questions and results and are often ignorant of the significance of data in the source material that passes through their hands. A comprehensive handbook would alter this situation.

It is not my task, as an ethnologist, to set tasks for historians. Nor do I have an overview of research that is possibly at hand but not yet published. Hungarian historians have clearly followed the aspirations of the *Annales* School. I wish that they would follow as intensively English and central European economic and social historical research into the modern transition period in foodways[42] by investigating more thoroughly the 19th- and 20th-century position in Hungary.

References

1 Benda (1973).
2 Sandgruber (1978).
3 Perjés (1963).
4 Vita (1964).
5 Kirilly *et al.* (1965); Perjés (1963–4).
6 Makkai (1971); Hofer (1987).
7 Zimányi (1969); Kiss (1973).
8 Makkai and Zimányi (1982).
9 Sápi (1966).
10 Wyczański (1969).
11 Makkai (1974); Makkai (1979).
12 Dávid (1965–6); Wellmann (1985).
13 Timár and Veres (1969–70); *Magyarország története* (1979), pp. 1130–1.
14 Teuteberg (1986b).
15 Nagyváthy (1820).
16 Le Play (1877).
17 Somogyi (1888).
18 Hortobágyi (1919).
19 Illés (1913).
20 Miskolczi (1977).
21 Farkas (1901).
22 Sós (1942); Sós (1959).
23 Vörös (1978), pp. 639–42.
24 Wiener (1902).
25 Losonczi, vol. 3 (1972).
26 *Magyarország története* (1978), pp. 468–74.
27 Keleti (1887a); Keleti (1887b).
28 Balassa (1960).
29 Kósa (1980).
30 Bálint (1962).
31 Kisbán (1989a).
32 Kisbán (1988a).
33 Kisbán (1966), Kisbán (1988b).
34 Kisbán (forthcoming).
35 Kisbán (1974); Kisbán (1988c).
36 Kisbán (1989b).
37 Wiegelmann (1971).
38 Kisbán (1975).
39 Kisbán (1984).

40 Kisbán (1986).
41 Kisbán (1987).
42 Burnett (1968); Teuteberg (1972); Teuteberg (1986a); Sandgruber (1982).

Literature

Balassa, Iván, *A magyar kukorica [Maize in Hungary]* (Budapest, 1960).
Bálint, Sándor, *A szegedi paprika [Paprika at Szeged]* (Budapest, 1962).
Benda, Gyula, *Statisztikai adatok a magyar mezögazdaság történetéhez 1767-1867 [Statistical Data on the History of Hungarian Agriculture]* (Budapest, 1973).
Burnett, John, *Plenty and Want. A Social History of Diet in England from 1815 to the Present Day* (2nd edn, Harmondsworth, 1968).
Dávid, Zoltán, 'Adatok a mezögazdasági termelés nagyságáról 1786-1789 [Data on the Amount of Agricultural Production]', in *Történeti Statisztikai Évkönyv, (1965–6)*, pp. 99–141.
Farkas, Jenö, 'Élelmezés Magyarországon [Diet in Hungary]', in Schächter Miksa (ed.), *Farkas Jenö Munkái* (Budapest, 1901), pp. 72–120.
Hofer, Tamás, 'Agro-Town Regions of Peripheral Europe. The Case of the Great Hungarian Plain', *Ethnologia Europaea*, 17(1987), pp. 69–95.
Hortobágyi, László, *Munkásháztartás. Egy magyar mezögazdasági munkás gazdaságának leirása és háztartásának statisztikája 1910/11 és 1917-ben [Labourer's Household. The Hungarian Agricultural Labourer: Household Budget and Statistics of One Family in 1910/11 and 1917]* (Budapest, 1919).
Illés, Imre, *Egy pozsonyi hivatalnok-család háztartási számadása [The Household Budget of a Clerk's Family in the City of Pozsony]* (Budapest, 1913).
Keleti, Karl, *Die Ernährungs-Statistik der Bevölkerung Ungarns. Auf physiologischer Grundlage bearbeitet* (Budapest, 1887a).
Keleti, Károly, *Magyarország népességének élelmezési statisztikája physiologiai alapon [Food-Consumption Statistics of Hungary on a Physiological Basis]* (Budapest, 1887b).
Kirilly, Zsigmondné et al., 'Production et productivité agricoles en Hongrie à l'époque du féodalisme tardif (1550–1850)', in Dénes Csatári et al. (eds), *Nouvelles études historiques publiées a l'occasion du XIIe Congrès International des Sciences Historiques*, vol. 1 (Budapest, 1965), pp. 581–638.
Kisbán, Eszter, *A magyar kenyér. Néprajzi tanulmány [Bread in Hungary. An Ethnological Study]* (Budapest, 1966).
Kisbán, Eszter, 'Vom Speck zum Schmalz in der ländlichen ungarischen Speisekultur', in *In memoriam Antonio Jorge Dias*, vol. 2, (Lisbon, 1974), pp. 283–96.
Kisbán, Eszter, 'Tagesmahlzeiten im Wandel am Beispiel Ungarns', in Niilo Valonen and Juhani U.E. Lehtonen (eds), Ethnologische Nahrungsforschung – Ethnological Food Research (Helsinki, 1975), pp. 115-25.
Kisbán, Eszter, 'Korszakok és fordulópontok a táplálkozási szokások történetében Európában [Periods and sequences of change in the history of popular eating habits in Europe]' *Ethnographia*, 95(1984), pp. 384–99.
Kisbán, Eszter, 'Food Habits in Change: The Example of Europe', in Alexander Fenton and Eszter Kisbán (eds), *Food in Change. Eating Habits from the Middle Ages to the Present Day.* (Edinburgh, 1986), pp. 2-10.
Kisbán, Eszter, 'Phasen des Wandels der Nahrungsgewohnheiten in Mitteleuropa. Ein Vergleich zwischen Nordwestdeutschland und Ungarn', in Günter Wiegelmann (ed.),

Wandel der Alltagskultur seit dem Mittelalter (Münster, 1987), pp. 179–98.

Kisbán, Eszter, 'Coffee shouldn't hurt. The introduction of coffee to Hungary', in Nils-Arvid Bringéus et al. (eds), Wandel der Volkskultur in Europa. Festschrift für Günter Wiegelmann zum 60. Geburtstag, vol. 1 (Münster, 1988a), pp. 429–43.

Kisbán, Eszter, 'Bread and Bread Bowls', in Alexander Fenton and Janken Myrdal (eds), Food and Drink and Travelling Accessories (Edinburgh, 1988b), pp. 50–60.

Kisbán, Eszter, '"May his pig fat be thick": Domestic conservation of fat in Hungary', in Astrid Riddervold and Andreas Ropeid (eds), Food Conservation (London, 1988c), pp. 26–31.

Kisbán, Eszter, 'Die Aufnahme des Zuckers in die bäuerliche Nahrungskultur in Ungarn', in Béla Gunda et al. (eds), Ideen, Objekte und Lebensformen (Székesfehérvár, 1989a), pp.281–9.

Kisbán, Eszter, 'From peasant dish to national symbol. An early deliberate example', Ethnologia Europaea, 19(1989b), pp. 95–102.

Kisbán, Eszter, 'An innovation in cereal food: noodles', in PACT News, ed. European University Centre for Cultural Heritage (Ravello, forthcoming).

Kiss, István N., 'Húsfogyasztás (katonai és közfogyasztás) a XVI-XVII. századi Magyarországon [Meat consumption (military and civil) in 16th- and 17th-century Hungary]', Agrártörténeti Szemle, 15(1973), pp. 92–114.

Kósa, László, A burgonya Magyarországon [The Potato in Hungary] (Budapest, 1980).

Le Play, Frédéric, 'Iobajjy ou paysans (à corvées) des plaines de la Theiss (Hongrie centrale)', in Frédéric le Play, Les Ouvriers européens. Vol. 2: Les Ouvriers de l'Orient (2nd edn, Tours, 1877), pp. 272–303.

Losonczi, Agnes, 'A táplálkozás társadalmi és emberi viszonyai [Social and human relations of alimentation]', Valóság, vol. 3 (1972), pp. 16–29.

Magyarország története [The History of Hungary], ed. Zsigmond Pál Pach (ed.), vol. 7: 1890–1918 (Budapest, 1978).

Magyarország története [The History of Hungary], ed. Zsigmond Pál Pach, vol. 6: 1848–90, (Budapest, 1979).

Makkai, László, 'Der ungarische Viehhandel 1550-1650', in Ingomar Bog (ed.), Der Aussenhandel Ostmitteleuropas 1450–1650 (Cologne, Vienna, 1971), pp. 483–506.

Makkai, László, 'La structure et la productivité de l'économie agraire de la Hongrie au milieu du XVIIe siècle', in Spoleczenstwo - Gospodarka - Kultura (Warsaw, 1974), pp. 197–209.

Makkai, László, 'A magyarországi mezőgazdaság termelési és fogyasztási strukturája a XVII. század közepén [The agricultural production and the structure of consumption in Hungary in the mid-17th century]', in Peter Gunst (ed), Mezőgazdaság, agrártudomány, agrártörténet (Budapest, 1979), pp. 253–63.

Makkai, László and Vera Zimányi, 'Les registres de dîme, sources de l'histoire de la production agricole en Hongrie dans la periode du feudalisme', in Joseph Goy and Emmanuel le Roy Ladurie (eds), Prestations paysannes, dîmes, vol. 1 (Paris, 1982), pp. 91–119.

Miskolczi, Ambrus, 'Adatok az erdélyi reformkori hivatalnok-értelmiség életformájához [On the lifestyle and budget of the civil servant in Transylvania in the 1830s]', Agrártörténeti Szemle, 19(1977), pp. 412–21.

Nagyváthy, János, Magyar házi gazdasszony [The Hungarian Housewife] (Pest, 1820).

Perjés, Géza, Mezőgazdasági termelés, népesség, hadseregélelmezés és stratégia a 17. század második felében [Agricultural production, population density, army catering and strategy 1650–1715] (Budapest, 1963).

Perjés, Géza, Terméseredmény-vizsgálatok [Crop results analysis]. *Történeti Statisztikai Évkönyv*, (1963–4), pp. 128–72.

Sandgruber, Roman, *Österreichische Agrarstatistik 1750–1918* (Vienna, 1978).

Sandgruber, Roman, *Die Anfänge der Konsumgesellschaft. Konsumgüterverbrauch, Lebensstandard und Alltagskultur in Österreich im 18. und 19. Jahrhundert* (Vienna, 1982).

Sápi, Vilmos, 'Landwirtschaftliche Gesindelöhne in Ungarn vom 16. Jahrhundert bis 1848', *Annales Universitatis Scientiarum Budapestinensis, Sectio Historica*, 8(1966), pp. 43–70.

Somogyi, Manó, *Az óbudai hajógyár munkásainak helyzete [On the Conditions of the Shipyard Workers in Óbuda]* (Budapest, 1888).

Sós, József, *Magyar néptáplálkozástan [Staple Diet in Hungary from a Physiological Viewpoint]* (Budapest, 1942).

Sós, József, *Népélelmezés* [Nutrition] (Budapest, 1959).

Teuteberg, Hans Jürgen und Günter Wiegelmann, *Der Wandel der Nahrungsgewohnheiten unter dem Einfluss der Industrialisierung* (Göttingen, 1972).

Teuteberg, Hans Jürgen und Günter Wiegelmann, *Unsere tägliche Kost. Geschichte und regionale Prägung* (Münster, 1986a).

Teuteberg, Hans-Jürgen, 'Der Verzehr von Nahrungsmitteln in Deutschland pro Kopf und Jahr seit Beginn der Industrialisierung (1850–1975). Versuch einer quantitativen Langzeitanalyse', in Hans Jürgen Teuteberg und Günter Wiegelmann, *Unsere tägliche Kost. Geschichte und regionale Prägung* (Münster, 1986b), pp. 225–79.

Timár, Eszter und Éva Veres, 'A kenyérfogyasztás statisztikai becslése [Statistical estimation of bread consumption]', *A Magyar Mezőgazdasági Múzeum közleményei*, (1969–70), pp. 237–56.

'Vita a Történettudományi Intézetben Perjés Géza könyvéről [Discussion on Géza Perjés' book in the Institute of History]', *Agrártörténeti Szemle*, 6(1964), pp. 512–47.

Vörös, Károly (ed.) *Budapest története a márciusi forradalomtól az őszirózsás forradalomig [The History of Budapest 1848–1918]* (Budapest, 1978).

Wellmann, Imre, 'La Hongrie face au defi agricole de l'Occident', in Glatz Ferenc *et al.* (eds), *Études historiques hongroises 1985, publiées à l'occasion du XVIe Congrès International des Sciences Historiques*, vol. 2 (Budapest, 1985), pp. 663–93.

Wiegelmann, Günter, 'Was ist der spezielle Aspekt ethnologischer Nahrungsforschung?', *Ethnologia Scandinavica*, 1(1971), pp. 6–16.

Wiener, Moszkó, *A magyar cukoripar fejlödése [The Development of the Hungarian Sugar Industry]*, 2 vols, (Budapest, 1902).

Wyczański, Andrzej, *Studia nad konsumpcja żywnosci w Polsce w XVI i pierwszej połowie XVII.w. [Studies on Food Consumption in Poland in the 16th and the first half of the 17th century]* (Warsaw, 1969).

Zimányi, Vera, 'Sopron város húsellátása 1567-ben, 1570-ben és 1593-ban [Meat supply of the city of Sopron in 1567, 1570 and 1593]', *Agrártörténeti Szemle*, 11(1969), pp. 435–68.

12 A methodological approach to the system of food consumption in 16th-century Poland

Andrzej Wyczański

In many European countries interest in the history of food consumption began with a description of the more conspicuous meals and feasts.[1] The reason for this description was their peculiarity and atypical character, which the authors deemed valuable to preserve for future generations. The picture, however, gave us some information about the manners of the high strata of society and about the social value of the quantity and choice of certain food products. For the investigation of normal food consumption this kind of information was without great importance.

The growth of studies of economic history steadily changed the situation. Although research into agricultural production did not give special attention to food consumption, it is one of the most important sources for food history. The same situation is seen in studies of commerce and trade. Scientific interest rarely resulted in drawing up a list of food products, not to mention the number of actual consumers and the quantities of goods consumed, information which was even more scarce. The positive exception in Poland was a study made by J. Rutkowski. This historian, gathering elements for research on the distribution of income in 16th-century Poland, made some investigations into the cost of running the great land estates. He researched the cost of the paid personnel, and besides salary he also studied the quantities of food products and the expenses incurred by them.[2]

The initiative of French scholars grouped around the journal *Annales* in the year 1961 changed the state not only of the research made in France, but also in other countries such as Great Britain, Italy and Spain.[3] The impact of the French work also found a reply in Poland – rather individual, however, and leading to different interpretations. The *Annales* concept, as we know, provoked many parallel studies of food consumption, which gave us the results in similar form, that is, pictures comparable with those from different countries and periods of time. These pictures, obviously, represent the average daily ration with a list of products, their quantities, their calorie values, and sometimes with their cost and nutritive structure. In principle the great conspicuous meals and feasts were excluded, being peculiar and not representing the everyday nutrition of the time in question. Evidently, data concerning other topics, such as the delivery of food to the majority of town populations or the special use of some fats and beverages also contributed to our knowledge about earlier food consumption, though not being the principle task of it.

The *Annales* initiative, as already mentioned, provoked scientific interest in France and other countries.[4] This review gathered together articles dealing with this subject, and scientific meetings were also devoted to these problems. The uniformity of the scientific aims and the uniformity of the results obtained gave hope for great success in the future, that is to say, the growth of investigations in this field and the possibility of their aggregation for a future synthesis on an international scale. The great number of works published during the years immediately following the *Annales* initiative seemed to fulfil this hope.

But after these early successes the development of food consumption studies initiated by *Annales* slowed; and some years later the studies nearly ceased altogether. Valuable results became limited and of lesser interest to historians, especially to those with socio-economic tendencies and those interested in the customs of the past. The reasons for this handicap were numerous. The first studies dealing with early modernity, scattered as to whom they described and where they appeared, were difficult to fit into a common picture. The sources which were used and the examples given were rather atypical, describing food consumption in the army, the navy, in monasteries, among patients in hospitals, pupils in schools, and so on. These peculiar diet systems were difficult to compare and cannot be regarded as the normal consumption for the times and regions described. Finally, the patron of the *Annales* initiative, Fernand Braudel, was interested more in the different food products and their technological processing than in their human consumption. That means that he looked primarily into the products' lists, quantities and nutritional values.[5] This being the case, the studies on the history of food consumption needed greater perspective for social and economic research.

Polish participation in the action of the *Annales* group was at first rather limited. One paper published in the *Annales* [6] and further articles scattered among the other periodicals and collections of essays did not represent a large contribution. The Polish authors considered the diet of hospital patients in Warsaw[7] and Elblag[8] and that of the workhouse inhabitants in Danzig in the 17th century.[9] The last-mentioned city had preserved rich archive materials which allowed a study of the town's foodstores[10] and the nutrition in the navy.[11] Besides the current food problems some historians were interested in aspects of beverages, such as beer, especially in Royal Prussia,[12] or brandy.[13] Finally, exotic fruit such as oranges and lemons were the subject of a short study.[14] With the above-mentioned research in general being dispersed and its results rather limited, there was no basis for a more integrated picture; only the study of daily food rations in 9th- to 16th-century Europe made by M. Dembinska[15] tried to present an overview of the present scientific situation. Some works also dealt with the food problems of the late 18th and the early 19th centuries in Poland,[16] but their content is beyond the scope of our paper.

Some years after the first *Annales* initiative a larger Polish research project was completed, which took the form of a book on food consumption in 16th- and 17th-century Poland;[17] the same problems were discussed in university lectures in Paris

Table 12.1 Average daily rations of the royal court in 16th-century Poland

	Quantity (g)	Energy value (kcal)
Rye bread	890	2056
Wheat bread	100	246
Grain (barley)	21	77
Grain (millet)	6	22
Peas	56	196
Beer (litres)	4.8	2016
Meat	580	986
Fish	8	11
Bacon	39	208
Butter	17	127
Cheese	26	39
Eggs, etc.	39	31
+5%		302
Total		6317
Protein	200	18.8%
Fat	124	11.7%
Carbohydrates	738	69.5%

Source: Wyczański (1985), p.142

during the academic year 1970–1 at the 'École des Hautes Études en Sciences Sociales', then 'VIe Section d'École Pratique des Hautes Études'. The Polish version of the book was more detailed and documented. Many years afterwards the French version was published by the 'Publications de la Sorbonne'.[18]

The lack of statistics of the urban population necessitated a search for the materials in archives in rural areas, especially the accounts preserved from the landed estates in 16th- and 17th-century Poland. This necessity also had a positive side, because about 80% of the population in 16th-century Poland lived in the countryside; hence, the investigation dealt with the majority of the population and their normal living conditions. Nevertheless, the accounts concerned the expenses made in the farmsteads, that is, the home farms, especially those of the royal estates, where there lived respectively rural salaried personnel, chiefly male and female servants, sometimes also the noble family of the royal administrator, the *staroste* or leaseholder. Finally, we could detect in this material the special accounts presenting the cost and the diet of the great state officer or even the king, who stayed for shorter or lengthier times on his estates. In the latter case, the stays concerned the royal castles rather than just courts and farmsteads.

Although the accounts pertained exclusively to the great estates, especially those of the king, they were able to give us a picture of the food consumption of different social classes all over the country. The common feature of these accounts was, however, their rather limited content, that is, they generally did not list minor garden products such as vegetables, fruit and the like – those products which were not

Table 12.2 Average daily rations of the gentry in 16th-century Poland

Products	Quantity (g)	Energy value (kcal)
Rye bread	1070	2482
Wheat bread	49	121
Grain (barley)	43	147
Grain (millet)	28	99
Grain (buckwheat)	39	136
Peas	91	318
Beer (litres)	2.6	1092
Meat	169	287
Fish	30	42
Bacon	30	160
Fat	2	17
Flax oil	4	36
Butter	17	127
Cheese	18	27
+5%		255
Total		5346
Protein	139.9	13.6%
Fat	81.4	7.9%
Carbohydrates	806.3	78.5%

Source: Wyczański (1985), p. 140.

entered since they normally were not sold. Since a detailed picture obtained from those materials has been published elsewhere, I wish to demonstrate exclusively those results which had a general and especially methodological significance.

The first one is the conclusion about the peculiar nutritive level and structure linked with the social strata of the consumers. Simplifying our picture, we could posit three different types of food consumption in 16th-century Poland, i.e. different levels and structures of the daily mean food rations related to the social class of the consumers.[19] The luxurious daily rations of the Polish royal court are broken down in Table 12.1. This represents luxurious consumption, both actually eaten and wasted food products, in part perhaps offered to occasional visitors, for instance in the case of the beer.

The picture of the gentry's average daily ration could be more realistic (Table 12.2). The rations are more than necessary, the overbalance of carbohydrates substantial as before, the quantities of protein and fat sufficient; we might suspect an inclination to luxurious meals and a tendency to waste part of the food.

Most interesting are the daily food rations of the peasant personnel of the farmstead. The typical picture we have constructed is presented in Table 12.3. The picture requires comment. From a quantitative point of view it is sufficient, even for those working hard in the fields, for instance the girls and boys, but its structure is rather poor. The excess of carbohydrates and the deficiency of fat are evident. However, this seems to be the case with the majority of the population in 16th-

Table 12.3 Average daily rations of peasants in 16th-century Poland

	Quantity (g)	Energy value (kcal)
Rye bread	920	2134
Wheat bread	22	53
Grain (barley)	16	54
Grain (millet)	17	60
Grain (buckwheat)	15	53
Peas	46	160
Beer (litres)	1.2	504
Meat	20	34
Fish	4	6
Bacon	30	160
Fat	3	25
Flax oil	5	45
Butter	4	30
Cheese	10	15
+5%		167
Total		3500
Protein	77.8 g	11.0 %
Fat	47.2 g	6.7 %
Carbohydrates	583.5 g	82.3 %

Source: Wyczański (1985), p. 120.

century Poland and was perhaps similar in many other European countries. This type of food consumption could characterize the general food needs of the great majority of the population at that time in Poland, and as such it could form the starting-point for macro-economic considerations.

Tables 12.1–12.3 suggest some general conclusions concerning the study of historical food consumption. The most important is that demonstrating the social differences in nutrition. The daily rations differ according to place in the social hierarchy of the time, and the difference is reflected in the quantity as well as the structure of the normal diet. In short, the quantity increases as one rises in the social hierarchy, as does the share of the more prestigious products, for instance meat and beverages, which corresponds to the higher cost and more luxurious character of food. This conclusion leads to two other remarks. At first it is impossible to compare the daily rations of different social origins. This comparison could not give results concerning the differences between countries or changes in the time, because the social differences always tend to be predominant. Consequently, all computations of daily rations must be very well rooted in the social structure of the population; without that it is not valuable for further investigation. Otherwise the same conclusion has a positive side, because we often could detect the social composition of a group of consumers by their diet.

The social approach suggests a reconsideration of the problem of ostentatious and luxurious meals and feasts. It is evident that this type of consumption is not a normal one and does not represent everyday nourishment, but it did exist. Consequently, we could not neglect such feasts as a social phenomenon, although the exaggerated descriptions do not constitute a sound basis for scientific investigation. Even an exact computation, if it exists, does not give reliable information about the quantities of the food eaten, the number of consumers, the differentiation of the tables and dishes, and the duration of the meal. Such a situation makes it impossible to include this type of meal in the computation of the average daily rations of any social group.

Sometimes, however, we could detect in old accounts the generally accepted kinds of unusual meals, the meals related to the celebration of Christian feasts, such as Christmas or Easter, which usually were periods of more abundant and expensive nourishment. Nevertheless, the real cost of these feasts is very difficult to calculate because the most expensive purchases, such as those of spices, were made from time to time, since spices were easy to store. We also know that a more expensive period besides these feasts was Lent, the time of harvest, when more fish was bought and when the hard work demanded especially good nourishment. These brief remarks are necessary in order to understand the fluctuation of food consumption levels outside of famine times hidden behind the figures for average daily rations.

For macro-economic reasons it is very important to choose a social group corresponding in its habits and professional activity to the majority of the population. In 16th-century Poland the peasantry accounted for about three-quarters of the population of the country. Not having the relevant documentation concerning the peasants' own farms, we could use, as we have said, the great estate accounts for the computation of the daily food rations of that part of the peasantry employed as permanent salary workers in the farmsteads. It is evident that to consider this kind of diet as the basis of the food needs of the whole population is to simplify matters somewhat. But since this type of ration corresponds to the consumption of the majority of the population, we could make some correction for the higher strata as well as deductions for the children, according to the demographic patterns of the time. At the same time, the choice of the most typical daily rations could allow us to make international comparisons and to observe the changes in food consumption of the time.

A deeper knowledge of food consumption, with its social and demographic differences, could form the basis for observations of a macro-economic nature. Our knowledge of agricultural production is always fragmentary; even the yields ratio could be disputed, as well as the size of fields, the distribution of the crops, and so on. As a consequence, the computation of production on the basis of the study of agriculture is a very dangerous one, with results extremely difficult to obtain. Errors could be somewhat reduced in magnitude if we tried to calculate agricultural production on the basis of the average food needs of the population, adding the data concerning the transfer of food goods across the border and that portion which was usually left for use as seed. Even where it is possible to make a computation only for part of the country, our knowledge could be enlarged in this way, and the picture of the old economy would be better presented and understood. For example, we made such a computation for the most important part of 16th-century Poland,

Food consumption in 16th-century Poland   219

Table 12.4 Average annual agricultural production in 16th-century Poland

	Production (kilotons)
Rye	968
Wheat	123
Barley	213
Peas	74
Millet	45
Buckwheat	46
Bacon and pork meat	31
Pig fat	4
Vegetable oil	5
Butter	8
Cheese	29
Beer (hl)	1,280,000
Animal stock	
Cattle (excluding calves)	2.5 mill.
Pigs	2.7 mill.

Source: Wyczański (1985), p. 190.

namely the region where about 3.4 million people lived (about 200,000 km^2). Annual agricultural production in the 1580s was probably at the levels shown in Table 12.4.[20]

Table 12.4 is not complete, lacking information on oats, for instance, and we could supplement the data by way of calculation made on the basis of the distribution of the seed in the fields. Also, we could estimate on a comparative basis the agricultural production of the rest of the country, but the agrarian structure being a little different we decided to abandon the computation in question.

Macro-economic questions usually deal with the problem of total production and trade, especially with the attempt to establish the level of national income, which allows us to estimate economic growth, or lack thereof, and to compare the economic development of different countries.[21] The national income was calculated for 17th-century England by Gregory King at the end of the 17th century, but in our opinion this kind of computation is better made on the basis of material production and calculated again by the modern historian. The value of agricultural production, roughly calculated, even supplemented by the cost of processing the products, is relatively easy to estimate. This value represents the majority of the national income at that time. Nevertheless, the contribution to the national income made by the part of the population engaged in trade and other employment cannot be omitted. The problem could be solved based on the principle that this part of population had to buy their food goods and consequently had to earn the income which allowed them to make those purchases. This solution enables us to calculate the additional part of the national income and to establish its totality. Obviously, the computation of the national income for the 16th century remains purely a theoretical achievement, and is very controversial indeed. But the results of this theoretical reasoning could nevertheless be of practical use, especially the fact that the level of the national income is linked directly with the size of that part of population not connected with agricultural production. We can roughly say that the more urbanized a country is, the higher the level of its national income.[22] And this principle, in spite of its crudeness, is important for the economic picture of the old European continent.

The consecutive steps of reasoning leading from the analysis of the individual diet to macro-economic problems, were always very sophisticated and could be criticized as dangerous and inaccurate. There were indeed many difficulties at different stages of the investigations and two problems especially need to be stressed. One problem is dealing with the quantity of products known in the natural form, such as beef, whose weight is not noted.[23] It is always ambiguous to draw conclusions about the quantities and different forms of meat and fat from the number of livestock. The propositions to use for establishing the relations in the archaeological data stemming from the Middle Ages and the data known from the 19th century are both controversial. Apparently, the problem of the ancient measures is easier to resolve, but we must take care to note not only formal measures because their social use could be misleading.[24] A similar inaccuracy is connected with the processing of the product, the waste which is inevitably produced in the process, their biological value, and so on. Without more detailed studies on cooking habits, we shall always be in a very difficult situation.

A more important problem, according to our experience, is the question of the social framework of food consumption. We have stressed above the problems of nutritional stratification and the errors linked with the generalization of atypical or socially unrecognized examples. But there is also the other side of the coin, strictly speaking the problem of the quantity of the consumers and their distribution within the group. The most spectacular example of the controversy was the dispute started by one Polish historian who proposed to compute the farmstead servants as having families.[25] In this respect the food products had to be calculated as the allowance paid to the much more numerous consumers. The basis of objections were observations of the 19th- and 20th-century salaried personnel who lived with their families and were paid in cash and in food products.

The social reality of the 16th century was, however, quite different. The farmstead personnel was composed of young girls and boys, and when one of them wished to marry, a contract had to be cancelled. The personnel lived in the farmstead, where there was a special room for the farm hands and sometimes a special kitchen for them. Their salary was composed of money and often clothes or shoes. It sometimes happened that the manager of the farmstead was married and his wife was the salaried manageress. In this case it was necessary to calculate the additional consumers, but this kind of the family among the older salaried personnel is easy to detect. The conclusion which we could draw from this controversy is the necessity of deeper study of the social group, which we should observe as the consumers of food products. The list of wages and knowledge about the organization of the farmstead, even of the use of the buildings, could be helpful in this investigation. And transferring social customs and social structure on to other times and conditions without checking their validity is not proper scientific procedure.

Some general remarks should be made to conclude this line of argumentation. The food consumption study could also be developed as part of the history of manners and human customs. In our opinion those needs do not exclude investigations made in the framework of social and economic history, because food consumption represents the counterpart to food production and it corresponds in great part to agricultural production. At the same time, the food consumption studies lead our interest towards the macro-economic problems presented above which are worth investigating with different scientific approaches. On the other hand, food consumption could not be studied without the social framework. The social structure is reflected in the types of food consumption and allows us to interpret its peculiarities and to understand its functions. Knowledge of the structure of a social group is also the basic condition for all computations of daily rations, the fundamental element of our food consumption studies. Finally, the previous social and economic analysis enables the correct cultural interpretation of the results, a very valuable task for the study of everyday life in earlier times.

References

1. See Karbowiak (1900); Michalewicz (1965).
2. Rutkowski (1938).
3. See Braudel (1961).
4. See also *Pour une histoire de l'alimentation* (1970).
5. Braudel (1979).
6. Wyczański (1962).
7. Karpiński (1977). See also Bogucka (1977).
8. Klonder (1988). See also Klonder (1983b).
9. Bogucka (1986).
10. Bogucka (1970).
11. Bogucka (1984).
12. Klonder (1983a).
13. Kuchowicz (1971).
14. Tazbir (1967).
15. Dembińska (1979).
16. For instance, Baszanowski (1984); Turnau (1967); Wyczański (1985); Baranowski (1960); Sobczak (1968).
17. Wyczański (1969).
18. Wyczański (1985).
19. Wyczański (1982).
20. Wyczański (1985).
21. Wyczański (1971).
22. Wyczański (1978).
23. See, for instance, Dembińska (1987).
24. Kula (1970).
25. Dembińska (1970).

Literature

Baranowski, Bohdan, 'Próba obliczenia rozmiarów produkcji i konsumpcji rolniczej w czasach Księstwa Warszawskiego i Królestwa Polskiego (1807-1830) [Attempts to calculate the agricultural production and consumption in the period of the Warsaw duchy and of the Polish kingdom]', *Kwartalnik Historii Kultury Materialnej*, 7 (1960), pp. 209-28.

Baszanowski, Jan, 'Konsumpcja zbóż, mięsa i masła w Gdańsku w połowie XVIII wieku [The consumption of grains, meat and butter in Danzig in the middle of the 18th century]', *Kwartalnik Historii Kultury Materialnej*, 32 (1984), pp. 491-523.

Bogucka, Maria, 'Urząd zapasów a konsumpcja Gdańska w pierwszej połowie XVII wieku [The provision office and consumption in Danzig in the first half of the 17th century]', *Kwartalnik Historii Kultury Materialnej*, 18 (1970), pp. 255-60.

Bogucka, Maria, 'Z badań nad konsumpcją żywnosciową mieszczan warszawskich na przetomie XVI - XVII wieku [Studies of the food consumption of the Warsaw townsmen at the turn of the 16th and 17th century]', *Kwartalnik Historii Kultury Materialnej*, 25 (1977), pp. 31-43.

Bogucka, Maria, *Gdańscy ludzie morza w XVI-XVII wieku [The Danzig seamen in the 16th and 17th centuries]* (Gdańsk, 1984).

Bogucka, Maria, 'Dom pracy przymusowej w Gdańsku w XVII wieku [The workhouse in Danzig in the 17th century]', *Kwartalnik Historii Kultury Materialnej*, 34 (1986), pp. 265-69.

Braudel, Fernand, 'Retour aux enquêtes', *Annales E.S.C.*, 16(1961), pp. 421-4.

Braudel, Fernand, *Civilisation matérielle, économie et capitalisme, XVe - XVIIIe siècle*, vol. 1: *Les Structures du quotidien: Le possible et l'impossible* (Paris, 1979).

Dembińska, Maria, 'Racje czy normy żywnościowe [Rations or standards of food consumption]', *Kwartalnik Historii Kultury Materialnej*, 18 (1970), pp. 277-94.

Dembińska, O., 'Dzienna racja żywonościowa w Europie w IX - XVI wieku [Daily food rations in Europe in the 9th-16th centuries]', in *Studia i Materiały z Historii Kultury Materialnej*, vol. 3 (Wrocław, 1979), pp. 7-114.

Dembińska, Maria, 'Wyżywienie oficerów w osiemnastowiecznym Poznaniu - arytmetyka a rzeczywistość (uwagi na marginesie artykulu B. Wiecławskiego) [The nourishment of the officers in 18th-century Poznań. Arithmetic and reality (Considerations on the margin of B. Wiecławski's Paper)]' *Kwartalnik Historii Kultury Materialnej*, 35 (1987), pp. 139-43.

Pour une histoire de l'alimentation, ed. Jean-Jacques Hémardinquer (Paris, 1970).

Karbowiak, Antoni, *Obiady profesorów Uniwersytetu Jagiellońskiego w XVI i XVII wieku [Professors' dinners at the Jagellonian University in the 16th and 17th centuries]* (Kraków, 1900).

Karpiński, Andrzej, 'Warunki życia pensjonariuszy szpitali warszawskich w XVI i pierwszej połowie XVII wieku [Living conditions in the Warsaw hospitals in the 16th and the first half of the 17th century]', *Kwartalnik Historii Kultury Materialnej*, 25 (1977), pp. 43-62.

Klonder, Andrzej, *Browarnictwo w Prusach Królewskich (2 polowa XVI - XVII wiek [Brewing in Royal Prussia from the second half of the 16th to the 17th Century]* (Wrocław, 1983a).

Klonder, Andrzej, 'Wyżywienie wojsk szwedzkich w Prusach Królewskich w dobie 'Potopu [The nourishment of the Swedish army in Royal Prussia in the period of the "Deluge"]', *Kwartalnik Historii Kultury Materialnej*, 31 (1983b), pp. 27-36.

Klonder, Andrzej, 'Wyżywienie w szpitalach Elbląga w pierwszej połowie XVII wieku [Diet in Elbląg hospitals in the second half of the 17th century]', *Kwartalnik Historii Kultury Materialnej*, 36 (1988), pp. 449-68.

Kuchowicz, Zbigniev, 'Uwagi o konsumpcji produktów destylacji alkoholowej w Polsce XVI wieku [Considerations on the consumption of distillation products in 16th-century Poland]', *Kwartalnik Historii Kultury Materialnej*, 19 (1971), pp. 667–78.

Kula, Witold, *Miary i ludzie [Measures and People]* (Warsaw, 1970).

Michalewicz, Witold, 'Z badań nad konsumpcją spożywczą w Polsce. Kuchnia Zygmunta III [Studies of food consumption in Poland. The cuisine of Sigismond III.]', *Kwartalnik Historii Kultury Materialnej*, 13 (1965), pp. 701–18.

Rutkowski, Jan, 'Ze studiów nad położeniem czeladzi folwarcznej w dawnej Polsce [Studies on the living conditions of farmstead servants in old Poland]', in *Studia historyczne ku czci St. Kutrzeby*, vol. 1 (Kraków, 1938), pp. 381–402.

Sobczak, Tadeusz, *Przełom w konsumpcji sponżywczej w Królestwie Polskim w XIX wieku [The turning-point in Food Consumption in the Polish Kingdom in the 19th Century]* (Wrocław, 1968).

Tazbir, Janusz, 'Konsumpcja cytrusów w Polsce XV–XVIII wieku [The consumption of lemons in Poland in the 15th to the 18th centuries]', *Studia z Dziejów Gospodarstwa Wiejskiego*, 9 (1967), no. 3, pp. 105–15.

Turnau, Irena, 'Polżywienie mieszkańców Warszawy w epoce Oświecenia [The nourishment of the inhabitants of Warsaw in the period of enlightenment]', *Studia z Dziejów Gospodarstwa Wiejskiego*, 9 (1967), no. 3, pp. 115–30.

Wieclawski, Boguslaw, *Zaopatrzenie i konsumpcja w Poznaniu w drugiej polowie XVIII wieku [The Supply and consumption of food in Poznań in the second half of the 18th century]* (Poznań, 1985).

Wyczański, Andrzej, 'La consommation alimentaire en Pologne au XVIe siècle', *Annales E.S.C.*, 17 (1962), pp. 318–23.

Wyczański, Andrzej, *Studia nad konsumpcją zywności w Polsce w XVI i pierwszej polowie XVII wieku [Studies of food consumption in Poland in the 16th and the first half of the 17th centuries]* (Warsaw, 1969).

Wyczański, Andrzej, 'Le revenu national en Pologne au XVIe siècle. Premier résultats', *Annales E.S.C.*, 26 (1971), pp. 105–13.

Wyczański, Andrzej, 'Peut-on comparer les niveaux économiques des pays aux temps préstatistiques?', in *Studi in memoria di Federigo Melis*, vol. 4 (Naples, 1978), pp. 549–65.

Wyczański, Andrzej, 'Rémarques sur la consommation alimentaire en Pologne du XVIe siècle – types de la consommation', *Kwartalnik Historii Kultury Materialnej*, 30 (1982), pp. 21–6.

Wyczański, Andrzej, *La consommation alimentaire en Pologne aux XVIe et XVIIe siècles* (Paris, 1985).

13 Ethnographical studies in the traditional food of the Russians, Ukrainians and Byelorussians between the 16th and 19th centuries: state of research and basic problems

Michail G. Rabinovich

Food is one of the vital aspects of any people's subsistence culture. It is not only connected with the ecological environment of a society under study, but also reflects its production, social and family system, as well as its level of social development, historical relations and, finally, its religion. As an old Russian adage puts it: 'A man is what he eats.' A hunter differs in eating habits from a fisherman or a farmer, a townsman from a peasant, a poor man from a rich man, a believer from an atheist, an adult from a child. But however, the state of research into traditional food does not reflect the importance of this issue.

Of course, it is impossible to demonstrate the whole state of research into food and meals of the numerous peoples of the USSR in what is necessarily a short paper. Therefore we will confine ourselves to a short description of the history and the present state of studies concerning the food of the East Slavic peoples (Russians, Ukrainians and Byelorussians). These peoples, connected by a common origin and history, constituted almost three-quarters of the population of the former USSR. They have much in common in their food, although there are also quite distinct local differences.

In our approach to the history of the Russian, Ukrainian and Byelorussian peoples, food is usually related to the field of material culture – or, as another definition puts it, the public way of life. This is, as we have already recognized, a restrictive method in many respects, because there is a much wider complex of questions connected with food. The points of view from which this problem is regarded are also very different. Some researchers concentrate their attention mainly on the assortment of products of which food consists, the manner of its preparation and consumption, the number, ingredients and character of meals. Others widen the scope of research by also investigating the ways of obtaining food, the aquisition and storage of products (in some cases agriculture is even combined with the food issue), and, in connection with that, household effects and eating utensils, the table settings, table manners, the division of tasks associated with food in family and society – its meaning for the way of life of family and society. The same complex of questions consists also of the investigation of ritual meals, which are usually studied in connection with customs and religion.

Accordingly, works devoted to food are usually entitled 'diet' or 'food and utensils'. Compared to the research into other fields of material culture, less progress was made in studies in food and studies in material culture on the whole were taken over by fields of ethnology. S. A. Tokarev emphasizes that the investigation of material ways of life began in Russia not before the second half of the 19th century, and progress was not made until the end of the 19th century. The increasing activities of ethnological museums in the 1890s sparked the ethnographic work in this field.[1] But even later problems concerning traditional food remained less investigated than those concerning dwellings or clothing, for example.

It is significant that the basic bibliography of ethnographical literature, drawn up by D. K. Zelenin at the beginning of the 20th century, does not contain a section on food, while there are sections on dwellings, clothing, music and folkcraft as well as on people's way of life. And in the survey of Soviet ethnographical literature up to 1932, which continues Zelenin's work, only a few publications on food are mentioned.[2] In Zelenin's comprehensive work on the folk culture of the East Slavs, the main information about food can be found in the chapter on 'Preparation of meals'. Many questions, such as about the construction of the oven, utensils, the assortment of traditional meals and drinks, as well as eating prohibitions of different kinds, are investigated. Ritual meals and their meanings are explained in the chapters on 'Life and family' and 'Rituals of different annual festivals'. But even up to now not all works on material culture include the field of 'Food' or 'Meals and Utensils'. They mainly deal with the fields of 'Dwellings' and 'Clothing'. And yet, already by the middle of the last century, researchers were aware of the necessity of investigating those problems that refer to the diet of people.

The 'Project for Collecting Local Ethnographic Data' (1846) was developed by the Ethnographic Commission of the Russian Geographical Society and included already in the chapter 'The way of private life' one point on studying food aspects, namely 'daily food, food on holidays, periods of fasting and meat days'.[3] As we can see, a complete discussion of the whole set of questions on food as already mentioned is still lacking. Only ingredients of meals are considered, but the changes which are connected with a social way of life and religion have now also become important.

The actual work in connection with the gathering of this information, however, brought with it an expansion of themes: by studying the replies of the society's correspondents we also find information about the order of meals and table manners inside the family as well as with guests.

As already stated, the establishment of this project was the result of a strict scientific treatment of the direction of the society's ethnographic research. To the leading group of scientists (N.I. Nadeshdin, W.I. Dahl, P.N. Melnikov, etc.) belonged those who believed that the Russian Geographical Society should not only take an interest in the 'exotic' and 'backward' peoples, but should first concentrate on Russians and other peoples of Russia. All the various classes 'who still led a simple, a Russian way of life' should be included.

The lively reaction to this project showed that this was an issue of great interest. The replies of the correspondents, mostly teachers and priests, became an important part of the research archives of the Geographical Society.

Mention should also be made of a few ethnographic articles from the second half of the 19th century. These are concerned with people's food from the point of view contained in the local ethnographic data project. For example, in his small monograph about the city of Toropez, M. I. Semevskiy wrote a few pages on the composition of the town's citizens' daily meals and of their meals on holidays.[4] N. Markevich widens this complex of investigated problems by introducing the preparation of meals and table manners.[5]

In particular, historians worked on the issue of the people's diet at that time. The well-known historian and writer, N. I. Kostomarov, for example, devoted a paragraph to meals and drinks of that time which also included elements of customs associated with eating. He also studied the diet of different groups of society – peasants and townsmen, poor and rich. In the book itself, however, he did not differentiate clearly between them because he wanted, above all, to show the richness and variety of the meals and their distinctive rituals.[6]

Not even I. E. Zabelin, an important researcher into the history of the Russian way of life, could ignore the history of food. He did not devote an entire work to this subject, but did make occasional mention of table manners and habits.[7] His basic thoughts were further developed by S. P. Bartenev, who explained in detail the ritual of the Tsar's banquets.[8]

It is so obvious how near the research, which exclusively builds upon written sources, is to ethnography.[9] The fact that V. O. Kluchevski thought it necessary to add numerous data about the Russian material culture of the 16th and 17th centuries to P. Kirkhmann's translated edition testifies to the amount of data historians had collected about the Russian way of life in the later Middle Ages. The book's first chapter is about meals.[10]

The projects developed by V. N. Tenishev in the late 19th and early 20th centuries were strictly sociological in nature and included some valuable material on the dietary habits of peasants and townsmen. All parts of this project included questions concerning the attitude of the investigated group of people towards this or that phenomenon. Thus, in the rather small chapter on meals, remarks on social differences follow the already traditional questions pertaining to ingredients of meals, their dependence on seasons or periods of fasting; there it has to be explained first what should be understood by meagre or opulent food, which special meals have to be prepared for special festivities, who is cooking, how the seating order is arranged, and whether the head of the family should or should not get the biggest and best portions. In the project about townsmen the questions also refer to two categories of financial circumstances. The relationship between the work of the housewife and the cook, the food of the family and servants is considered. Furthermore, it is demonstrated which meals are regarded as tasty, how greed is expressed, who has the most prestigious position, what kinds of conversation can be held at the table, and so on.

Many letters followed the first project, which today are kept in the archives of the State Ethnological Museum of the USSR in Leningrad and are widely used by ethnographers. The second project is kept in the same museum, but it was never published because V. N. Tenishev died suddenly in 1902 without having finished his work on the project.[11]

At the end of the 19th and the beginning of the 20th centuries, the material for this investigation (for instance, the *Project for the Study of Townsmen among the Educated Class*) was seldom used for studies in food because of the reasons already mentioned. A certain stimulation of research into this question can only be recognized at the beginning of the 20th century in connection with the increasing growth of cities and their meaning for the social life of the country. Also during this time, more in-depth research into the way of life of industrial workers took place, including their households as well as their food. Several essays on this issue were published as well. The researchers' attention was concentrated on workers of special professions and in a particular area.[12] And even the first attempts to summarize and analyse the material on the food issue on a bigger scale go back to the early 20th century.[13] However, food was the least researched of the questions in material culture. In this field archaeology was ahead of ethnography during the first decades following the Revolution.

Both archaeology and ethnography developed considerably. The archaeologists pointed out the complexities in food studies based on archaeological finds and Old Russian written traditions. In some respects this could be traced to the necessity of a correct interpretation of archaeological finds. Thus, it became necessary to compare them with the content of written sources, old descriptions and present folklore traditions. Already before the war not only detailed studies but also more general work about Old Russian culture, had been undertaken, although these had to wait until after the War to be published. The chapter on food here was written by N. N. Voronin.[14] The complex method of research allowed the writer not only to reproduce the old utensils, which were necessary for cooking and eating, but also to uncover the old secrets of preparing meals. Thus, he laid the foundations for research into the Russian cuisine. For us the results are very important in this particular case because the roots of the food and utensils of the Russians, Ukrainians and Byelorussians of the 16th to 20th centuries stretch back into the deep past.

The main object of ethnographical studies in the 1920s and 1930s remained the peasantry. But similar studies were beginning to include industrial workers as well. Museum funds were replenished considerably with expedition material and offered source material allowing more general conclusions, which became much more important during the post-war period. The most important results of popular food studies were achieved between the 1930s and the 1980s.

The progress made by the elaboration of this food issue was so rapid that many monographs on the inhabitants of several villages and cities carried special sections on this theme. The monograph by L. A. Anokhina and M. N. Shmeleva, *Culture and Way of Life of Kolkhoz Peasants in the Area of Kalinin*,[15] for example, consists in one chapter on material culture of one section on 'Food'. There, they deal not only with the ingredients of meals and their preparation but also with eating habits at various meals.

Further essays of general character on the food of the Ukrainians and Byelorussians were published. They mainly deal with the food of the rural population or with traditional meals and utensils. Many general ethnographic works about the material culture of the people as the whole include one section on 'Food and utensils'. Studies have advanced since it became possible to publish these (necessarily short) sections by N. A. Dvornikova, L. A. Demidenko, L. P. Shevchenko, V. K. Bondarchik, etc., in the volume *Peoples of the USSR, Eastern Europe* of the well-known series *Peoples of the World*.[17] These articles were most important not only in completing a general survey on folk culture, but also for further generalizations. The chapter on 'Food and utensils' in L. A. Molchanova's monograph *Material Culture of the Byelorussians*[18] belongs here as well as her historio-ethnographic monograph on material culture of the Byelorussians in the 16th and 17th century[19] and M. G. Rabinovich's essay on 'The Traditional Meal of the Russians up to the End of the 19th Century' (in German).[20] This last-mentioned essay also concerns the history of the establishment and organization of Russian cuisine as well as the character of meals.

Subsequent food studies include monographic descriptions of several groups of the East Slavic population – the coast-dwellers (T. A. Bernstham), the inhabitants of the Chudskoye Lake area (E. V. Rikhter), the Central Volga area (E. P. Busygin), the Kuban (N. A. Dvornikova), Siberia and Altai (L. M. Saburova, V. A. Lipinskaya).[21] These sections are more extensive than the articles mentioned above. Apart from general characteristics of the Russian cuisine, these essays also mention local peculiarities (for example, the extent to which meals consisted of meat), the relation to Slavic and non-Slavic neighbouring peoples or the consumption of sour fish by the Russians in Sibiria.

The research into food has reached a point where its results are also used in larger, summary works on cultural history. In most of the books in the series *Essays on Russian Culture* there are special chapters on food.

Referring to the chronological frame of this paper we wish to draw attention to part I of the *Essays on Russian Culture of the 16th Century*: one chapter by N. A. Gorskaya is called 'Food' while there is another chapter by L. N. Vdovina called 'Food and utensils'.[22] Both chapters refer mainly to written sources and their explanations of the preparation of meals are of special interest. Questions of table manners are not broached, however. In the single volumes of this edition which are devoted to the 18th century, there is no special chapter on this; nevertheless, information on the subject of food is contained in a chapter on the city.

In most of the editions mentioned above from the end of the 19th and beginning of the 20th centuries, food of the people was understood to mean exclusively the diet of the peasants, for ethnography at that time was confined to studies on the peasantry, which is viewed as the sole keeper and carrier of national cultural traditions. The investigations, discussed above, into the diet of the workers, were thus a rare exception. The change of focus in this field of East Slavic ethnography is connected with the work of V. Y. Krupyanskaya and her school. Krupyanskaya, who had begun with the investigation of the workers' way of life, extended her studies further and produced works on the ethnography of the cities, treating as well the food of different classes in the urban population. Although in the first of such investigations the authors, in the corresponding chapter, are concerned mainly with the diet of workers,[23] it was, nevertheless, they who showed the inappropriateness of treating the workers separately from the remainder of the urban population, and as a result all later studies of this kind also contain sections devoted to the diet and meals of different classes of the urban population. This is true both of the past as well as of the present. In a special paragraph in Chapter III, 'Material Culture', of their monograph on the cities of the central regions of the Russian Federation, L. A. Anokhina and M. N. Shmelieva treat the food of the inhabitants of the cities Kaluga, Yefremov and Yelez.[24] The authors go much further in their investigation, however, by tracing as a totality the role and meaning of the problem of food in urban life. Thus, for example, city-dwellers' widespread habit of buying their food in small shops on credit caused special connections which were reflected in various spheres of activity and everyday life of the city-dwellers and were characteristic not only of pre-revolutionary Russia but also of many countries of the world even today. A considerable number of the sources are taken up by the authors' direct observation as well as documents from their expeditions.

One investigation of the developmental history of food, of the evolution of the combination of dishes, as well as of the table manners and eating customs of Russian townsmen of the distant past, has been undertaken in recent decades by M. G. Rabinovich, based on written traditions as well as interpretative art and archaeological material. His two monographs on the ethnography of the Russian feudal city (from the 9th to the 19th centuries) contain both an overview of the 'Table of a townsman' (here he treats the composition of a meal, types of dishes, the number, times and character of normal, festive and ritual meals among the common and upper-class townspeople and their utensils) and a paragraph on the family in which the table manners and eating customs are described along with their role in society and in the family ('Bratchiny', receptions, evening gatherings and parties, wedding banquets, meals celebrating the birth or baptism of a child or a funeral feast).[25]

Comprehensive works concerning the food of a whole nation did not appear until the last three decades. These include the monograph of L. F. Artyukh on Ukrainian national cuisine,[26] in which antiquity and the present are joined by means of numerous examples taken from everyday food and ritual meals, and the already mentioned work of L.A. Molchanova on the diet of the Byelorussians.[27]

The comparative investigations of the food of the East Slavic peoples, both among themselves and with neighbouring peoples, are very promising. They are of particular importance for studies on ethnic processes. A book by L. F. Artyukh has recently appeared which undertakes a comparative analysis of the diet of the Ukrainians and the Russians.[28] The comprehensive investigation entitled *Ethnography of the East Slavs: Outlines of their Traditional Culture* contains a sketch of meals and household effects in which the foodstuffs which formed the diet of the people, the preparation of meals, and kitchen and table utensils among the Russians, Ukrainians and Byelorussians are discussed comparatively using charting methods.[29]

The methods of the studies which have been undertaken in the last two or more decades in the area of food and meals are reflected continuously in the general method of the Russian ethnographic science of the given period. We have already spoken about the application of methods of direct observation (which are very characteristic of ethnography), of elicitation of information and of the complex investigation of different historical sources and areal studies.

The last-mentioned method was developed in the ethnography of P. I. Kushner in the process of setting up ethnographic maps for practical use. He drew ethnic boundaries of peoples on the basis of a card catalogue of different phenomena: the peculiarities of language, and the spiritual and material culture of the neighbouring peoples. Kushner wrote that 'the method of preparing a meal represents as a rule a good criterion for the recognition of an ethnic group'; however, this is especially effective when ascertaining the territories of peoples whose cultures are fundamentally different from each other. It is necessary to investigate and catalogue the meal, the culinary art, and the totality of household effects connected with the preparation and storage of food: 'Normally the art of cooking entails the most ethnic attributes. It is necessary to study ordinary meals and the products most in use.'[30] He wanted to develop these principles further by working on a historio-ethnographic atlas, in which he planned to catalogue, above all using the same method for all the categories, agriculture, living space, clothing and food. Maps of food of the sort Kushner wanted have not come into being for organizational reasons; nevertheless, a general method for drawing food charts has been set up, in which quantitative criteria play a major role. After a representative selection those points were determined where expeditionary investigations were carried out in every occupational unit of a particular territory (within the boundaries of an earlier administrative district or in a square area of a particular size), and every charted phenomenon was measured according to the frequency of its various types and in this respect compared with others. In this way the prevailing phenomena, which occur next to others, and solitary phenomena were elicited. They were later entered onto the map with corresponding designations. By comparing the charts, which were drawn up for particular historical periods, it was possible to determine with greater clarity the changes in areal distribution of the phenomena as well as their mutual interactions and relations.[31] In the internationally coordinated *Historio-Ethnographic Atlas of Europe*, V. A. Lipinskaya drew up, among other provisional maps, one which concerns the consumption of vegetable oils and meat products.[32]

One investigation of the population's food is also found in particular aspects in disciplines which border on ethnography. Thus specialists in the history of religion and historians who write about the way of life investigate ritual feasting. Here mention must be made of the thorough investigation by V. Y. Propp, *The Russian Agricultural Festival*, which contains many important ideas about the religious meaning of ritual foods and their constituent ingredients, and which goes into the manner of their preparation.[33] It may be mentioned in passing that ritual meals are also taken up, in varying depth, in the ethnographic works mentioned above. A certain revival of research pertaining to this topic has occured in the last few decades, and it can also be traced to the introduction of various new non-religious practices in the USSR.

Already by the end of the 1970s a task force was set up in the Ethnographic Institute of the Academy of Sciences of the USSR which undertakes investigations in the ethnography of the city. In the programme for this group[34] – applicable not only to East Slavic peoples but also to all cities in the Soviet Union – one paragraph (VIII) concerns the investigation of the problem of feeding the townsmen. Its eleven points provide for the study of the foodstuffs in connection with the ethnic and religious peculiarities of a region's population, of bought products and those made at home, and of prohibitions relating to particular meals, and – in connection with peculiarities in the preparation of particular meals – of the number and character of meals (at home and in restaurants), of the similarities and differences in the diet of rural and urban populations, of novelties introduced in connection with urbanization, of the city's role in the formation of a national cuisine, of the reflection of inter-ethnic contacts in the food of cities, of the handling and storage of products, and of kitchen and food implements, as well as kitchen and table utensils and utensils for festive occasions. Particular attention is devoted to the craving for recognition with respect to various aspects of food.

Finally, such a specialized area of research as advice of various kinds for the practical use of Russian cuisine in everyday life deserves attention. Books on cookery and housekeeping constitute a whole literature, and in mentioning a few of them here we are but scratching the surface: for the 18th century, the book by S. Drukovtsev (which is the first Russian work of this sort) as well as that by V. Levshin; for the 19th century, the work of Katharina Avdeeva; for the 20th century, that of N. I. Kovalev.[35] The special nature of these books for our subject is that while their authors were acquainted with an extraordinarily large number of meals, since they adapted their recipes to contemporary taste and customs, they were not so very careful about the historical accuracy of the recipes, and even less so about table manners.

Future assignments for the ethnographic study of the food of the Russians, Ukrainians and Byelorussians can be formulated as follows: a deepening of our knowledge about the special local characteristics of traditional food, especially of the food of different social and occupational groups; interrelations in the food of rural and urban populations in connection with the problems of urbanization; interaction with neighbouring peoples; influence of the development of trade and the food industry on the food of rural and urban populations; traditions and innovations in eating customs and habits; and prestige and symbolism in food and eating customs.

References

1 Tokarev (1966), pp.406–9.
2 Zelenin (1913); Zelenin (1932); Zelenin (1927).

3 'Programma' (1846); Rabinovich (1971b).
4 Semevskiy (1864).
5 Markevich (1860).
6 Kostomarow (1860).
7 Zabelin (1869); Zabelin (1905).
8 Bartenev (1916).
9 Rubinshteyn (1941).
10 Kirkhmann (1867).
11 *Programma* (1898), issue 381, pp.167ff; Rabinovich (1968).
12 Davidovich (1912).
13 Klinovetska (1911).
14 Voronin (1948); Artsikhovskiy (1944), pp.93ff.
15 Anokhina and Shmeleva (1964), pp.156–69.
16 See, for example, Georgijevskij and Shemakinskij (1963), Molchanowa (1960).
17 Dvornikova (1967); Demidenko and Shevchenko (1964); Kollektiv (1964).
18 Molchanova (1968), pp.183–225.
19 Molchanova (1981), pp.43–59.
20 Rabinovich (1971a).
21 Bernstham (1978); Busygin (1966), pp.360–84; Dvornikova (1964); Lipinskaya (1981); Lipinskaya (1987).
22 Gorskaya (1970); Vdovina (1979).
23 Krupyanskaya (1953); Krupyanskaya (1971), pp.140–7; Krupyanskaya (1974), pp. 243–9.
24 Anokhina and Shmeleva (1977):
25 Rabinovich (1988), pp. 213–64, 288–92; Rabinovich (1978), pp. 197–265; Rabinovich (1986).
26 Artyukh (1982); Artyukh (1986).
27 See also Korzun (1963).
28 Artyukh (1982).
29 Lipinskaya (1987).
30 Kushner (1951), pp.68, 74. See also Rabinovich (1968).
31 *Istoriko etnografitscheskij atlas Russkije* (1967, 1970).
32 Lipinskaya (1987), p.303, 305.
33 Propp (1963).
34 See Rabinovich and Shmeleva (1981), p. 32, paras 38–48.
35 Drukovtsev (1779/1783); Levshin (1793); Avdeeva (1851); Kovalev (1984).

Literature

Anokhina, L. A. and M. N. Shmeleva, *Kul'tura i byt kolkhoznikov Kalininskoy oblasti [Culture and way of life of Kolkhoz Peasants in the area of Kalinin]* (Moscow, 1964).

Anokhina, L. A. and M. N. Shmeleva, *Byt gorodskogo naseleniya sredney polosy RSFSR v proshlom i nastoyashchem na primere gorodov Kaluga, Yelets, Yefremov [Life of the urban population in the central region of the RSFSR in the past and present. The examples of Kaluga, Elec and Efremov]* (Moscow, 1977).

Artsikhovskiy, A. V., *Drevne-russkiye miniatyury kak istoricheskiy istochnik [Old Russian miniatures as historical sources]* (Moscow, 1944).

Artyukh, L. F., *Ukrainska narodna Kulinariya [The national Ukrainian cuisine]* (Kiev, 1977).

Artyukh, L. F., *Narodne kharchuvaniya ukraintsiv ta rossiyan pivnichnoskhidnikh rayoniv Ukraini [Food of the Ukrainian and Russian people in the north-eastern areas of the Ukraine]* (Kiev, 1982).
Artyukh, L. F., 'Izha ta kharchuvaniya v Kiivskiy Rusi' [Food and dishes in the Kiev realm], in *Etnografiya Kiyeva ta Kiivshchini* (Kiev, 1986).
Istoriko-etnograficheskiy atlas 'Russkiye' [Historio-ethnographical atlas] (Moskow, 1967, 1970).
Avdeeva, K. A., *Polnaya khozyayistvennaya kniga [The complete account book]*, vols I-IV (St Petersburg, 1851).
Bartenev, S. P., Moskovskiy Kreml' v starinu i teper', Kniga II, Gosudarev dvor. Dom Ryurikovichey [The Moscow Kremlin in past and present, vol. 2: the reigning dynasty. The royal family of the Rjurikides] (Moscow, 1916)
Bernstham, T. A., *Pomory: formirovaniye gruppy i sistema khozyaystva [The Pomoranians: formation of the ethnic group and its economic system]* (Leningrad, 1978).
Busygin, E. P., 'Russkoye naseleniye Srednogo Povolzh'ya [The Russian population of the central area around the Volga]', *Kazan* (1966), pp. 360–84.
Davidovich, M., 'Peterburgskiy tekstil'nyi rabochiy v ego byudzhetakh [The textile workers of Petrograd as reflected in their budget]', *Zapiski Russkogo geograficheskogo obshchestva*, (February–March 1912).
Demidenko, L. A. and L. P. Shevchenko, 'Pishcha i utvar [Food and utensils]', *Narody Yevropeyskoy tschasti SSR*, 1(1964), pp. 677–85.
Drukovtsev, S., *Povarenniye zapiski [Kitchen notes]* (Moscow, 1779; 2nd edn, 1783).
Dvornikova, N. A., 'Pishcha i utvar [Food and utensils]', in *Kubanskiye stanitsy. Etnicheskiye i kul'turno-bytovye protsessy na Kubani* (Moscow, 1967), pp. 393–406.
Georgiyevskiy, M. I. and O. E. Shemakinskiy, *Ukrainski stravi [Ukrainian food]* (Kiev, 1963).
Gorskaya, N. A., 'Pishcha [Food]', in *Ocherki russkoy kul'tury XVI v. [Essays on Russian culture of the 16th century]*, vol. I (Moscow, 1970), pp. 217–24.
Kirkhmann, P., *Istoriya obshchestvennogo i chastnogo byta, dopolneno V. Klyuchevskim [History of the social and private life, completed by V. Kljucevskij]*, vol. I (Moscow, 1867).
Klinovetska, S., *Stravi i napitki Ukraini [Food and drink of the Ukraine]* (Kiev, 1911).
Kollektiv avtorov, rokovod, W. K. Bondarchik, 'Pishcha i utvar [Food and utensils]', *Narody Jevropeyskoy tchasti SSR*, 1(1964), pp. 848–52.
Korzun, I. P., *Pishcha i pitaniye kolkhoznogo krest'yanstva Belorussii (istoriko-etnograficheskoye issledovaniye) [Food and diet of the Kolkhozniks in Byelorussia. A historio-ethnographical study.]* (Avtoreferat kandidatskoy dissertatsii, Kiev, 1963).
Kostomarov, N. I., *Ocherk domashney zhizni i nravov velikorusskago naroda v XVI i XVII stoletiyakh [Sketch of domestic life and customs of the great Russian people during the 16th and 17th centuries]* (St Petersburg, 1860).
Kovalev, N. I., *Rasskazy o russkoy kukhne. O blyudakh, ikh istorii, nazvaniyakh i pol'ze imi prinosimoy, a takzhe ob utvari, posude i obychayakh stola [Account of the Russian kitchen. Meals and their history, designation and use. Cutlery, dishes and table-manners]* (Moscow, 1984).
Krupyanskaya, V. Y., 'Opyt etnograficheskogo izucheniya ural'skikh rabochikh vo vtoroy polovine XIX v. [Empiric ethnographical survey of the working-class in the area of the Ural mountains in the second half of the 19th century]', *Sovjetskaya etnografiya* (1953), part 1.
Krupyanskaya, V. Y., 'Pishcha [Food]', in V. Y. Krupyanskaya and N. S. Polishchuk, *Kul'tura i byt rabochikh gornozavodskogo Urala (konets XIX – nachalo XX. v.)* (Moscow, 1971), pp. 140–7.

Krupyanskaya, V. Y., 'Pishcha [Food]', in V. Yu. Krupyanskaya, O. R. Budina, N. S. Polishchuk and N. V. Yukhneva, *Kul'tura i byt gornyakov i metallurgov Nizhnego Tagila (1917–1970)* (Moscow, 1974), pp. 243-9.

Kushner, P. I., 'Etnicheskiye territorii i etnicheskiye granitsy [Ethnic regions and ethnic borders]', *Trudy Instituta etnografii AN SSSR*, new series, 15 (1951), pp. 68–74.

Levshin, V., *Narodnaya povarnya [The national cuisine]* (Moscow, s.a. (1793)).

Lipinskaya, V. A., 'Pishcha russkikh sibiryakov [The diet of the Russian farmers in Sibiria]', in *Etnografiya russkogo krestiyanstva Sibiri XVII – serediny XIX vv.* (Moscow, 1981).

Lipinskaya, V. A., 'Pishcha i utvar [Food and utensils]' in *Etnografiya vostochnikh slavyan. Ocherki traditsionoy kul'tury* [Historic Ethnographic Atlas of Europe] (Moscow, 1987), pp. 292-312.

Lipinskaya, V. A., *Russkoye naseleniye Altayskogo kraya. Narodnye traditsii v material'noy kul'ture XVIII-XX vv. [The Russian population of the Altaian national tradition in the material culture]* (Moscow, 1987).

Markevich, N., *Obychai, pover'a, kukhnya i napitki malorossiyan [Customs, superstitious belief, cuisine and drinks of the Ruthenians]* (Kiev, 1860).

Molchanova, L. A., 'Izha ta domashne nachinnya bilo-rus'kogo selyanstva do revolutsii [Diet and kitchen-tools of the Byelorussian farmers until the revolution]', *Narodna tvorchist ta etnografiya,* (1960), no. 1.

Molchanova, L. A., *Material'naya kul'tura belorusov [Material culture of the Byelorussians]* (Minsk, 1968).

Molchanova, L. A., Ocherki material'noy kul'tury belorusov XVI -XVII vv. [Sketches of the material culture of the Byelorussians during the 16th and 17th centuries] (Minsk, 1981).

Narody Yevropeyskoy chasti SSSR [The peoples of the European part of the USSR], vol. 1 (Moscow, 1964).

'Programma dlya sobiraniya mestnykh etnograficheskikh svedeniy [Programme for the collection of local ethnographical knowledge]', in *Arkhiv geograficheskogo obshchestva SSSR,* Fond 1, op. 1, (1846), no. 4.l.60.

Programma etnograficheskikh svedeniy o krest'yanakh Tsentral'noy Rossii, sostavlennaya knyazem V. N. Tenishevym na osnovanii ego knigi 'Deyatelnost' cheloveka' [Programme of ethnographical knowledge concerning central Russian peasants. Compiled by the Duke V. N. Tenisev based on his book *Human Activities*] (Smolensk, 1898).

Propp, V. Y., *Russkiye agrarnye prazdniki [The Russian agricultural festival]* (Leningrad, 1963).

Rabinovich, Michail G., 'Istoriko-etnograficheskiy atlas "Russkiye". Printsipy i metody sostavleniya [Historio-ethnographical atlas *Russkiye*. Principles and methods of its conception]', in *Istoriya, kul'tura, fol'klor i etnografiya slavyanskikh narodov. VI. mezhdunarodnyi s'ezd slavistov* (Moscow, 1968).

Rabinovich, Michail G., 'Etnograficheskoye izucheniye goroda v Rossii v kontse XIX – nachale XX v. (programma V. N. Tenisheva) [Ethnographical investigation of Russian towns at the end of the 19th and beginning of the 20th century]', *Ocherki russkoy etnografii, fol'kloriki i antropolgii vol. 4* (Moscow, 1968).

Rabinovich Michail G., 'Traditional dishes of the Russians until the end of the 19th century', *Ethnologia Europaea,* 5 (1971a).

Rabinovich, Michail G., 'Otvety na programmu Russkogo geograficheskogo obshchestva kak istochnik dlya izucheniya etnografii goroda [Answers to the programme of the Russian Geographical Society as a source for the investigation of town ethnography]', *Ocherki po istorii russkoy etnografii, fol'kloristiki i antropologii, vyp. U.* (Moscow 1971b).

Rabinovich, Michail G., *Ocherki etnografii russkogo feodal'nogo goroda. Gorozhane, ikh obshchestvennyi i domashnyi byt [Ethnographical sketches of the Russian feudal town. The urban population, its social and private life]* (Moscow, 1978). *Ocherk 2, Obshchestvennyi byt. Piry i bratchiny [Sketch 2, social life. Banquets and brotherhoods], Ocherk 3, Glavnye cherty domashnego byta. Rasporyadok dnya. Priyemy. Vechorki. Brak, Rodil'niye obryady, Imeniny [Sketch 3, main characteristics of private life, agenda, receptions, evening gatherings and parties, marriage, birth, name day]* (Trizna. M. 1978)

Rabinovich, Michail G. and M. N. Shmeleva, 'K etnograficheskomu izucheniyu goroda [Ethnographical investigation of towns] *Sov. etnografiya* (1981–3), p. 32, paras 38–48.

Rabinovich, Michail G., 'Eating habits in Russian towns in the sixteenth to nineteenth centuries: the main phases of development', in *Food in Change* (Edinburgh, 1986), pp. 104–10.

Rabinovich, Michail G., *Ocherki material'noy kul'tury russkogo feodal'nogo goroda, ocherk 3: Stol gorozhanina [Sketches on the material culture of the Russian feudal town, Sketch 3: the table of the town dweller]* (Moscow, 1988), pp. 213–64.

Rikhter, E. V., *Russkoye naseleniye zapadnogo Prichudiya [The Russian population of the western pricudie]* (Ocherki istorii, material'noy i dukhovnoy kul'tury), s.l., s. a.

Rubinshteyn, N. L., *Russkaya istoriografiya [Russian Historiography]* (Moscow, 1941).

Saburova, L. A., *Kultura i byt russkogo naseleniya Priangariya, Konets XIX-XX vv. [Culture and life of the Russian population in the Angara area during the 19th and the 20th centuries]* (Leningrad, 1967).

Semevskiy, M. I., *Toropets - uyezdnyi gorod Pskovskoy gubernii [Toropec – an Ujazd-town in the Gouvernement Pskov]* (St Petersburg, 1864).

Tokarev, S. A., *Istoriya russkoy etnografii (dooktyabr'skiy period) [History of Russian ethnography up to the October Revolution]* (Moscow, 1966).

Vdovina, L. N., 'Pishcha i utvar [Food and Utensils]' *Ocherki russkoy kul'tury XVII v. [Essays on Russian Culture of the 16th Century]*, Vol. I (Moscow 1979), pp. 219–33.

Voronin, N. N., 'Pishcha i utvar [Food and Utensils]', in *Istoriya kul'tury Drevney Rusi*, vol. I (Moscow, Leningrad ,1948), pp. 93–4.

Zabelin, I. E., *Domashniy byt russkago naroda, t.II. Domashniy byt russkikh tsarits v XVI i XVII st. [The private life of the Russian people during the 16th and 17th centuries]* (Moscow, 1869).

Zabelin, I. E., *Istoriya goroda Moskvy [History of the City of Moscow]* (Moscow, 1905).

Zelenin, D. K., 'Bibliograficheskiy ukazatel' literatury o vneshnem byte narodov Rossii 1700–1900 [Bibliography on the social life of the Russian people 1700–1900]* (St. Petersburg, 1913).

Zelenin, D. K., *Russische (ostslavische) Volkskunde [Russian (eastern Slavonic) folklore]* (Berlin, Leipzig, 1927).

Zelenin D. K., 'Obzor sovetskoy etnograficheskoy literatury za 15 let [Summary of the Soviet ethnographical literature of the last 15 years]', *Sovetskaya etnografiya* (1932), no. 5–6.

14 Development and possibilities of historical studies of meals and nourishment in Bohemia

Lydia Petránová

Beginnings of historical studies

As elsewhere in Europe, the history of meals in Bohemia has long been studied by cultural historians. At the end of the 19th century they included especially the ethnographically-oriented historians, L. Niederle, C. Zíbrt and Z. Winter. Like O. Henne am Rhyn and W. H. Riehl they directed their attention to various forms of private lifestyle.

Zíbrt, after years of study, put sources on Czech cuisine from ancient times to the 18th century in a European context. He used reports by Arab and Jewish merchants from the 10th century, reports from medieval chronicles, moral tracts, accounts of court kitchens, descriptions of banquets, reference works from the 14th to the 18th centuries dealing with meals and kitchen equipment, recipe collections, and the oldest printed cookbooks. He issued an extensive edition of these sources accompanied by a cultural-historical commentary in 1927.[1]

Having an impressive knowledge of comparative material, he evaluated Czech terms and so-called Czech recipes in the oldest German cookery-books, pointed to the importance of Italian patterns and to the cosmopolitan nature of central European cookery-books of the 16th and 17th centuries. He proved that the oldest Czech cookery-book by Pavel Severin (1535) had been spread in Polish translation which is referred to as the oldest Polish cookery-book.[2] He was the first to notice the striking absence of Czech cookery-books in the 17th century. Even though Zíbrt tried to illustrate the meals of various social strata, his work is most complete in characterizing the meals of town-dwellers. This is due to the lexicographic sources which he used and which come from the bourgeois environment (he quotes thematic entries from eleven reference works). New partial studies refine the findings of C. Zíbrt, but do not substantially extend the range of sources gathered by him.[3]

Niederle dealt with meals within the framework of Slavic antiquity and his works on the life of the Slavs in the Middle Ages, in which he combined archaeological, ethnographic and linguistic sources.[4] Winter gathered in particular diverse illustrative data on meals, beverages, clothing and other necessities from municipal and juridical books and chronicles.[5]

The above-mentioned studies are precious today especially for the material contained in them; their authors succeeded in collecting a large quantity of data from written sources thanks to diligent heuristic work. The methods used are questionable: in most cases the authors do not go beyond quantitative data and usually stop at a general description without assessing the quality of nourishment.

Development of ethnographically-oriented studies

The roots of ethnographic interest in meals and nourishment can be indirectly sought in a prominent female figure of the Czech national enlightenment period, M. D. Rettigová (1785–1845). The latest literature sees her importance not only in the literary field (in addition to other books, she is the author of the most famous and most frequently published Czech cookery-book), but also in the sphere of education.[6] From an ethnographic viewpoint, it is important that Rettigová distinguished popular meals of the countryside from those taken in towns when she recommended her cookery-book, published for the first time in 1825, for 'towns and townlets, parsonages, mills and gamekeepers' lodges', while writing a different work for countryside households.[7]

The end of the 19th century saw, in addition to historical studies connected with farming education and the ethnographic programme, the development of studies of contemporary meals, especially in the countryside. These studies were carried out mainly on the basis of field research and various surveys. They were most important for the material gathered which, however, has not yet been analysed adequately by modern methods. The first such survey was conducted by a commission of the Vienna Ministry of Agriculture in the years 1898–1900 in which, among other things, the composition of the food of peasant families was determined. Meals were also given attention in a survey carried out by the Research Institute of Farming Cooperatives in the 1930s, and in the 1940s a so-called school survey was conducted, the aim of which was to study the level of nourishment of elementary school pupils. In 1940 M. Ulehlová-Tilschová organised an inquiry entitled 'We are Seeking the Roots of Folk Nourishment' which was carried out by the newspaper *Lidové noviny*. In connection with the traditional views of ethnographic studies as studies of the culture of village folk, these people's meals were also studied in surveys by the *Národopisná spolecnost ceskoslovenská* (Czecheslovak Ethnographic Society) and *Ustredí lidové umelecké vyrpby* (Folk Art Production Centre) after the Second World War. The material gathered in these surveys has not yet been fully used in research.

The only all-embracing work on popular meals issued thus far is the scientific monograph by Ulehlová-Tilschová, *Ceská strava lidová*, completed in 1944.[8] The rich variety of contemporary material collected by the author was put into historical context. She kept to the traditional division of meals according to the raw materials used and to the division of meals into those taken on workdays, festive days, fasting-days, to mark various ceremonies and on special occasions. The work also explains customs connected with meals. In her last work Ulehlová-Tilschová considered nourishment from a regional viewpoint, but that work is popular in nature.[9]

Unlike Slovakia, the Czech lands do not have a solid work on popular food in various regions which can act as an ethnographic atlas.[10] But there exist a number of valuable regional monographs devoted to popular diet in particular ethnographic regions in Bohemia and Moravia.[11] A general survey is contained in two books on Czechoslovak national history and geography.[12] The study of so-called traditional popular nourishment in the ethnographic sense means the study of the nourishment of the countryside society in the 19th and the first half of the 20th centuries. J. Stastná studied the nourishment of industrial workers within the development of a new direction in the so-called workers' ethnography of the Prague School of Professor A. Robek.[13] Ethnographic studies of food concentrate on social, ethnic and regional differences in the composition of meals, in their names and means of preparation, and on the social role of food in the family and wider groups. They also deal with substitute and emergency food.[14] Nutritional and calorie values are considered only marginally, and statistical methods are not used. Many studies of this kind are contained in ethnographic periodicals, especially *Cesky lid* (published since 1892), *Národopisny vestník ceskolovensky* (published since 1906) and others. The latest ethnographic publication on nourishment is the well-researched monograph by J. Stastná and L. Pracharová on popular pastries.[15]

Studies on food hygiene

After the First World War modern medical views on food hygiene began to be adopted in Czechoslovakia. Closely connected with this was an interest in the state of the popular diet.[16] From the ethnographic viewpoint an important figure in this movement was M. Ulehlová-Tilschová, who combined in her numerous works, methodically based on the works of German researchers (K. Hintze and others), the study of the history of what people eat with instruction and education.[17] After the Second World War this author participated, in theoretical and organizational work, in building the system of public catering.[18]

Specialized medical studies of food hygiene and problems of nourishment in postwar Czechoslovakia were the main task of the *Ustav pro vyzkum vyzivy lidu.* (People's Nutrition Research Institute) in Prague-Krc, founded in 1951, and then abolished in 1971. These questions have been take up by Spolecnost pro racionální vyzivu (Rational Nourishment Society) which publishes the monthly *Vyziva lidu* (*The People's Nourishment*, begun in 1946). The Society is headed by S. Hejda, author of the modern popular scientific monograph, *Kapitoly o vyzive*.[19] Issues pertaining to hygiene issues in food and catering are now monitored by the Institut hygieny a epidemiologie, centrum hygieny a vyzivy (Institute of Hygiene and Epidemiology, Centre of Hygiene and Nourishment) in Prague. One specialized institute within Czechoslovakia now exists only in Slovakia: Vyzkumny ústav vyzivy lidu (The People's Nourishment Research Institute).

Historical studies of consumption statistics

In the framework of the European trends, the consumption statistic came into being in this country at the beginning of the century as a new field of science with its own identification of the subject of study and with a more reliable quantification method. As early as 1913, statistical surveys were organized, according to Swiss and German models, by a predecessor of the later *Zemedelsky ústav ucetnicko spravovedny* in Prague. It followed consumption in peasant families which consumed their own produce as well as bought food. It gathered data which can be processed by statistical methods, but which have not yet been used in professional historical research, on the yearly consumption and production of farmers.

Already usable in the study of household budgets are the results of Austrian surveys contained in *Tafeln zur Statistik der Österreichischen Monarchie* between the years 1828 and 1865 (a complete set is owned in Czechoslovakia only by the library of Ustrední úrad lidové kontroly a statistiky (Central Office of People's Control and Statistics)) and the results of other regular surveys conducted in the years 1857, 1869, 1880, 1900 and 1910. The regular statistical surveys carried out since the beginning of the existence of Czechoslovakia (the first was conducted in 1921) methodically followed the statistical surveys of Austria, but they have been gradually expanded in connection with the needs and progress of world statistics.

The problems of consumption statistics were studied by economic historians, especially those dealing with the history of farming, who tried to quantify the consumption in kind of farming families and particular components of the food of farm servants in large homesteads. These included K. Príbram, F. Teply, V. V. Skorpil, V. Cerny, E. Janousek, V. Pesák, P. Burdová in the Czech lands, and S. Jansák and others in Slovakia.[20] The authors of these monographs concentrated on regional problems and studied individual large farms in the 16th to the 18th centuries. They based their studies especially on accounts and standard contained in sources collected at large estates which fixed food rations for labourers and servants. However, imperfect methods and only partial results led to pessimistic views of the possibility of synthesizing consumption statistics, especially as regards nourishment. The Commission for the History of Farming, set up in 1932, therefore did not include studies of the consumption in its programme, though it stressed the importance of research into the history of prices and wages for studying the material conditions of the life of country people.

Study of the history of prices and wages

In 1958 a working group on the history of prices and wages was set up at the Philosophical Faculty of Prague University with the aim of gathering further data and analysing and critically assessing sources for the study of the material conditions of life in the 16th to 19th centuries. Proceeding from the experience gained by historians in other European countries (especially in the interwar period), the group wanted to do more than merely collect typical data on prices, wages and currency. Such data may be impressive for their quantity, but they can be used only on a limited scale if broader connections are not known. That is why the group focused on monographic processing of the selected range of problems of the history of economic and social life. Within this program it also studied the prices of consumer goods and the consumption of food as a starting point for gaining information on the cost of living, costs on the reproduction of the labour force, material conditions of life and the overall standard of living in the past. Works published by the group deal mainly with the production and consumption of grain for bread, data which were drawn from production sources and standards. Jaroslav Honc investigated the average annual capacity of mills at large estates in southern Bohemia in the year 1590 and compared it with the estimated annual quantity of ground grain per farm.[22] The same author also studied the annual consumption of rye and bread in domestics' rations, in allowances in kind, in old peasants' rations and in hospital rations for the years 1452–1845.[23] Studies on wages, prices and consumption of grain for bread have been published in two volumes of *Acta Universitatis Carolinae*.[24] The consumption of grain by serfs' households in the second half of the 16th century and at the beginning of the 17th century has been studied in connection with estimated market production by J. Petrán.[25] An analysis on the nourishment of the people in southwestern Slovakia in the 18th century has been published by a member of the working group, S. Kazimír.[26] The working group tried to compare their own results and methods with European research developments.[27] In the mid-1980s the work of the group was suspended.

Problems of contemporary historical studies

The present-day historical research trying to get quantitive data on the amount and composition of diet, strives to get comparable results with those obtained abroad.

Difficulties in the study of the consumption and composition of food further in the past are encountered by archaeologists and historians of agriculture who, in cooperation with palaeobotanists and zoologists, concentrate on consumption in the Middle Ages and in early modern times.[28]

Broader studies of diet and meals continue within the research group for the history of material culture and the culture of everyday life, coordinated by the Chair of Czechoslovak History of the Philosophical Faculty of Prague University. Up to now two volumes of the first part of a handbook on the problem have been published. They also briefly survey problems of nourishment and food at the end of the Middle Ages.[29] The second in preparation will embrace the period up to the year 1800. The research so oriented is concerned with the differences in the quantity and quality of people's diet and that of higher social strata (as evidenced especially by aristocrats' travel and court accounts), the culture of meal-serving, meals served on workdays, festive days and at various ceremonies, changes in nourishment throughout the year, fireplaces, kitchen inventories, and so on. In addition to official written sources, it

Table 14.1 Annual and daily rations of rye bread in Bohemia, 1635–1726

Year	Locality or owner of the estate	Recipient	Rations (pounds)	Daily (kg)	Yearly rations (kg)
1635	Rakovník	Soldier	2 daily	1.03	375.5
1648	Herman Cernín	Shepherd	12 weekly	0.88	321.8
1726	Vysoké Myto	Farm domestics	12 weekly	0.88	321.8
1648	Herman Cernín	Farm domestics	11 weekly	0.81	295.0
1726	Vysoké Myto	Hireling	11 weekly	0.81	295.0
1648	Pardubice	Farmhand	1.5 daily	0.77	281.6
1648	Herman Cernín	Farm-maid	10 weekly	0.73	268.2
1726	Vysoké Myto	Farm-maid	10 weekly	0.73	268.2
1726	Vysoké Myto	Farm-maid	10 weekly	0.73	268.2
1648	Herman Cernín	Shepherdess	9 weekly	0.66	241.4
1648	Herman Cernín	Herdswoman	9 weekly	0.66	241.4
1726	Vysoké Myto	Herdswoman	9 weekly	0.66	241.4
1726	Vysoké Myto	Shepherdess	9 weekly	0.66	241.4
1655	Vlasim	Farmhand	1.25 daily	0.64	234.7
1726	Vysoké Myto	Small herdswoman	8 weekly	0.59	214.6

1 Czech pound = 514.35 g
Source: Honc (1971), p. 207.

uses cookery-books, recipe collections, herbaria and other literary sources, as well as iconographic, archaeological and ethnographic sources. This form of study is only in its initial stages, and is at present not systematic and in need of adequate methods. Better developed is the study of consumption and composition of popular food in the past, as is evident from the survey.

The quantity and different degrees of reliability and importance of the sources of studies of the popular diet make the application of a single method of processing and a single approach difficult. Just as in other countries in Europe, Czechoslovak authors use two main types of sources for studying consumption from the 16th century through the first half of the 19th century: normative ones, which mostly contain regulations, and records which contain accounting items. Both types of sources document domestics' rations, which constituted part of their wages; allowances in kind of those farm workers who took their meals in their own households; rations of former landlords having their own households; and rations of inmates of hospitals, orphanages, paupers' homes, prisoners, soldiers, etc. (see Table 14.)

The most common source of knowledge of the volume of consumption has thus far been the standard on domestics' rations which contain economic instructions from the 16th to 18th centuries and which have been partially published by J.

Kalousek and treated by V. Cerny.[30] They are easily accessible and establish per-capita standards for certain time periods. Components of the consumption usually listed by our sources are rye, wheat, barley (or rye and wheat flour and peeled barley), peas, butter, cheese, salt and meat. A comparison of the structures of individual standards shows that even though they differ largely in individual items, the final energy value is quite balanced. Smaller quantities of bread were levelled off by higher rations of peeled barley and the like.

Comparison with accounts of allowances in kind shows that the strong criticism of consumption standards made by some historians is not justified. Agreements on extra allowances in kind arranged as a supplement to the worker's wage contract if he did not eat at the farm and did not have accommodation at the farm, list rations in kind (mainly rye, wheat, barley, peas, cheese, butter, beer and timber) which he was to receive from the farm's stocks. The number of agreements preserved on allowances in kind is much smaller than that of accounts, and sometimes allowances in kind were turned into cash. Agreements on rations for former landlords used to be part of the agreements on the sale or transfer of homesteads as early as the 16th century and were entered in real estate records which contain figures on the quantities of grain and peas that the new landlord had to give annually to his predecessor and that man's wife until the end of their lives, in addition to other duties (providing rooms for the old married couple, a plot for growing vegetables and flax, or possibly for one's cow and poultry, and so on).

A valuable source for the study of food consumption are hospital accounts; these have not yet been fully exploited. The oldest preserved in Czechoslovakia come from the 14th century. The method of processing them encounters the same problems as the analysis of farm produce accounts. They can be confronted with the standards quoted frequently in the foundation documents of and subsidies to hospitals. However, none of these institutional sources can be a reliable substitute for modern consumption statistics.

Also used in the historical studies of consumption are the travel accounts of feudal lords, kitchen accounts of royal and noble courts, monastery accounts, standards on travel allowances, data on nourishment in garrisons, prisons, paupers' homes, orphanages and so on, which, however, are most incomplete and sporadic in the Czech lands.[31] A method for processing them has not been developed, and the data are mostly used in conjunction with results attained on the basis of processing other sources.

While the food of landlords and other higher social strata was more varied and richer, norms and accounts for folk meals are rather monotonous. Normative sources and records do not list some components which were undoubtedly contained in meals, such as fruit, vegetables, spices and others. Therefore rash generalizations must be avoided, especially in attempts to calculate the calorie values of daily rations. Czechoslovak historians, like historians in other countries, distinguish between the energy and nutritional values of food at present and in the past. Calculations are especially difficult for meat, since sources do not usually state its quality or weight. Nevertheless, J. Honc, who primarily studies these problems, does not reject

Table 14.2 Recommended monthly rations for Bohemian farm domestics, 1701

Persons	Rye flour (l)	Meat (kg)	Peas (l)	Peeled barley (l)	Pearl barley (l)	Salt (kg)	Butter (kg)
1	46.8	1.03	5.8	2.9	5.8	0.93	0.26
2	93.6	2.06	11.7	5.8	11.7	1.87	0.51
3	140.4	3.09	17.5	8.8	17.5	2.80	0.77
4	187.2	4.1	23.4	11.7	23.4	3.74	1.03
5	233.9	5.14	29.2	14.6	29.2	4.67	1.28
6	280.8	6.2	25.1	17.5	35.1	5.60	1.54
7	327.5	7.2	40.9	20.5	40.9	6.54	1.80
8	374.3	8.2	46.8	23.4	46.8	7.48	2.05
9	421.1	9.25	52.6	26.3	52.6	8.40	2.31
10	467.9	10.3	58.5	29.2	58.5	9.34	2.57
11	514.7	11.3	64.3	32.2	64.3	10.30	2.83
12	561.5	12.3	70.2	35.1	70.2	11.20	3.08
13	608.3	13.4	76.0	38.0	76.0	12.10	3.34
14	655.1	14.4	81.9	40.9	81.9	13.10	3.60
15	701.9	15.4	87.7	43.9	87.7	14.00	3.86
16	748.7	16.5	93.6	46.8	93.6	14.90	4.11

Source: Grynwald (1701), p. I 3.

quantitative indicators and takes the view that the calculation of the energy and nutritional values of food, however problematic, can serve as a means for international comparative studies, as long as the results are viewed only as a means of orientation.

A table from 1701, included in a farming calendar for the year 1702,[32] can serve as an example (Table 14.2). This is so far the oldest known standard for an exact number of persons, recommended by central authorities but not binding on big landlords. The calorie value of this standard is close to the average annual per-capita consumption as stated in the confiscation documents of 1622, constituting 98 per cent of it. In confiscations after the Battle of the White Mountain, commissioners calculated the average per-capita norm irrespective of whether the person was a nobleman or a serf (the average would be about 4,350 kcal per day by present value tables). In this light the proposed norm of 1,701 kcal for domestics would be relatively good if it did not show a profound discrepancy in the nutritional composition of food, mainly in the ratio between meat and grain. It prescribes meat comprising a mere 14.2% compared with calculations in the confiscation documents. This norm also shows higher consumption of grain to the detriment of meat when compared with all available instructions of large private farms from the years 1556–1648, while none of these amounts to more than 88.5% or less than 78.5% of the 1701 norm. Even though the sources are incomplete, it can be concluded that standards calculated by central authorities were higher in value than the private norms of farm domestics' nourishment; and that in the course of the 17th century the consumption of meat declined sharply while the consumption of grain rose. This conclusion confirms findings on the declining production of stock-farming in Europe as noted by agrarian historians such as E. Le Roy Ladurie concerning France in the 16th century, and it partly agrees with the conclusions of D. Saalfeld concerning the situation in Germany. Important for the composition of food in Bohemia was the transition to using barley malt instead of wheat malt in the second third of the 17th century.[33]

Studies of the development of kitchen equipment and of fireplaces

Interest in the development of kitchen interiors and fireplaces increased in Czechoslovakia in the past two decades as two areas of science began to develop: research of the building's history and archaeology of the final stage of the Middle Ages. New discoveries and methods of these areas of science brought a number of new achievements, but ethnographic work is still of major importance. Ethnographic research since the beginning of the 1920s into the archaic forms of fireplaces in less developed regions is of primary importance. This is true especially of works by K. Chotek, D. Stránská, A. Plessingerová, J. Vareka, S. Svecová. The standard study was written by V. Prazák in 1966.[34] He accepted methods of ethnic theory and defended the autochthony of Czech cultural development. His developmental typology is divided into four historical eras connected with characteristic forms and constitutes a single line of development from a fireplace on the ground in the living room up to the most perfect forms. More recent authors place ever greater emphasis on the economic and social aspects of the development of popular architecture, and have abandoned the notion of ethnic determination of phenomena. The question of the historical development of fireplaces has thus appeared to be much more complex. The latest formulation of this question by J. Langer comes from the year 1987.[35] He proved that there existed at least two lines of development in the Czech lands (in the countryside and in towns), but he pointed out that even this attempt at typology is not exhaustive since the two lines intertwined and sometimes reverted to previous forms.

Revolutionary innovations were introduced in Bohemia in connection with developments in central Europe. The latest work on the transition from smoky rooms to open-hearth kitchens was written by J. Petrán.[36] Transition from the open hearth to the stove had been placed till then in connection with English inventions from the end of the 18th century, but some reports seem to prove that transitional, less perfect forms of the stove already existed earlier.[37] Kitchen stoves generally spread throughout Bohemia in the 1840s and later.

Equipment in noblemen's kitchens and the aristocrat's way of serving meals are studied by experts in historical architecture and art historians, but they have not yet been treated in a comprehensive way in Czechoslovakia.[38]

Town-dwellers' kitchen equipment and table utensils were consistently listed by heritage inventories from the 16th century. These inventories are gradually being studied by students in their dissertations within a broader research project concern-

Historical studies of meals and nourishment in Bohemia 245

ing the history of the culture of everyday life. They have also been partially used in the cooperative work of ethnographers and post-medieval archaeologists.[39] The systematic study of the inventories should provide a survey of social stratification for instance, of the direct relationship between the quantity of pewterware in the 16th and 17th centuries and the profit of the farmstead. But they also contain valuable details on the functioning of kitchens.[40]

Conclusion

The studies of the history of meals and food in Bohemia has quite a long tradition, but not all the available sources have as yet been fully used. A palpable shortcoming is the absence of a summary bibliography. There exists only a partial bibliography on the growth of the food industry.[41] The history of meals and nourishment is studied simultaneously by economic and social historians, cultural historians, ethnographers and physicians. Using the methods of their field they are trying to gain results comparable with the results of research workers in other countries.

References

* Technical reasons made it impossible to print all correct signs in the Czech titles.
1 Zíbrt (1927); Zíbrt (1917); Zíbrt (1916); Zíbrt (1907); Zíbrt (1910); Zíbrt (1914); Zíbrt (1890).
2 Zíbrt (1926); Dembinska (1963); Dembinska (1984).
3 Rohanová (1987).
4 Niederle (1911).
5 Winter (1892); Winter (1888); Winter (1913); Winter (1909).
6 Wünschowá (1986).
7 Rettigová (1825); Rettigová (1838).
8 Ulehlová-Tilschová (1945).
9 Ulehlová-Tilschová (1970).
10 Stastná (1966a); Stastná (1966b).
11 Vollgruber (1906); Bachmann (1907); Kaizl (1944); Ludvíková; (1961); Ludvíková (1968); Stika (1980); Hosková (1986); Kubálková (1972); Stastná (1978).
12 *Ceskoslovenska Vlastiveda II* (1937), pp. 584–5; *Ceskoslovenská Vlastiveda II* (1936); *Ceskoslovenska Vlastiveda III* (1968), pp. 185-95.
13 Stastná (1977); Stastná (1981b); Stastná (1975a); Stastná (1975b); Stastná (1974–75).
14 'Prostredky k nasycení' (1972); Zásterá (1902); Stoklasa (1916); Stastná (1985); Stastná (1981a); Stastná (1983); Stastná (1962).
15 Stastná and Pracharová (1988).
16 Babák (1922); Merhout (1924); Eiselt (1922); Pelc (1940); Karásek (1940); Poupa (1956); Masek (1957); Houska (1971); Podzimková-Rieglová (1937); Charvát (1946); Kabelková (1968).
17 Ulehlová-Tilschová (1944); Ulehlová-Tilschová (1947); Hons and Ulehlová-Tilschová (1951); Hons and Ulehlová-Tilschová (1961).

18 Halacka (1953). Specialized literature first registered interest in catering at enterprises and factories under German occupation which was due to wartime limited food supplies and a decline in the value of food, Kleinert (1944); Lison (1944).
19 Hejda (1985).
20 Pribram (1916); Teply (1926); Skorpil (1923); Cerny (1930); Janousek (1967); Pesák (1940); Burdová (1952).
21 Honc (1962).
22 Honc (1959).
23 Honc (1971).
24 'Problémy cen' (1971); 'Problémy cen' (1977).
25 Petrán (1964).
26 Kazimír (1968).
27 Maur (1971).
28 Vyziva (1986); Opravil (1974); Opravil (1985).
29 Petrán (1985).
30 Cerny (1930); Kalousek (1905–13).
31 Honc (1973); Secky (1930).
32 Grynwald (1701); Table 2.
33 Vilikovsky (1936).
34 Prazák (1966); Chotek (1937); Stránská (1947); Plessingerová (1964); Plessingerová (1963); Vareka (1971).
35 Langer (1987).
36 Petrán (1985).
37 Erb (1770).
38 Stolnicení (1988).
39 Petránová (1987).
40 As an example we can cite baked clay bowls used for horseradish grinding which are listed in inventories up to the 18th century, but which have not been found by ethnographers in their fieldwork. The high consumption of horseradish in Czechoslovakia up to the 18th century, when changes in farming brought also changes in the food base and enrichment with vitamins, is also proved by special small horseradish bowls included in every table set in that period. The name of the baked clay bowls also indicates the way of treating horseradish before the introduction of graters.
41 Kuttelvaser (1986).

Literature

Adámek, Karel, *Krize hospodárského prumyslu [The Economic Crisis of the Industry]* (Chrudim, 1906).
Babák Eduard, *Vyziva rostlinami [Vegetable Diet]* (Prague, 1917).
Babák, Eduard, *O vyzive [On Nutrition]* (Prague, 1922).
Bachmann, Johann, *Speise und Trank im Egerlande [Meals and Drinks in Egerland]* (Prague, 1907).
Barthová, Ludmila, *První ceská vegetárska kucharka [The First Czech Vegetarian Cookery Book]* (Prague, 1908).
Bendl, L., *Pestování lécivych a kuchynskych rostlin v zahrade [The Herbs of the Garden]* (Prague, 1943).

Benesová, Milada, *Nakládání, zavování a pouzívání vseho ovoce a zeleniny [The Preserving, Sterilizing and Use of all Kinds of Vegetables and Fruits]* (Prague, 1914; 12th edn, 1946).
Bohmannová, Andrea, *Umení stolovat [The Art of Banqueting]* (Prague, 1981).
Bohmannová, Andrea, *Dvanáct rozprav kolem stolu [Twelve Talks about the Dinner Table]* (Prague, 1982).
Bozdech, V., 'Prehled vyvoje ceskoslovenské lihovarnické techniky do roku 1945 [A Survey of the Technical Development of Czech Distilling up to 1945]', *Spolecnost pro dejiny ved a techniky* 10 (1965), pp. 129ff.
Brizová, Józa, *Varime detem [We cook for Children]* (Prague, 1967).
Brozová, J. and D. Tucná, *Prostreny stul [The Set Table]* (Prague, 1964).
Burdová, P., 'Pomery námezdne pracujících v zemedelství na Mnichovohradistsku po tricetileté válce [The Living Conditions of the Agricultural Labourers in Mnichovo Hradiste after the Thirty Years' War]', *Sborník archivních prací*, 4(1952), pp. 99–119.
Cerny, V., *Hospodárské instrukce. Prehled zemedelskych dejin v dobe patrimonijního velkostku v XV.–XIX. století [Economic Instructions. Survey of an Agricultural History in the Time of Patrimonial Rule from the XV. to XIX Century]*, (Prague, 1930).
Ceskoslovenská Vlastiveda II Clovek [Czechoslovak National History and Geography, vol. II: The Man] (Prague, 1930).
Ceskoslovenská Vlastiveda II. Národopis [Czechoslovak National History and Geography, vol. II: Ethnology], (Prague, 1968).
Ceskoslovenská Vlastiveda III. Lidová kultura [Czechoslovak National History and Geography, Folk Culture], (Prague, 1936).
Charvát, Josef, *Vyziva pracujících [The Food of the Employees]* (Prague, 1946).
Chotek, Karel, 'Lidová kultura hmotná cs. lidu [Material Folk Culture of the Czechoslovak People]', *Ceskoslovenská vlastiveda*, II(1937), pp. 148–85.
Clovek, spolecnost a vyziva (Prague, 1971).
Dejiny hmotné kultury I/1-2 [History of the Material Culture], ed. J. Petrán, (Prague, 1985).
Dembinska, M., *Konsumpcja zywnosciowa w Polsce sredniowiecznej [Food Consumption in Medieval Poland]* (Wroclaw, 1963).
Dembińska, M., 'Kuchnia sredniowieczna, nowozytna czy "narodowa"? Uwagi na marginesie ksiazki Le Cuisinier François [The Medieval, the Modern or the Popular Cuisine?]', *Kwartalnik Historii Kultury Materialnej*, 32 (1984), pp. 555.
Detské kucharení [Cookery Book for Children] (Prague, 1901).
Doryzio, S., *Moje skrze ctyricetileté vykonání známá kucharská kniha pro mensí a vetsí tabule [Cookery Book for Small and Big Tables arisen from my Forty-Year-Experience]* (Brno, 1820).
Drahorádová-Lvová, Sína, *Brambory jako samostatny pokrm, predkrm [Potatoes as Main-Dish and Hors-d'Oeuvre]* (Prague, 1939).
Dumková, Hana, *Ceská kucharka [Bohemian Cookery Book]* (Prague, 1882).
Dumková, Hana, *Cokoládová jídla a nápoje [Meals and Drinks from Chocolate]* (Prague, 1884).
Eiselt, Rudolf, *O vyzive a nemocech z vyzivy [On diet and dietetical Diseases]* (Prague, 1922).
Erb, K., *Unterricht der neuerfundenen Koch-, Brat-, Back- und Oefen-Maschinen, welche zu Ersparung der Hälfte, auch zwey Drittheil Holzes die beste Wirkung machen [Lessons on the new Kitchen Machines which save two Thirds of Firewood]* (Vienna, 1770).
Farsky, Frantisek, *Víno medové [Mead]* (Prague, 1902).
Fialová, Juliana, *Moderní kucharka pro zenu i muze [Modern Cookery Book for Women and Men]* (Prague, 1958).
Fragner, Jirí, *Tekuté ovoce a zelenina [Fruit- and Vegetable Juice]* (Prague, 1958).

Frolec, Václav, *Tradicní vinarství [Traditional Viniculture]* (Brno, 1974).

Grynwald, Petr, *Novy hospodársky a kancalársky kalendár s pripojenou hvezdárskou praktykou ke cti sv. Václava k létu Páne 1702 [New Economy - and Chancellery Calendar]* (Prague, 1701).

Guth, Jirí Stanislav, *O hostinách a hodokvasech jindy a jinde [On Banquets and Feasts in Former Times and Other Regions]* (Prague, s.a.).

Guth, Jirí Stanislav, *O jídle a pití jindy a jinde [On Dishes and Drinks in Former Times and Other Regions]* (Prague, 1918).

Guth-Jarkovsky, S. J., *Kterak slusne jísti a dobre se chovati u stolu [Decent Behaviour and Good Manners at the Table]* (Prague, 1923).

Halacka, Karel and Marie Ulehlová-Tilschová, *Hygiena a sanitace ve spolecném stravování [Hygiene and Sanitary Systems in Canteens]* (Prague, 1953).

Hartmann, J., *Zemedelské prumysly ceskoslovenské v krizi [Czechoslovak Agricultural Industry in the Time of Crisis]* (Prague, 1933).

Hausgirgová, F., *Nová ceská kucharka [New Bohemian Cookery Book]* (Prague, 1863).

Hájek z Hájku, T., *Herbár aneb bylinár ... P. O. Mathiola [Herbary or Collection of Herbs]* (Prague, 1562; new edn, Prague, 1924).

Hájek, Frantisek, *Vyroba medoviny [The Production of Mead]* (Prague, 1899).

Hejda, Stanislav, *Kapitoly a vyzivé [Chapters on Nutrition]* (Prague, 1985).

Hodac, Ervín et al., *Staroceská kuchyne [Old-Bohemian Cuisine]* (Prague, 1970).

Honc, Jaroslav, *Spotreba chlebového obilí a rusení rajonizace mlynu na rozmberskych panstvích v roce 1590. Vedecké práce CSAZV z dejin zemedelství a lesnictví [The Consumption of Corn and the Abolition of the Mill-Rayons in Rozmberk Dominions in the Year 1590]* (Prague, 1959).

Honc, Jaroslav, 'Prehled literatury k dejinám cen a mezd v Ceskoslovensku za léta 1788-1962 [Bibliography on the History of Prices and Wages in Czechoslovakia, 1788–1962]', *Zápisky katedry ceskoslovenskych dejin a archivního studia*, 6 (1962), pp. 27ff.

Honc, Jaroslav, 'Rocní spotreba zita a chleba v celedních dávkách, deputátech, vymencích a ve spitálních dávkách v letech 1452-1845 [The Yearly Consumption of Rye, Bread and other Foodstuffs in Domestic Servants' Rations, Allowances in Kind, Rations of Retired Farmers and Rations in Hospitals 1452–1845]', *Acta Universitatis Carolinae, Philosophica et Historica*, 1(1971), pp. 177–210.

Honc, Jaroslav, 'Cestovní úcet diplomatické mise Viléma Rozmberka do Polska r. 1588/89 a budget slechtické domácnosti a dvora [Journey Costs of the Vilem Rozmberk Mission to Poland in 1588–89 and the Budget of an Aristocratic Household and of the Court]', *Archivum Trebonense*, 2(1973), pp. 44-83.

Hons, Vilém and Marie Ulehlová-Tilschová, *Vyziva a potrava [Diet and Foodstuffs]* (Prague, 1951).

Hons, Vilém and Marie Ulehlová-Tilschová, *Správná vyziva a potrava [Adequate Diet and Foodstuffs]* (Prague, 1961).

Hoskova, M., *Tradice lidové stravy na severní Morave [The Tradition of the Popular Diet in Northern Moravia]* (Gottwaldov, 1986).

Houska, Václav et al., *Vyvoj zemedelství a vyzivy v Ceskoslovensku (1920-1969) [The Development of Agriculture and Diet in Czechoslovakia, 1920–1969]* (Prague, 1971).

Hradilová, M., *Konzervování potravin [Preservation of Foodstuffs]* (Kromeríz, 1935).

Hroch, Miroslav and Josef Petrán, *Das 17. Jahrhundert. Eine Krise der feudalen Herrschaft? [The 17th Century: A Crisis of Feudalism?]* (Hamburg, 1981).

Hrubá, Marie, *Nase kucharka [Our Cookery Book]* (Prague, 1957).

Hrubá, Marie and Frantisek Raboch, *Kucharka nasi vesnice [Cookery Book of Our Village]* (Prague, 1965).
Hruska, Frantisek, *Nynejsí rizení hospodarení s potravinami [Contemporary Impacts on Food Economy]* (Prague, 1940).
Janácek, Josef, *Pivovarnictví v ceskych kralovskych mestech v 16. století [The Brewing Trade in Bohemian Royal Cities during the 16th Century]* (Prague, 1959).
Janousek, Emanuel, *Historicky vyvoj produktivity práce v zemedelství v období predbelohorském, [Historical Development of Agricultural Productivity before the Battle at the White Mountain (near Prague)]* (Prague, 1967).
Jeníček, Vladimír, Josef Kraus and Jirí Horniecky, *Zemedelství a vyziva roku 2000 [Agriculture and Diet in the Year 2000]* (Prague, 1975).
Jeníček, Vladimír, *Potraviny pro sest miliard [Foodstuffs for Six Billions]* (Prague, 1982).
Jirásek, V., *Rostliny na nasem stole [Vegetables on our Dinner Table]* (Prague, 1958).
Jones, Alois, *Na sálek kávy [A Cup of Coffee]* (Prague, 1969).
Kabelková, Zdenka, *Vyziva lidu. Doporúcujicí soupis literatury pro sirsí verejnost [Diet of the People: A Recommended Bibliography]* (Brno, 1968).
Kaizl, Ladislav, *Lidová vyziva I. Strava v Podkrkonosi [Diet of the People. Vol I: Food in the Giant Mountains (Riesengebirge)]* (Prague, 1944).
Kaizl, Ladislav, 'Ovoce ve staroceské kuchyni [Fruit in the Old Bohemian Cuisine]', *Vyzivá lidu*, 7 (1952), pp. 116ff.
Kalousek, J., 'Rády selské a instrukce hospodárské [Farming Instructions]' *Archiv cesky* XXII (1905); XXV (1906); XIX (1908); XXV (1910); XXIX (1913).
Kamenicky, Karel, *Ochrana ovoce a zeleniny pred zkázou [Protection of Fruit and Vegetables against Spoilage]* (Prague, 1943).
Karásek, Frantisek, *Základy nauky o vyzive cloveka [Principles of Human dietetics]* (Prague, 1940).
Kazimír, S., 'Strava ludu na juhozápadnom Slovensku v 18. storocí [Diet of the People in South-western Slovakia during the 18th Century]', *Slovensky národopis*, 16 (1968), pp. 571–88.
Kleinert, A., *Betriebsverpflegung [Subsistence in Factories]* (Prague, 1944).
Klimentová, Maryna, *Co máme vedet o priprave pokrmu [What We Ought to Know about the Preparation of Dishes]* (Prague, 1956).
Koblic, Josef, *Chléb a pecivo pro diabetiky [Bread and Pastries for Diabetics]* (Prague, 1935a).
Koblic, Josef, *Zitná káva a zitné konservy [Substitute Coffee and Preserved Rye]* (Prague, 1935b).
Konyásová, Katerina, *Kniha kucharská, v které se pro pamet lidskou o rozdílnych krmich ... [Cookery Book for the Remembrance of Various Dishes]* (Prague, 1712).
Kraus, Josef, Petr Tucek and Josef Volosin, *Vyziva jako surovinovy problém [Diet as a Problem of Resources]* (Prague, 1984).
Krzemienska, Barbara, 'Uzitkové rostliny a rostlinná vyziva rane stredovekych Cech [Useful Plants and Vegetables in Early Medieval Bohemia]', *Vznik a pocatky Slovanu*, 4 (1963), pp. 122ff.
Kubálková, Hana, *Strava vesnického lidu na stredním Polabí [Diet of the Rural Population at the Middle Elbe]* (Podebrady, 1972).
Kuchar, Jan, *Uprava hostiny. Posluha u stolu, úprava stolu, kladení ubrousku, krájení drubeze a zveriny [The Arrangement of a Banquet. Service, Setting of the Table, Carving of Poultry and Game]* (Prague, 1881).
Kucharství o rozlicnych krmích. Jana Kantora [Jan Kantor's Art of Cooking], ed. Cenek Zíbrt (Paris, 1895).

Kunc, Ludvík, 'Rolnické olejny na Hané a Záhorí [Rural Oil Presses in Hana and Zahori/ Moravia]', *Casopis Moravského muzea,* 44 (1959), pp. 127–50.

Kutnar, Frantisek, *Malé dejiny brambor [A Short History of the Potato],* (Havlickuv Brod, 1963).

Kuttelvaser, Zdenek, 'Poznámky k vyvoji pivovarské technologie do konce 19. století [Some Remarks on the Development of the Brewing Technology until the End of the 19th Century]', *Vedecké práce Zemedelského muzea v Praze,* 13 (1973), pp. 163–93.

Kuttelvaser, Zdenek, Marie Curdová, *Vyberová bibliografie dejin ceského potravinárského prumyslu, 1–2 [Selected Bibliography on the Czech Food Industry, Vol. 1–2],* Bibliografie a prameny Národního technického muzea v Praze 23-24 (Prague, 1986).

Langer, Jirí, 'Prispevek k typologii topenist [A Contribution to the Typology of Fireplaces]', *Archaeologia historica,* 12 (1987), pp. 233–43.

Laxa, Otokar, *Máslarství [Production of Butter]* (Prague, 1924).

Laxa, Otokar, *Syrarství [Making of Cheese]* (Prague, 1924).

Lánská, Dagmar et al., *Koreni pro kazdé vareni [Spices for every Art of Cooking]* (Prague, 1979).

Lánská, Dagmar and Bohumír Hlava, *Vitamíny z domova i zdaleka [Vitamins from Home and Abroad]* (Prague, 1982).

Lison, Oldrich, *Závodní stravování [Subsistence in Factories]* (Prague, 1944).

Lom, Frantisek, 'Vyvoj osevních ploch obilnin a sklizní od 16. století v Cechách [The Development of Corn Crop Areas and Harvests in Bohemia since the 16th Century]', *Historie a muzejnictví,* 2 (1957), pp. 161ff.

Lom, Frantisek, 'Vyvoj zemedelství a zemedelského vzdelání v Cechách [The Development of Agriculture and Agricultural Education in Bohemia]', *Sborník Vysoke skoly zemedelské,* (1958), pp. 21–107.

Lom, Frantisek, *Vyvoj zemedelskych ved a pokrok v zemedelstvi na uzemí CSSR [The Development of the Agricultural Sciences and the Progress in Agriculture in Czechoslovakia]* (Prague, 1968).

Ludvíková, Miroslava, *Lidová strava na Brnensku 1890-1915 [Diet of the People in the Brno Area, 1890–1915]* (Brno, 1961).

Ludvíková, Miroslava, *Lidová strava na Kloboucku a Zdánicku [Diet of the People in the Klobouky and Zdanice Area (Moravia)]* (Gottwaldov, 1968).

Luhanová, Zdenka and Jirí Hruby, *Spolecné stravování pracujících v zemedelstvi [Cooperative Subsistence of Agricultural Workers]* (Prague, 1960).

Macalík, Basil, 'Dejiny veprového dobytka na Hané [A History of Hog-Breeding in Hana (Moravia)]', *Vestník ceskoslovenské akademie zemedelské,* 2 (1962), p. 561.

Masek, Josef, *Zásady správné vyzivy [Principles of Adequate Diet]* (Prague, 1957).

Masek, Josef, *Clovek, spolecnost a vyziva [Man, Society and Nutrition]* (Prague, 1971).

Maur, Eduard, 'Problémy stravy v soucasné francoruzské historiografii [Problems of Diet in Contemporary French Historiography]', *AUC, Phil. et Hist.,* 1(1971), pp. 211–21.

Maur, Eduard, 'Cesky komorní vekostatek a trh v druhé polovine 17. století [Cameral Estates and the Market in the Second Half of the 17th Century]', *Sborník historicky,* 22 (1975), pp. 66ff.

Medková, Jirina, 'Z ceho se kdy pilo víno [How People Used to Drink Wine]', in *Sborník ke 100. vyrocí zalození Moravského umeleckoprumyslového muzea v Brne* (Brno, 1973), pp. 133–45.

Merhout, A., *Základy správné a úsporné vyzivy lidu [Principles of Adequate and Economical Nourishment of the People]* (Prague, 1924).

Ministerstvo pro zásobování lidu a soubor zákonu, narízení i vynosu zásobování se tykajících *[The Ministry of National Catering and the Body of Laws, Regulations and Orders]* (Prague, 1920).
Mlékarství moravské *[The Moravian Dairy Industry]* (Brno, 1930).
'Náhrazky tuku a oleju ve válecné dobe [Fat and Oil Substitutes during the War]', *Obzor prumyslovy*, 2 (1916).
Nemec, Bohumil, *Dejiny kulturních rostlin nejdulezitejsích [History of the Most Important Cultivated Plants]* (Prague, 1908).
Nemec, Bohumil, *Dejiny ovocnictví [History of Fruit Growing]* (Prague, 1955).
Neubauer, Leopold, *Vídenská kucharská kniha aneb ponavrzení, jak se masitá a postní jídla bez velkého nákladu vsak predce dobré chuti pripraviti mohou [Viennese Cookery Book. How to Prepare Meat- and Fasting Dishes Cheaply but Tasty]* (Brno, 1792).
Neudeckerová, A., *Bavorská kucharka v Cechách [Bavarian Cuisine in Bohemia]* (Pardubice, 1810).
Niederle, L., *Slovanské starozitnosti I-XI [Slovanian Antiquities]* (Prague, 1911).
Noback, G., *Die Bierbrauerei in Österreich-Ungarn, deren Statistik und volkswirtschaftliche Bedeutung [The Brewing Trade in Austria-Hungary, its Statistics and Economical Significance]* (Prague 1871).
Nove rozmnozená knízka kucharská [The Newly Spread Cookery Book] (Prague, 1729).
Opravil, E., 'Zajímavy nález rostlinnych pochutin a drog z poc. 17. stol. z Uherského Brodu [The Find of Herbal Delicacies and Drugs in Uhersky Brod at the Beginning of the 17th Century]', *Cesky lid*, 61 (1974), pp. 220ff.
Opravil, E., 'Rostlinné zbytky z odpadní jímky v Tábore c.p.6. [The Herbal Finds in Tabor]', *Archeologické rozhledy*, 37 (1985), pp. 186–94.
Opravil, E., 'Rostlinné makrozbytky z historického jádra Prahy [The Herbal Finds in Prague]', *Archeologica Pragensia*, 7 (1987), pp. 237–71.
Pátek, Jaroslav, *Racionalizace zemedelské vyroby mechanizací v ceskych zemích v první polovine 20. století [The Rationalization of the Agricultural Production through Mechanization in Czechoslovakia in the First Half of the 20th Century]* (Prague, 1971).
Pelc, Hynek and Marie Podzimková, *Brambory ochrana proti kurdejím [Potatoes – Protection against Scurvy]* (Brno, 1934).
Pelc, Hynek, *Pokus o srovnání vyzivy v rodine zemedelské, delnické a úrednické [An Attempt of a Comparison of Diet in a Farmer's, a Worker's and an Officer's Family]* (Prague, 1940).
Pesák, Václav, 'Panství rodu Smirickych v letech 1609-1618 [The Estate of the House of Smiricky in the Years 1609–1618]', *Sborník archivu ministerstva vnitra*, 13 (1940), pp. 166ff.
Petrán, Josef, *Zemedelská vyroba v Cechách v 2. polovine 16. a pocátkem 17. století [The Agricultural Production in Bohemia in the Second Half of the 16th and at the Beginning of the 17th Century]* (Prague, 1963).
Petrán, Josef, *Poddany lid v Cechách na prahu tricetileté války [Subordinate People in Bohemia at the Beginning of the Thirty Years' War]* (Prague, 1964).
Petrán, Josef, 'Ceny obilí a trzní okruhy v Cechách v 18. a pocátkem 19. století [Corn Prices and Market Areas in Bohemia during the 18th and the First Half of the 19th Century]', *Acta Universitatis Carolinae Philosophica et Historica*, 3 (1977), pp. 9–49.
Petrán, Josef et al., *Dejiny hmotné kultury I/1-2 [History of the Material Culture]* (Prague, 1985).
Petránová, Lydia and Josef Vareka, 'Vybavení venkovské zemedelské usedlosti v dobe predbelohorské (na pozadí poddanskych inventáru) [The Inventory of Furnishings of a Farmer's House before the Battle at the White Mountain]', *Archaeologia historica*, 12 (1987), pp. 277–83.

Pleskotová, Pavla, *20 000 let vareni [20000 Years of Cooking]* (Prague, 1976).
Plessingerová, Alena, 'Vyvoj topeniste, jeho vyuzíváni a vyznam ve slovenskych obcích pod Javorníky [Development of Fire-Places, Their Use and Meaning in Slovak Villages near the Javorniky-Mountains]', *Sborník Národního muzea v Praze*, A-17 (1963), pp. 149–236.
Podzimková-Rieglová, Marie, *Soucasné typy nasí lidové vyzivy [Contemporary Forms of Our Popular Diet]* (Prague, 1937).
Potravní kodex ceskoslovensky [Food Codex of Czechoslovakia] (Prague, 1937).
Poupa, Otakar, *Cteni o vyzive [A Reader on Nutrition]* (Prague, 1956).
Prazak, Vilém, 'Vyvojové epochy a stupne topenist v ceském a slovenském lidovém obydlí [The Stages of Development of Fire-places in Czech and Slovak Folk Flats]', *Cesky lid*, 53 (1966), pp. 321–48.
Pribram, Karl, 'Der Mehlverbrauch der Bevölkerung Österreichs in der Friedenszeit [The Flour Consumption of the Austrian Population in Times of Peace]', *Statistische Monatsschrift* new series, 21 (1916), pp. 679ff.
'Problémy cen, mezd a materiálních podmínek zivota od 16. do poloviny 19. století [The Problems of Prices, Wages and Material Living-conditions from the 16th to the 19th Century]', ed. Josef Petrán, *Acta Universitatis Carolinae, Philosophica et Historica*, 1 (1971).
'Problémy cen, mezd a materiálních podmínek zivota lidu v Cechách v 17.-19. století II [The Problems of Prices, Wages and Material Living-conditions from the 17th to the 20th Century]', ed. Josef Petrán, *Acta Universitatis Carolinae, Philosophica et Historica*, 3 (1977).
Procházka, J., *Dejiny konzervování potravin na území CSR [History of Food Preservation in the Territory of Czechoslovakia]* (Prague, 1931).
'Prostredky k nasycení v dobe hladu pred 200 lety [Means of Repletion during the Famine Period 200 Years ago]', *Cesky lid*, 59 (1972), pp. 192.
Rajchart, Miroslav and J. Kraus, *Spolupráce clenskych zemí RVHP v zemedelství a vyzive [The Cooperation of the COMECON-States in Agriculture and Nutrition]* (Prague, 1979).
Rettigová, Magdalena Dobromila, *Dobrá rada slovanskym venkovankám aneb pojednání kterak lze ony pokrmy sprosté lacine a chutne pripraviti a tak se bud pro budoucí svou domácnost neb pro sluzbu cviciti [Good Advice for Slavonic Country Women...]* (Hradec Králové, 1825).
Rettigová, Magdalena Dobromila, *Domácí kucharka, aneb pojedání o masitych a postních pokrmech pro dcerky ceské a moravské [The Cookery Book for the House: A Treatise about the Meat and Fasting Dishes for Bohemian and Moravian Girls]* (Hradec Králové, 1838).
Rettigová, Magdalena Dobromila, *Kaficko a vse co je sladké [Coffee and Sweets]* (Prague, 1843).
Rodovsky Z Hustiran, Bavor, *Kucharství, to jest knízka o rozlicnych krmích, kterak se s chuti a uzitecne strojiti mají [The Art of Cooking. A Booklet about Various Dishes]* (Prague, 1591).
Rohanová, Miroslava, 'Príspevek k poznání ceskych tistenych kucharskych knih 16.-18. století [A Contribution to the Understanding of Czech Printed Cookery Books from the 16th to the 18th Century]', *Praha, Státní Knihovna CSR, Miscellanea*, 4 (1987), no. 1, pp. 55–83.
Rozmarová, Olga Ruzena, *Vzorná ceská kuchyne a domácnost [A Model Bohemian Cuisine and Household]* (Prague, 1916).
Rozmarová, Olga Ruzena, *Ceská kuchyne [Bohemian Cuisine]* (Prague, 1922).
Sakarová, Bozena and Jiri Hruby, *Vyziva jako ekonomicky problém [Nutrition as an Economic Problem]* (Prague, 1967).
Schneider, J., *Veda v kuchyni [Science in the Kitchen]* (Prague, 1937).
Secky, Rudolf, 'Jak byli v Cechách za starych dob stravováni lidé ve spitálech [How People in Bohemian Hospitals Were Fed in the Past]', *Cesky lid*, 30 (1930), pp. 99ff.
Severyn Mladsí, Jan, *Kucharka [Cookery Book]* (Prague, 1542).

Severyn Z Kapí Hory, Pavel, *Kucharství o rozlicnych krmech, kterak se uzitecne s chutí strojiti maji [The Art of Cooking. The Book about Various Dishes]* (Prague, 1535)

Skorpil, Václav V., 'Celádka [The Domestic Servants]', *Casopis pro dejiny venkova*, 10 (1923), pp. 192.

Slanina, Antonín, *Stravování zemedelcu ve srovnání se stravováním uredníku, zrizencu a delniku [The Diet of Agricultural Workers Compared to that of Officers, Clerks and Industrial Workers]* (Prague, 1933).

Soukup, Václav, *Zelinárská kuchyne [Vegetable Cuisine]* (Prague, 1948).

Stastná, Jarmila, 'Zmeny v tradicní lidové strave a její stav v soucasnosti [Changes in the Traditional Popular Diet and Its Present Condition]', *Cesky lid*, 49 (1962), pp. 1–8.

Stastná, Jarmila, 'Navrh na vyber témat pro Národopisny atlas CSSR lidová strava', [Themes for the Ethnographical Atlas CSFR – Folk Food] *Vestnik NSC* (1966a), pp. 1–2, 35.

Stastná, Jarmila, 'Vysledky dotazníkové akce k lidové strave [Results of the Survey about Folk Food]', *Vestník NSC* (1966b), pp. 3–4, 47–55.

Stastná, Jarmila and V. Kyliánková, 'Strava horníku na Pribramsku ve druhé polovine 19. a na pocátku naseho století [The Diet of Miners in the Pribram Area in the Second Half of the 19th Century]', *Vlastivedny sborník Podbrdska*, 8–9 (1974–75), pp. 286–311.

Stastná, Jarmila, 'Nákupy, zpusoby stravování a strava prazského delnictva [Purchases, Way of Life and Food of Workers in Prague]' *AII Etnografie prazského delnictva. Maketa sv. III* (Prague, 1975a), pp. 103–240.

Stastná, Jarmila, *Prazské delnické potravní spolky ve druhé polovine 19. století [The Alimentary Associations of Workers in Prague during the Second Half of the 19th Century]* (Prague, 1975b).

Stastná, Jarmila, *K nekterym vysledkum studia stravy prazského delnictva [On the Nutrition Research of Workers in Prague]* (Prague, 1977).

Stastná, Jarmila., 'K vyzkumu stravy na Pribramsku [On the Nutrition Research in the Pribram Area]', *Vlastivedny sborník Podbrdska*, 13 (1978), pp. 93–95.

Stastná, Jarmila, 'Poddanské povinnosti ve vztahu ke strave venkovského obyvatelstva Cech (konec 18. a první polovina 19. století) [Duties of Vassals and Folk Food in Bohemia at the End of the 18th and during the First Half of the 19th Century]', *Cesky lid*, 68 (1981a), pp. 145–55.

Stastná, Jarmila, 'Strava a stravování prazskych delníku [The Diet of Workers in Prague]', in A. Robek *et al.* (eds), *Stará delnická Praha* (1981b), pp. 183–216.

Stastná, Jarmila, 'Strava venkovského a mestského obyvatelstva Cech koncem 18. a v první polovine 19. století a její sociální diferenciace [The Diet of the Urban and Rural Population of Bohemia and Their Social Differences at the End of the 18th and during the First Half of the 19th Century]' in *Lid a lidová kultura národního obrození* (Prague, 1983), pp. 157–65.

Stastná, Jarmila, 'Prostredky ke zmírnení bídy a hladu obyvatel na Vysocku v padesátych letech 19. století [The Means for Mitigating Hunger and Want in Vysocko Area in the 1850's]', *Zpravodaj koordinované síte vedeckych informací*, 2 (1985), pp. 100–9.

Stastná, Jarmila and Ludmila Pracharova, *Lidové pecivo v Cechách a na Morave [Folk Pastry in Bohemia and Moravia]* (Prague, 1988).

Stekl, Josef, *O vyzive cloveka zdravého a nemocného [On the Diet of Healthy and Ill People]* (Prague, 1914).

Stika, J., *Lidová strava na Valassku [Folk Diet in Walachia-Moravia]* (Ostrava, 1980).

Stoklasa, Julius, *Vyziva obyvatelstva ve válce [The Diet of the People During the War]* (Prague, 1916).

Stolniceni a vytvarné umeni peti staleti (exhibition in Nelahozeves, 1988).
Stránská, Drahomíra, 'Poslední kurloky na Tesínsku [The Last "kurloky" in Tesín Area]', *Slezsky sbornik*, 45 (1947), pp. 16–32, 234–42.
Teply, Frantisek, *Príspevky k dejinám ceského zemedelství [Contributions to the History of Czech Agriculture]* (Prague, 1926).
Tesar, F., *Technicky vyvoj ceského pivovarnictví [Technical Development of Czech Brewing]* (Prague, 1940).
Tobolková-Kotíková, Zuzana, *Prostreny stul a jeho dejiny [The Set Table and its History]* (Prague, 1949).
Ulehlová-Tilschová, Marie *Vyziva ve svetle veku [Diet and its Characteristics in that Time]* (Prague, 1944).
Ulehlová-Tilschová, Marie, *Ceská strava lidová [Bohemian Folk Diet]* (Prague, 1945).
Ulehlová-Tilschová, Marie, *Vyzivnost a hygiena potravin [Nutritive Value and Hygienic Condition of Food]* (Prague, 1947).
Ulehlová-Tilschová, Marie, *Varíme úcelne pro zdravé a nemocné [We Cook Appropriately for Healthy and Ill People]* (Prague, 1953).
Ulehlová-Tilschová, Marie, *Chutovy mistopis [Topography of Taste]* (Prague, 1970).
Usnesení strany a vlády o opatreních v zemedelské vyrobe, vykupu, masném prumyslu a obchodu ke zlepsení zásobování obyvatelstva masem a masnymi vyrobky v roce 1953 [Decision of Party and Government on steps in Agricultural Production, Meat Industry and in Improving the Trade of Supplying People with Meat and Meat Products in 1953] (Prague, 1953).
Vareka, Josef, 'Poslední dum s polodymnou jizbou na Moravskoslezském pomezí [The Last House with a Fire Place Without Flue on the Border of Moravia and Silesia]', *Národopisné aktuality*, 8 (1971), pp. 109–23.
Venzmer, Gerhard, *Tvé zdraví a vitaminy [Your Health and Your Vitamins]* (Prague, 1940).
Vetvicka, Milos and Vladimír Sorm, *Dejiny druzstevního hnutí. 1 - Spotrební druzstevnictví [History of the Cooperative Society Movement, 1. Consumer Cooperative Societies]* (Prague, 1959).
Vilikovsky, Václav, *Dejiny zemedelského prumyslu v Ceskoslovensku od nejstarsích dob do vypuknutí svetové krize hospodarské [History of Agricultural Industry in Czechoslovakia from the Beginning to the Outbreak of International Economic Crisis]* (Prague, 1936).
Viskup, Pavel, *Lékar kucharem [A Doctor is Cooking]* (Prague, 1934).
Vyziva lidu. Casopis spolecnosti pro racionální vyzivu [Folk Diet. Journal of the Association for Rational Diet] (Prague, 1946ff.).
Vlcek, Karel, *Vyvoj druzstevního mlékarství [Development of Cooperative Milk Production]* (Brno, 1947).
Vlk, Miloslav, 'O slechtickych jídelních souborech [Table Sets of the Nobility]', *Umení a remesla*, 85 (1985), pp. 47–51.
Vlk, Miloslav and Jan Assmann, *Stolniceni a vytvarné umeni peti staleti [Tables and the Plastic Arts of Five Centuries]* (Nelahozeves, 1988).
Vokácová, Vera, 'Prostreny stul [The Set Table]', *Tvar*, 15 (1964), pp. 138–54.
Vokácová, Vera, *Noze, lzíce, vidlicky ze sbírek Umeleckoprumyslového muzea v Praze [Knives, Forks and Spoons in the collections of the Museum of Art and Industry in Prague]* (Prague, 1981).
Vollgruber, F. E., *Vom Essen und vom Trinken [On Eating and Drinking]* (Prague, 1906).
Vonka, Rudolf Jordan, *Od hroudy k chlebu [From Clod to Bread]* (Prague, 1939).
Vrabec, Vilém, *Studená kuchyne [Cold Cuisine]* (Prague, 1942).
Vrabec, Vilém, *Teplá kuchyne [Warm Cuisine]* (Prague, 1943).

Vyziva a rozvrh dne [Diet in the Day's Time Table], Sborník referatu z 12. celostátního sjezdu Spolecnosti pro racionální vyzivu (Prague, 1962).

Wiesner, J., *O vyzive v hospodarském roce 1947–48 [On diet in the Financial year 1947/48]* (Prague, 1948).

Winter, Zikmund, *Zac bylo zivobytí za starodávna? [How much Were the Costs of Living in the Past?]* (Prague, 1888).

Winter, Zikmund, *Kuchyne a stul nasich predku [Cuisine and Table of our Ancestors]* (Prague, 1892).

Winter, Zikmund, *Remeslnictvo a zivnosti 16. veku v Cechách [The Business of the Craftsmen and Trade in Bohemia in the 16th Century]* (Prague, 1909).

Winter, Zikmund, *Sat, strava a lékar v XV. a XVI. veku [Clothing, Diet and the Physician in the 15th and 16th Century]* (Prague, 1913).

Wünschová, F., 'Spisovatelka a kucharka [The Woman as Author and Cook]', in M. D. Rettigová (ed.) *Domácí kucharka* (Prague, 1986), pp. 9–32.

Zácek, Zdenek, *Vune korení [Aroma of Spices]* (Prague, 1974).

Zácek, Zdenek, *Nad sálkem plnym vune [A Cup of Aroma]* (Prague, 1977).

Záhlava, Frantisek, *Intenzívní reprodukce zdroju vyzivy [Intensive Reproduction of Food Sources]* (Prague, 1987).

Zástera, Karel, 'Jídelní lístky lidu ceského za doby hladu a bídy [Czech Folk Menus in the Time of Hunger and Want]', *Cesky lid*, 11 (1902), pp. 130–2.

Zeman, A., *K historii plzenskych pivovaru [History of the Breweries in Pilsen]* (Plzen, 1959).

Zíbrt, Cenek, *Poctivé mravy a spolecenské rády pri jídle a pití po rozumu starych Cechuv [Manners and Social Orders of Eating and Drinking]* (Prague, 1890).

Zíbrt, Cenek, *Z dejin piva a pivovarnictví v zemích ceskych [On the History of Beer and Brewing in the Czech Countries]* (Prague, 1894).

Zíbrt, Cenek, 'Lidová kuchyne a kucharství staroceské [Old Bohemian Art of Cooking and Cuisine]', *Cesky lid*, 16 (1907), pp. 167–72.

Zíbrt, Cenek, 'Vavákova zpráva o zemskych jablkách z roku 1771 [Vavak's Report on Potatoes from 1771]', *Cesky lid*, 19 (1910) pp. 304ff.

Zíbrt, Cenek, 'Slovanské kyselice [A Slavonic Dish "kyselice"]', *Cesky lid* 29 (1914), pp. 91–4.

Zíbrt, Cenek, *Starocesky perník [Old Bohemian Ginger-Bread]* (Karlín, 1916).

Zíbrt, Cenek, *Ceská kuchyne za dob nedostatku pred sto lety [Bohemian Cuisine in the Time of Want one Hundred Years Ago]* (Prague, 1917).

Zíbrt, Cenek, *Polské Kuchmistrzostwo prekladem staroceského kucharství Pavla Severina z r.1535 [The Polish Cookery Book "Kuchmistrzostwo" – a Translation of Pavel Severin's old Bohemian Cookery Book]* (Lvov, 1926).

Zíbrt, Cenek, *Staroceské umení kucharské [Old Bohemian Art of Cooking]* (Prague, 1927).

'Zpráva o porusování potravin v nasem mocnárství od 1. září 1898 do 31. srpna 1899 [Report on Food Adulterations in our Monarchy from 1st September 1898 to 31 August 1899]', *Casopis chemicky*, 10 (1900), p. 130.

15 Nutritional needs and social esteem: two aspects of diet in Sweden during the 18th and 19th centuries

Mats Essemyr

Introduction

Like many elements of everyday life food consumption changed remarkably after the Industrial Revolution. The traditional ways in which people were fed, clothed, housed and put to work gave way to modern ones. Industrialization affected people's living conditions as no other event had ever done before.

The importance of the industrial (and closely connected agrarian) revolution has to be seen not only in relation to quantities – to how the economic growth is created – but also in relation to the qualitative new situation that emerged from it. Using Fernand Braudel's concept, the slow-moving sphere of everyday life, which had remained more or less unaffected since the end of medieval times, gave way to a new qualitative situation.[1] In general, economic historians today are reluctant to use the term 'revolution', since it presupposes a quick and sudden change. Instead, we now look at the industrial and agrarian revolution as a stepwise transformation over a long period of time.[2] Yet even if the alteration of diet in many cases took half a century or more, it must be reckoned as a rapid and profound change in comparison to dietary changes in earlier periods.

This perspective seems to be valid for most European countries and regions. Although industrial transformation did not happen at the same time in all countries it had in all cases a deep influence on diet by the time it took effect. In England important dietary changes took place during the first part of the 19th century.[3] In Sweden, the industrial transformation occurred between 1880 and 1914, thus affecting diet in many ways.

Still, in posing this framework it does not follow that nothing of interest happened during the pre-industrial period. Rather, it raises two main questions which I will tackle, using recent research results on the historical development of food consumption in Sweden.

First, we certainly find major economic and social changes during the period prior to industrial transformation. In Sweden, the period 1720–1850 can be regarded as the time when important preconditions for industrial take-off were established. Population grew and was subject to economic and social stratification, creating a rural proletariat, which later became the industrial working class.[4] Capital formation took place, not only within the early industries, but also among the yeomanry in the agrarian sector, enabling an increase in investment to take place.[5] Natural resources, wood and iron, were much more extensively used. During the first part of the 19th century, new models of organization and technology for industrial and agrarian production were adopted from abroad. Hence Swedish society was not the same in 1870 as it had been in 1720. If we can show that no fundamental change in diet occurred during this period, we must examine the factors that made the dietary system so stable during pre-industrial times.

Second, if we can show that diet in Sweden, after the establishment of industrial society, had gone through structural changes, we have to discuss the factors involved in this process. This means we have to pick out some explanatory factors describing the differences between industrial and pre-industrial production and consumption systems.

Supply and Demand, 1720–1914: A Macro-Perspective

As in most European countries, reliable figures on aggregate agricultural production in Sweden in earlier times are lacking. However, various limited studies indicate a growth of cereal production from the beginning of the 18th century.[6] At least up to 1820, this was to a great extent due to a transition from pasture to arable land.[7] The cultivation of barley and especially rye increased steadily during the 18th century, as the number of cattle decreased due to fodder shortage. The increase in total aggregate food supply might therefore have been somewhat smaller than the increase in cereal production.

From the first decades of the 19th century, Sweden became a net exporter of grain, especially of oats.[8] The enclosure movement, together with improvements in agricultural techniques, caused the productivity of cereal production to rise. Although the transition from pasture to arable land continued during the first part of the 18th century, the growth of cereal production seems to have increased more than animal production decreased. In the 1820s and 1830s the cultivation of potatoes spread rapidly over the country. As in many other countries, the crop had been introduced much earlier as a horticultural product. The crop seems to have encountered massive resistance among the common folk during the 18th century. It was not until the severe crop failures in the 1770s and 1790s that this resistance was to some extent broken.[9] Still, in the first phase of the expansion, potatoes were used mainly for distilling purposes. When domestic distilling was prohibited in 1855, the advantages of the crop had been so widely recognized that production continued to grow rapidly, but now for the purpose of direct consumption.

From the 1870s to 1914 animal production grew steadily. Not only did the number of cattle and pigs grow, increasing the production of beef and pork, but the production of dairy products also reached higher yields. This was mainly due to an

Figure 15.1 Population growth in Sweden pro mille, 1749–1914 (per 7-year moving averages)
Source: *Historical Statistics of Sweden*, ed. National Central Bureau of Statistics, part 1 (Stockholm, 1969), Table 28.

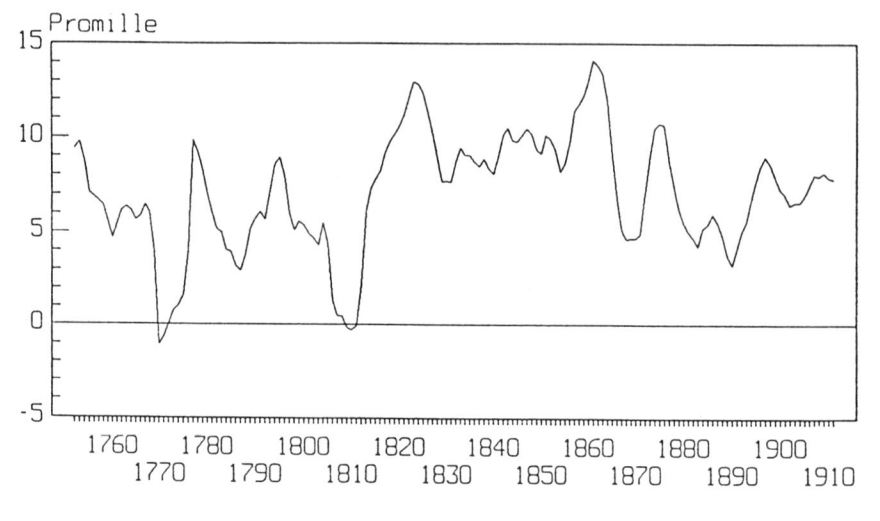

intensification of agricultural production. As the property rights system and labour organization in agriculture had been settled, technical improvements now could be adopted more easily. The growing use of artificial fertilizers and the transition to cultivation of fodder crops instead of pasturing seem to be factors of great importance for the simultaneous growth of cereal production and cattle breeding. To some extent, artificial fertilizers reduced the dependence on manure in cereal production, and fodder cultivation gave more fodder per acre than using the land for pasture. Hence, both sides of agriculture production were now able to expand with fewer restrictions on each other.

The aggregate demand for food can be described by the development of population. The Swedish population is estimated to have been *c.* 1,760,000 people in 1749. In 1914 it amounted to 5,680,000.[10] During the course of the 18th and 19th centuries, there were considerable variations in annual growth rates, as can be seen in Figure 15.1.

Up to 1810, annual variations were very marked. They were caused mainly by crop failures, diseases, and food shortages related to wartime conditions. Between 1810 and the mid-19th century, population growth was very strong. The population increased by *c.* 50% between 1810 and 1855. During the latter part of the 19th century and up to 1914, population growth was still at a high level, though the rate of growth slowed down remarkably, helped by two major periods of mass emigration (in the 1860s and 1880s).

As in most countries, the industrial transition in Sweden was preceded by a massive increase in population. This was more or less a precondition for the industrial transition. The historical problem is to understand how people were fed under pre-industrial conditions. This problem falls into two parts: first, what do we mean by 'fed', and second, what were the means of obtaining food?

Feeding People

'Man cannot live on bread alone' is an aphorism from the Bible which in its deeper meaning summarizes the concept of the necessities of life. Apart from daily bread, which symbolizes the nutritional needs of human beings, man will always have a desire for culture and social recognition. But it can be easily shown that bread, and food items in general, have not only nutritional but also cultural and social aspects. The nutritional aspects of food are more or less a question of the content of nutritional elements necessary to survive, such as energy, protein, fats, carbohydrates, vitamins and minerals. Every food item can be reduced to these elements. Hence, in this respect the problem of feeding people is a problem of producing and consuming enough of these nutritional elements as determined by the nutritional needs of the population.

However, one does not eat nutritional elements, but specific food items. In this respect diet is not only a matter of the arithmetic of calories but also a social and cultural view of food items. It can be shown that food items essentially are defined in a social context. Studies in ethnology and ethnography have shown that consumption of nettles and bark in earlier times was restricted to periods of severe food shortage. Although they do contain nutritional elements these items were regarded as emergency food, to be considered separately from normal food. Also, meat from dogs and horses seems to have been rejected by the majority of the people as a result of popular conceptions.[11]

Yet feelings related to diet seem to be relevant not only for such extraordinary items. It is not difficult to find evidence for divergences in the social esteem of items of normal food. The hostility towards the potato in the 18th and 19th centuries is an outstanding example. In Sweden, as in Britain, the drive towards the substitution of bread for potatoes led to vociferous protests among the population.[12] People obviously looked upon bread cereals as better food than potatoes.

I think that these differences in the esteem attached to food items were valid for many of the commonly used foodstuffs in earlier times. Altogether it can be looked upon as a structure of stratification of food items. Its historical relevance is shown by the general trends in relative prices and real wages. During periods of increased real wages such as the late Middle Ages, the 17th century and the period after 1850, the decline in prices for animal foodstuffs was less sharp than for vegetable ones. Within each group we can see the same tendency: the decline in meat and butter prices was less sharp than the decline in prices of fish, for example, and hence wheat prices were more stable than potato prices.[13] It has also been shown that households with higher incomes have a tendency to greater consumption of 'luxury' goods, which are not entirely necessary to stay alive.[14] Therefore, it seems to be a general

Table 15.1 Daily per-capita energy intake among agricultural workers in Sweden, 16th to 18th centuries

Century	Energy intake original	revised
16th	4837	4171
17th	3304	3523
18th	3978	3980

Source: Morell (1986), p. 11 (original revised).

truth that ,when they are able to do so, people tend to escape from the arithmetic of calories and use more of their resources to satisfy needs arising from the social and cultural approaches to diet. To conclude, the problem of feeding people is a problem of balancing between what is needed and what is wanted. These tasks have not always been solved simultaneously.

The arithmetics of calories

From this point I will present results concerning the nutritional standards of various groups of the Swedish population in the 18th and 19th centuries. The groups are agricultural workers, hospital inmates, iron-work labourers and sawmill workers.

Agricultural workers

As early as in the 1930s Eli Heckscher presented estimates of the calorie intake among the Swedish rural labour class in the 18th and early 19th centuries. Based on records of payments in kind on a large number of estates, he calculated the consumption of groups of female and male domestic servants. The energy intake was between 3200 and 4500 kcal per day per consumption unit (c.u.), from which $c.10\%$ came from animal food items. A consumption unit refers to the average consumption of males between the age of 15 and 65. The calorie intake was somewhat higher than in the 17th century, but much lower compared with the 'barbaric prosperity' of the 16th century. On the other hand, the proportion of calorie intake accounted for by animal products is supposed to have fallen during the course of the early modern period.

The latest critics of Heckscher have revised his figures substantially. Morell has shown that Heckscher's conversions of the old Swedish measures were based on incorrect factors. This led to an overestimation of consumption in the 16th century and to an underestimation of consumption in the 17th and 18th centuries. Although the share of animal products is likely to have decreased as a long-term phenomenon, the differences in the absolute level of calorie intake were below what Heckscher suggested (see Table 15.1).[15]

Nutritional needs and social esteem: two aspects of diet in Sweden 261

Figure 15.2 Enköping Hospital, 1759–81: per-capita energy intake (kcal per day)
Source: Morell (1987), p. 207.

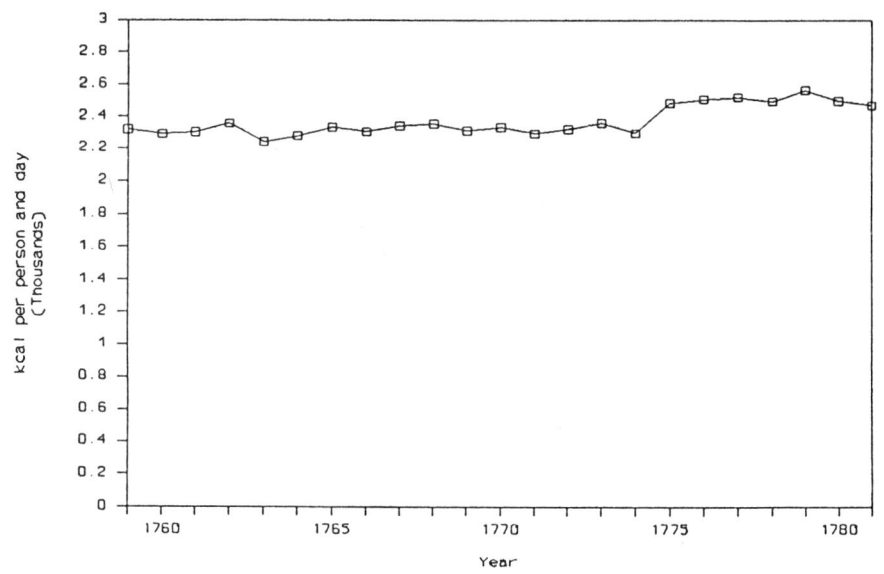

Modern recommendations of energy intake for males doing work with normal intensity are *c*.3,000 kcal per day. As agricultural work must have been more intense, the energy intake among the peasants in Sweden seems to have been on a par with what they needed.

Hospital Inmates [15]

In his dissertation Morell presents very long-term series on food consumption at four 'hospitals' in Sweden. These institutions were not hospitals in the modern sense of the word, but rather lodgings for paupers, people incapable of work, and the infirm and elderly. Supported by the central government, the hospitals became an integrated part of the general policy against pauperism. The hospitals under examination were all located in central Sweden, a region dominated mainly by agriculture and to some extent by forestry and metalworking.

As the hospitals used communal feeding it has been possible to produce dietary and nutritional figures at an individual level. In the following, we shall focus on the energy and protein intake.

At the hospital in Enköping during the latter part of the 18th century the energy intake was between 2,200 and 2,500 kcal per day (Figure 15.2) and daily protein intake 75–90 g (Figure 15.3). Apart from a minor increase in the 1770s, the trend was stable during the whole period.

Developments at the hospital in Falun follow the same pattern. Between 1659 and 1750, daily energy intake was about 1500–2500 kcal (Figure 15.4) and daily protein

Figure 15.3 Enköping Hospital, 1759–81: per-capita protein intake (g per day)
Source: Morell (1987), p. 215.

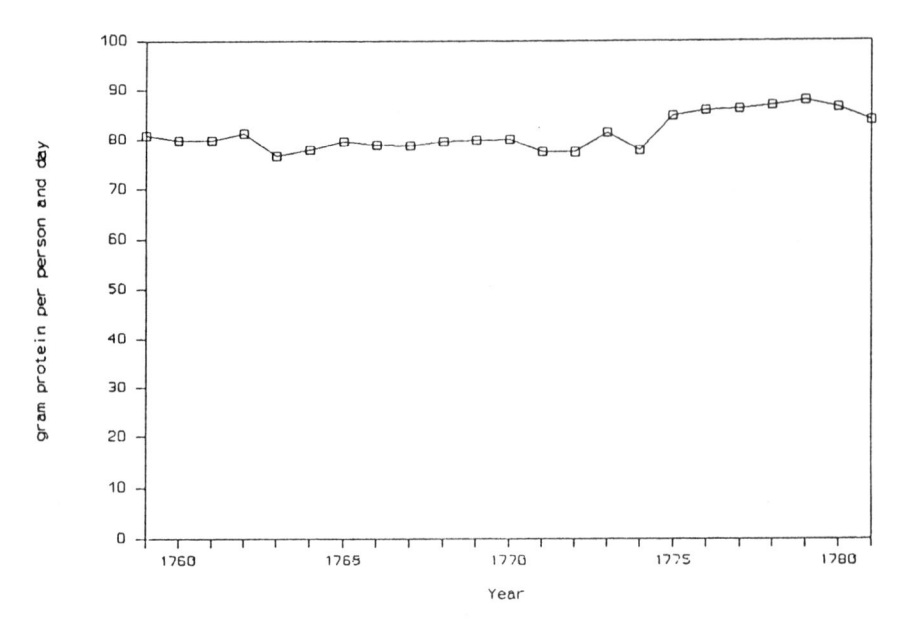

Figure 15.4 Falun hospital, 1659–1750: Per-capita energy intake (kcal. per day)
Source: Morell (1987), pp. 208-9.

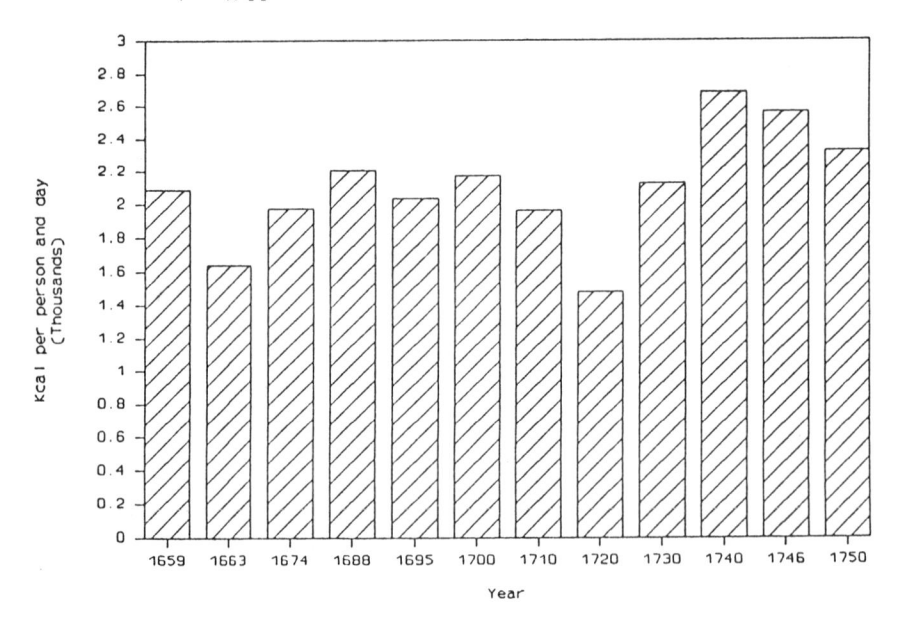

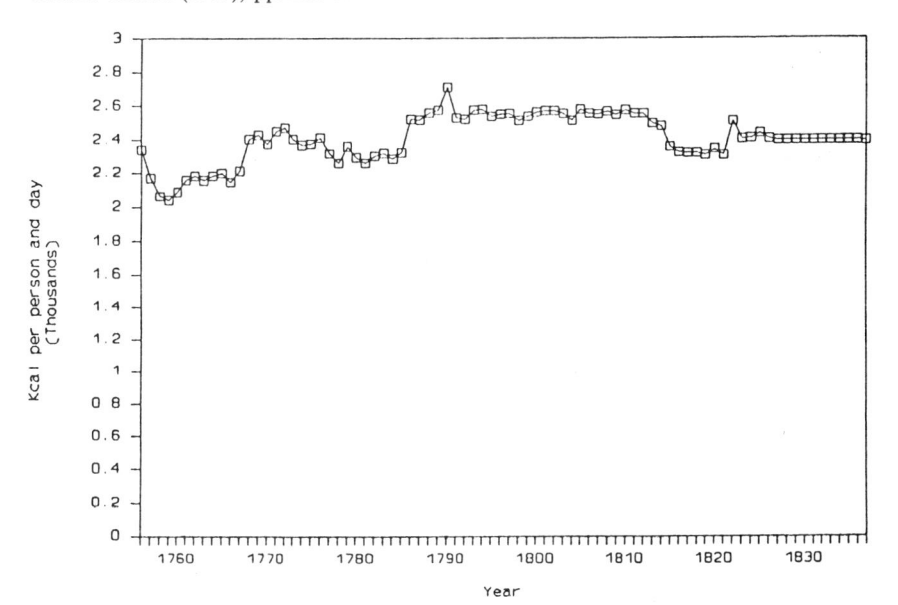

Nutritional needs and social esteem: two aspects of diet in Sweden 263

Figure 15.5 Falun hospital, 1659–1750: Per-capita protein intake (g per day)
Source: Morell (1987), pp. 216-17.

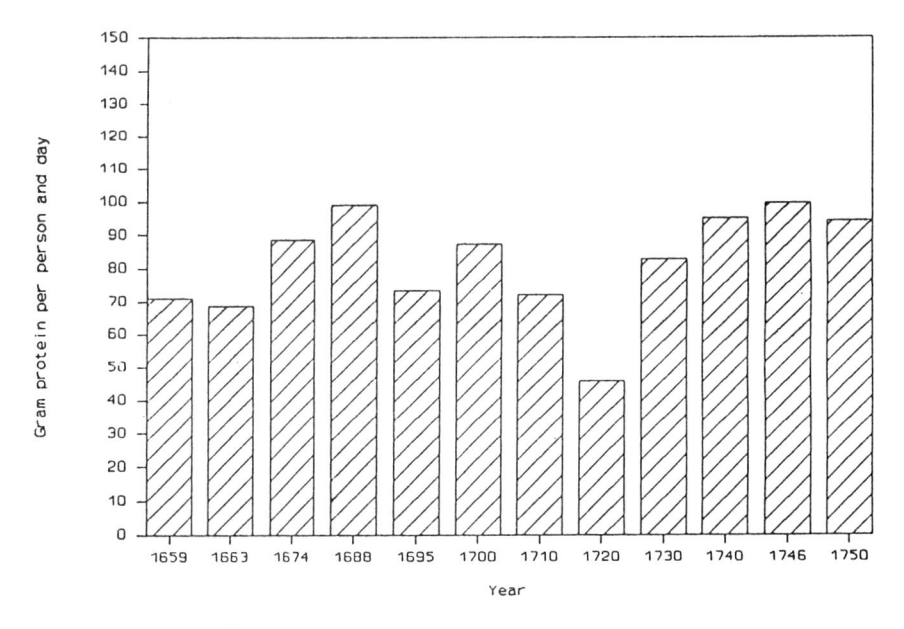

Figure 15.6 Falun hospital, 1756–1837: Per-capita energy intake (kcal per day)
Source: Morell (1987), pp. 208-9.

Figure 15.7 Falun hospital, 1756–1837: Per-capita protein intake (g per day)
Source: Morell (1987), pp. 216-217.

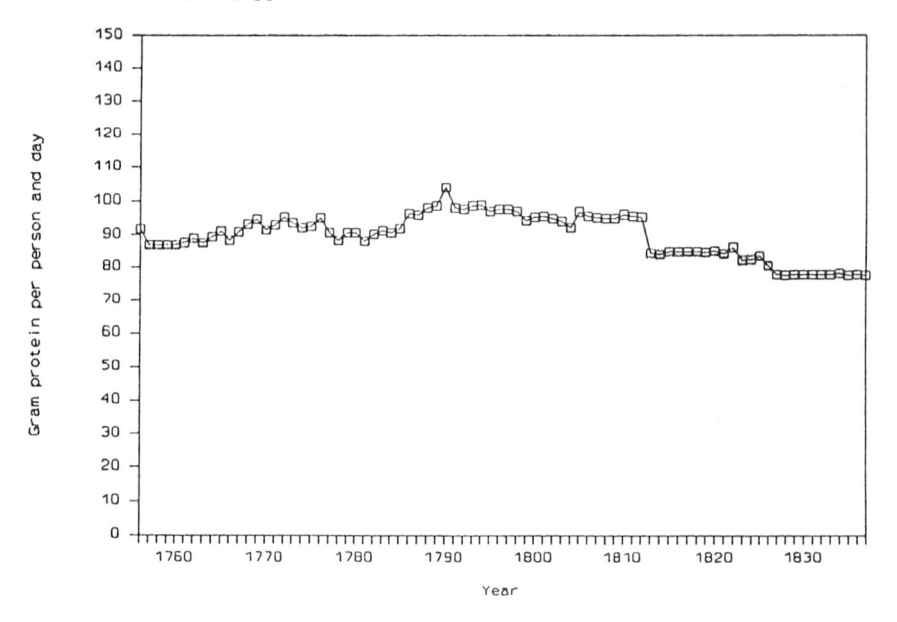

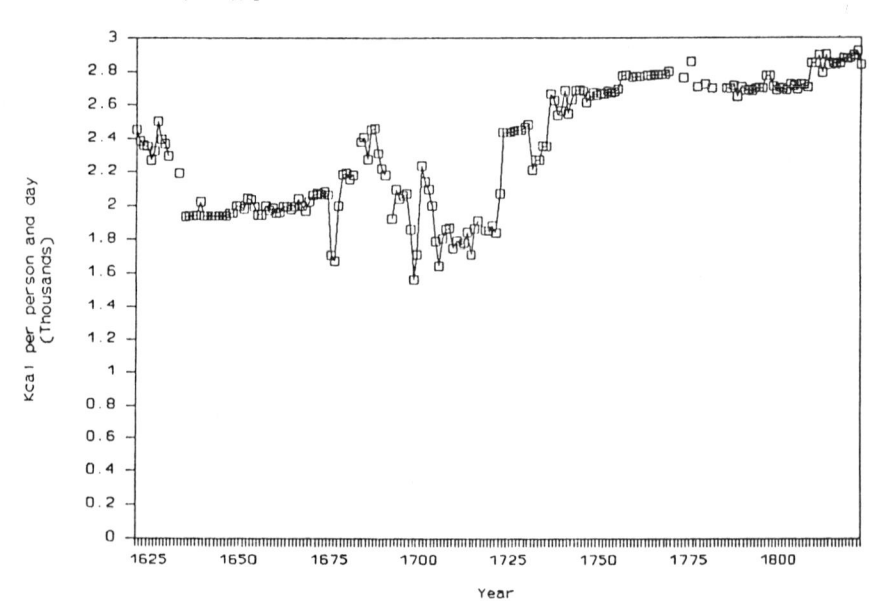

Figure 15.8 Västerås hospital, 1621–1823: Per-capita energy intake (kcal per day)
Source: Morell (1987), p. 211.

Nutritional needs and social esteem: two aspects of diet in Sweden 265

Figure 15.9 Västerås hospital, 1621–1823: Per-capita protein intake (g per day)
Source: Morell (1987), p. 220.

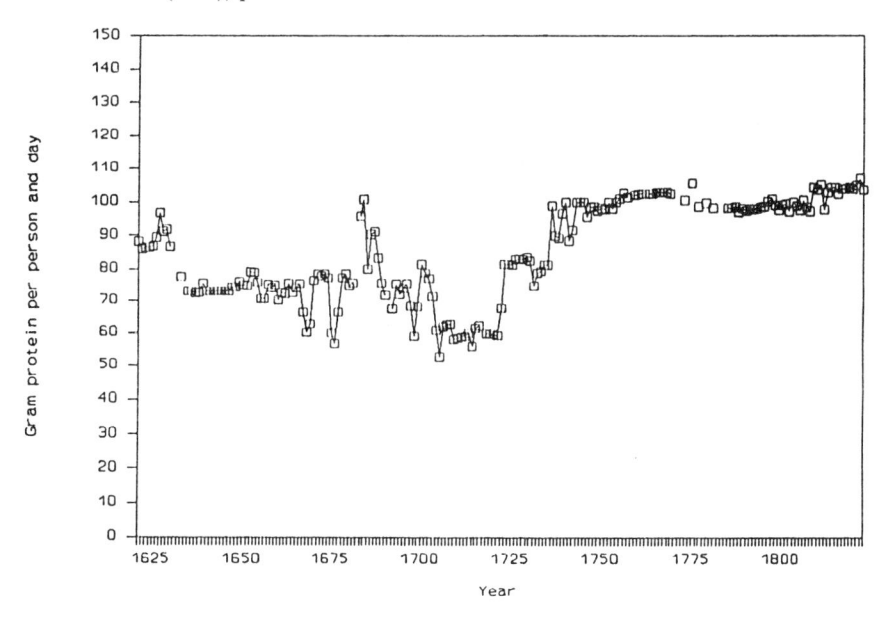

Figure 15.10 Weckholm hospital, 1696–1872: Per-capita energy intake (kcal per day)
Source: Morell (1987), p. 210.

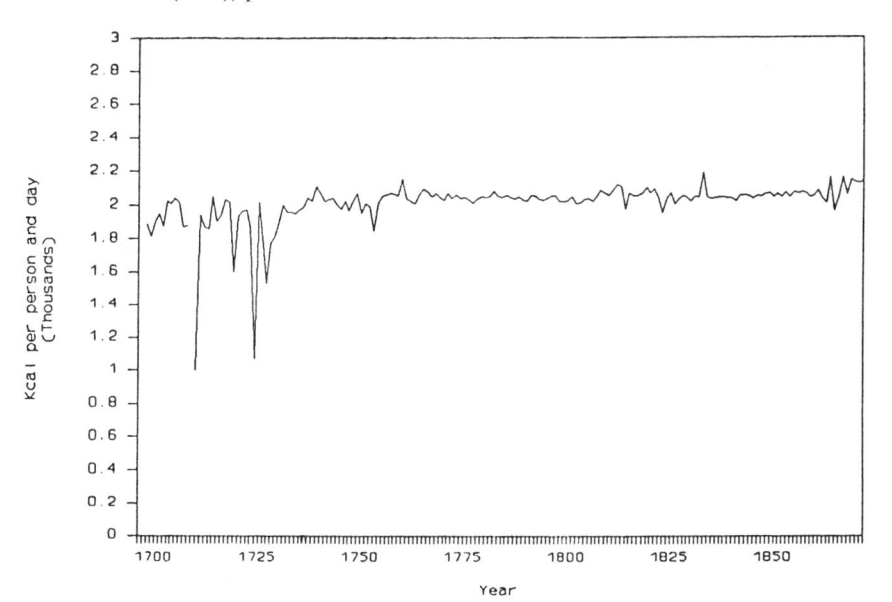

Figure 15.11 Weckholm hospital, 1696–1872: Per-capita protein intake (g per day)
Source: Morell (1987), p. 210.

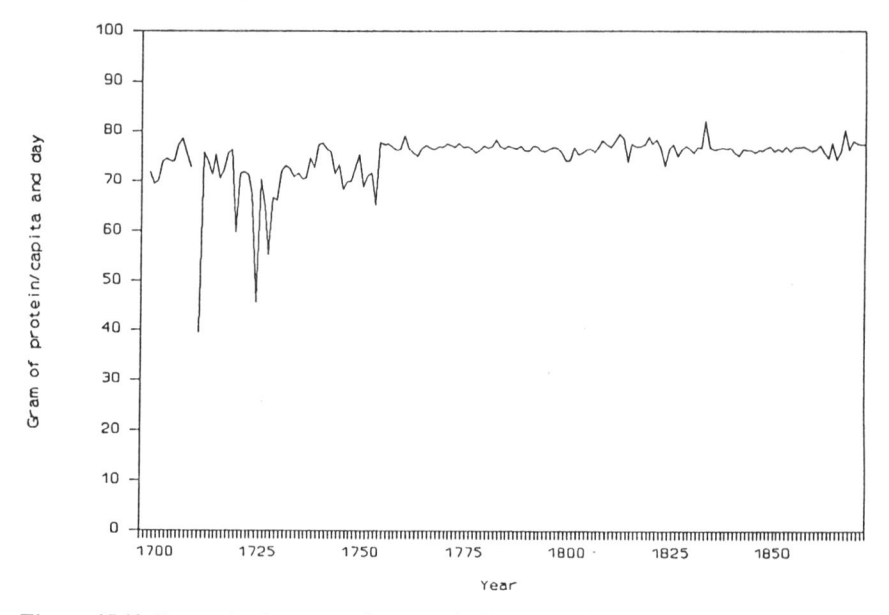

Figure 15.12 Energy intake among forgemen in Forsmarks bruk, 1730–1880 (kcal per day)
Source: Essemyr (1988), p. 144.

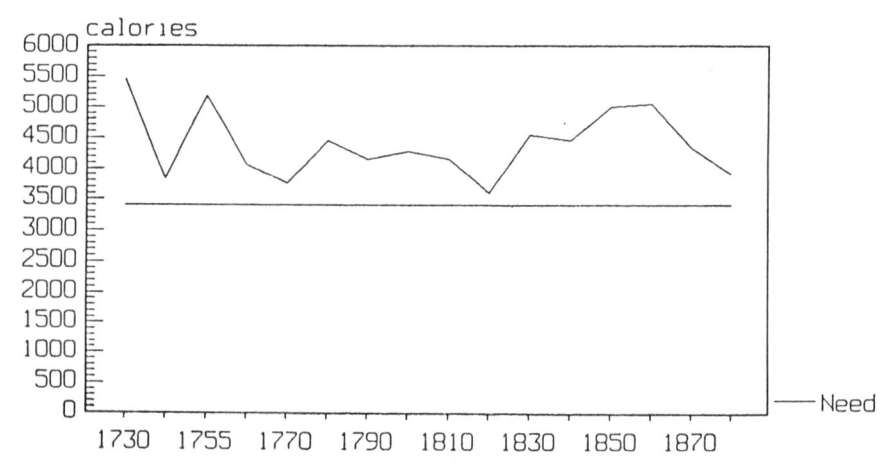

intake about 50–100 g (Figure 15.5). The lowest figures relate to the 1720s, a period of severe food shortage in Sweden. During the latter part of the 18th century and up to 1837, the situation became somewhat better, daily energy intake lying between 2000 and 2700 kcal (Figure 15.6) and daily protein intake between 80–110 g (Figure 15.7). On the whole, though, levels did not vary substantially.

At the hospital in Västerås, daily energy intake seems to have been around 2000

Figure 15.13 Protein intake among forgemen in Forsmarks bruk, 1730–1880 (g per day)
Source: Essemyr (1988), p. 148.

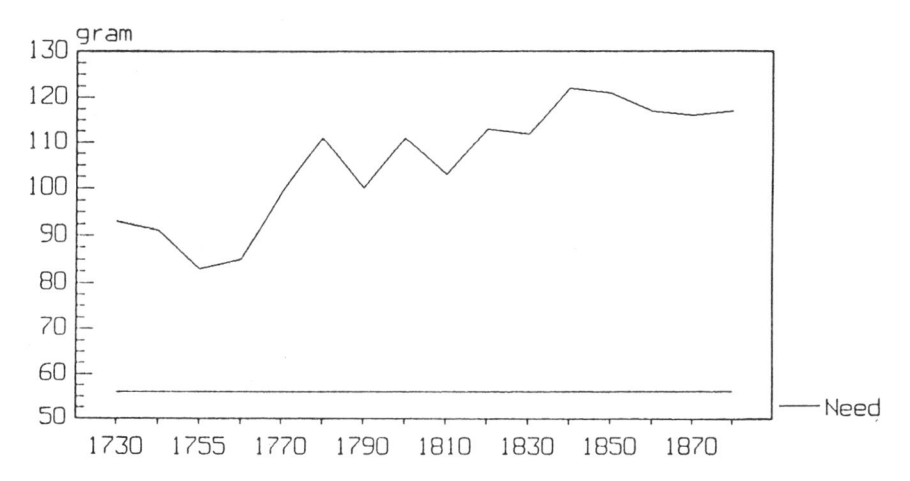

kcal during the early years of the 17th century (Figure 15.8). Protein intake was just over 70 g (Figure 15.9). From the last years of that century and up to 1725, we can see a decline, energy intake falling to $c.1500$ kcal and protein to $c.50$ g. During the following 25 years, both energy and protein reached higher levels, 2,800 kcal and 100 g protein. These levels are sustained for the rest of the period.

The figures for the hospital at Weckholm confirm a state of severe food crisis in the first decades of the 18th century. During two distinct years daily energy and protein intake fell to levels around 1,000 kcal and 40 g respectively (Figures 15.10 and 15.11). However, apart from these years the trends were remarkably stable. Up to the 1870s, daily energy intake was around 2,000 kcal and protein intake around 80 g.

Despite the very long timespan and the differences in the ways in which the hospitals were supplied with food, energy and protein intake per capita were nearly the same level at all four locations and for most of the period. In general, the energy intake seems to have been between 2,000–2,400 kcal/day and the protein intake between 70–100 g/day.

It would of course be of great interest to compare these figures of the actual intake with estimations of the energy and protein needs of the hospital inmates. Although it is impossible to give accurate levels of needs, as they are highly individual, Morell estimates the energy need to have been mainly that of older women who carried out no or just a limited amount of work; thus, these estimates seem fair enough. Hence the study suggests that the inmates' nutritional standard in general was satisfactory during the course of the 18th and 19th centuries, at least in terms of energy and protein. Apart from the food crisis in the 1720s food consumption managed to satisfy needs.

Iron-work Labourers[16]

A group that has received particular interest from Swedish economic historians are the iron-work labourers. Although few in number in relation to other groups, they were of significant importance for the development of Swedish industry and export. Built up mainly for wartime purposes during the Thirty Years War, the iron-work industry was transformed into an export industry during the 18th century, producing much of Europe's bar-iron. The plants were mainly located in central Sweden, close to ore resources, water, wood for fuel, and ports. It was an early rural industry, depending heavily on local resources and a loyal group of skilled workers. The iron-works referred to in the following was a traditional vallon iron-works located in Forsmark.

In comparison with the hospital inmates, iron-work labourers were all men who performed extremely hard work. The working day lasted twelve hours, giving them an extremely high energy need. Taking into account the periods when easier or no work was carried out, daily energy needs among the forgemen are estimated to have been 4100–4900 kcal. Daily protein needs, which depend mainly on body weight, are estimated at 60 g.

We can see from Figure 15.12 that, though energy intake sometimes fell below the level of minimum needs, it was in general satisfactory. As far as protein intake is concerned, it not only exceeded the need by far, it also increased steadily from the mid-18th century to the end of the 19th century (Figure 15.13).

As for the other two groups, the conclusion is that the iron-work labourers' food consumption in general was good enough to satisfy their nutritional needs, at least as far as energy and protein are concerned.

Sawmill workers

The timber industry, located along the coast in northern Sweden, expanded rapidly during the second part of the 19th century. As demand grew from countries which had industrialized earlier, such as Britain, and from domestic urban regions, production of sawn timber increased fourfold between 1860 and 1890. Consequently, a modern industrial proletariat was formed within the industry. It had but few similarities with the socially and economically stratified working class of the iron-works. The sawmill workers were to a great extent a socio-economically homogeneous group, and their formation was caused mainly by the modern industrial transition. For methodological reasons, it is not possible to present any time series on the development of energy and protein intake among the sawmill workers. Instead, their consumption is given for single years (Table 15.2). Information is given for two different plants.

We can see that energy supply was low in the 19th century, especially given the hard work that the sawmill workers carried out, but clearly it was not at starvation levels. Also, it is highly probable that the figures do not cover all sources of food supply, and hence that the energy intake – at least for Kubikenborg in the 19th century – is somewhat underestimated.

Table 15.2 Daily per-capita energy intake among sawmill workers in Sweden

Plant	Year	Energy intake (kcal)
Stocka	1877	3,100
Kubikenborg	1881	2,617
Kubikenborg	1896	2,999
Kubikenborg	1899	2,887
Kubikenborg	1913	4,267

Sources: Fjellström (1986), Table 2-3 (Stocka); Cornell (1982), p. 282 (Kubikenborg)

Table 15.3. Daily per-capita energy and protein intake in Sweden, 1913–14, 1922 and 1933

Year	Group	Energy intake (kcal)	Protein intake (g)
1913–14	Worker	3,300	97
	Civil servant	3,200	94
1922	Forgeman	3,100	92
	Worker	3,900	114
	Civil servant	3,900	120
1933	Worker	3,500	95
	Civil servant	3,500	96
	Crofter	3,900	111

Source: Essemyr (1983), p. 2; Hirdman (1983), pp. 66–7.

20th century

In 1913–14 the Swedish Board of Health introduced regular household surveys which covered information about diet and food supply. This makes it possible to present some data concerning the prewar and interwar periods (Table 15.3).

As we can see, daily energy intake was between 3,100 and 3,900 kcal and protein intake between 90 and 120 g.

To conclude this presentation of research on nutritional standards in Sweden, two things seem obvious. First, the standard of nutrition was fairly good in the sense that food consumption fulfilled nutritional needs, at least with respect to energy and protein. It must be mentioned, however, that various studies indicate deficits of other nutritional elements, such as vitamin C and calcium. Second, apart from short-term food crises, the level of energy and protein intake did not change significantly between the pre- and post-industrial periods. Hence, one can ask if food consumption really was affected by industrialization at all, or if it remained as it had been. Let us look at the other side of the problem.

What was on the plates?

The question here is: what did people eat to reach this favourable standard of nutrition? Which types of food were consumed and in what quantities? By answering these questions, we can throw light on the problem of the development of the social esteem of the diet.

It is difficult to find any relevant measure for analysing this side of the problem. However, I will use the share of energy intake provided by animal products, together with more qualitative information about food items consumed, as indicators of social values related to diet.

Agricultural Workers

Heckscher's studies indicate a widespread consumption of animal products in the 16th century. Not only were different sorts of fish a common food on Swedish estates, but also vast quantities of meat and butter were consumed. These highly appreciated items were reduced sharply in quantity during the 17th and 18th centuries. Cereals such as rye and barley, used for baking and malting, replaced them as the staple diet. Although the consumption of herring increased substantially during the last decades of the 18th century, many of the highly esteemed food items had disappeared from the agricultural workers' plates after the 16th century. As a result, the share of energy intake provided by animal products declined gradually (Table 15.4).

Table 15.4 Percentage share of energy intake provided by animal products in the diet of Swedish agricultural workers, 16th-18th centuries

century	original	revised
16th	28.5	25.9
17th	14.2	3.2
18th	10.9	13.4

Source: Morell (1986), p. 11.

Hospital inmates

At the hospitals there was a marked trend towards less variety in the diet during the course of the 17th and 18th centuries. A lot of items, many of them animal products, disappeared from the diet. The previous fare consisting of fish, meat, offal and vegetables was transformed into a diet consisting mainly of porridge, rye bread, malt and Baltic herring. It has been shown that the average per-capita consumption from 1759 to 1781 at the four hospitals under investigation amounted to 318 kg of cereals, 43 kg of vegetables and root crops, 27 kg of meat including offal, 46 kg of fish, and hardly any milk and butter at all.[17]

Figure 15.14 Enköping hospital, 1759–1781: percentage share of energy intake provided by animal products (in kcal)
Source: Morell (1987), p. 187.

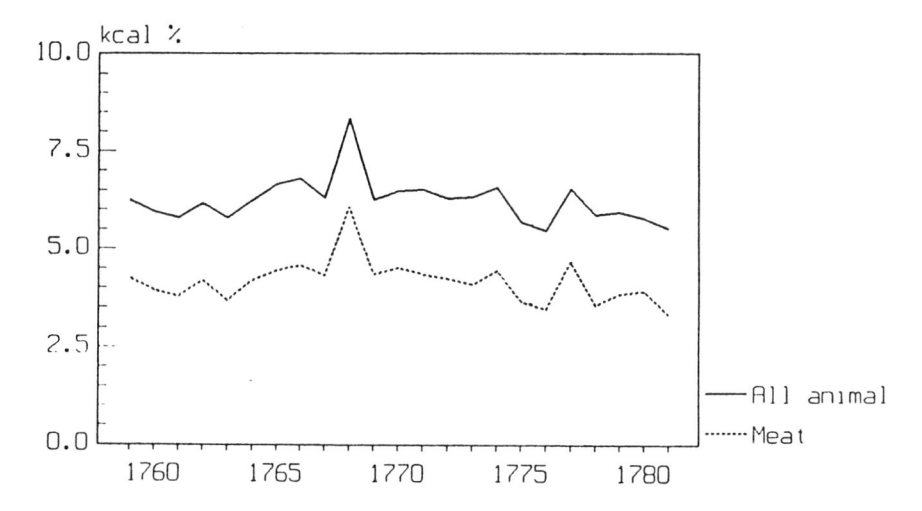

Figure 15.15 Falun hospital, 1756–1837: percentage share of energy intake provided by animal products (in kcal)
Source: Morell (1987), p. 190.

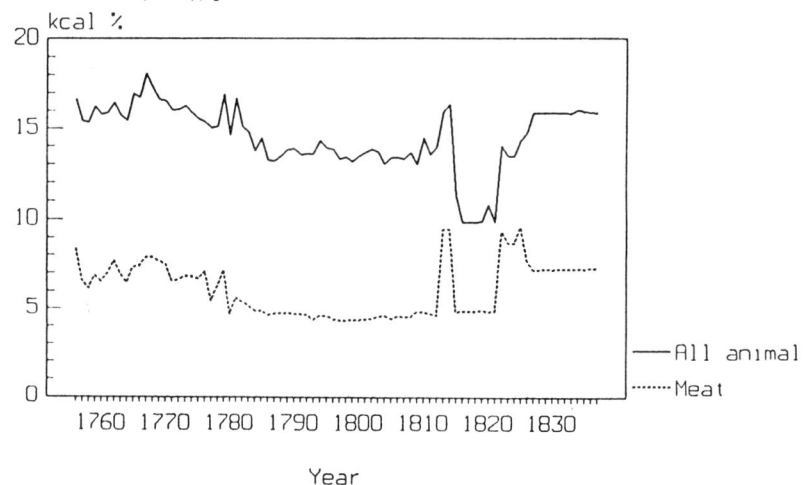

Although the figures are somewhat disparate, it can be seen from Figures 15.14–15.17 that there was a slight fall in the share of energy intake from animal products for those hospitals beginning at a high level. Also at those hospitals where meat had accounted for a large share of the total animal product intake, it went down much more quickly than at the other hospitals.

Figure 15.16 Weckholms hospital, 1696–1872: percentage share of energy intake provided by animal products
Source: Morell (1987), p. 192.

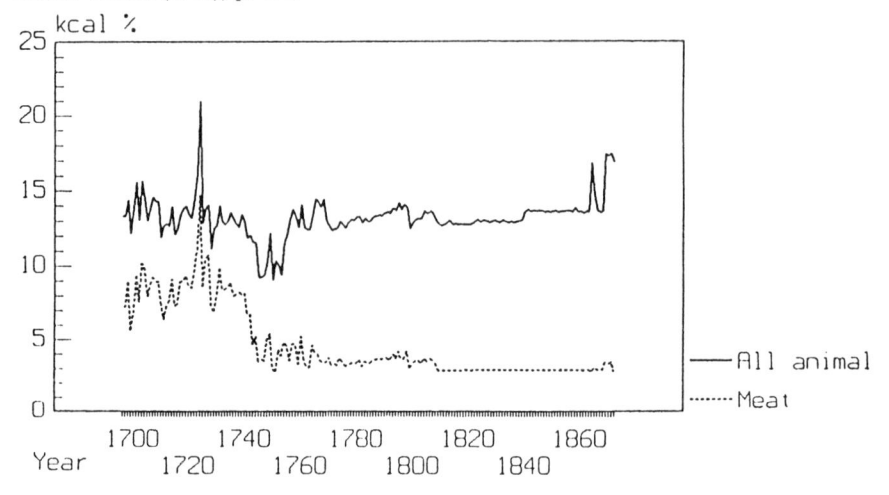

Figure 15.17 Västerås hospital, 1621–1823: percentage share of energy intake provided by animal products
Source: Morell (1987), p. 195.

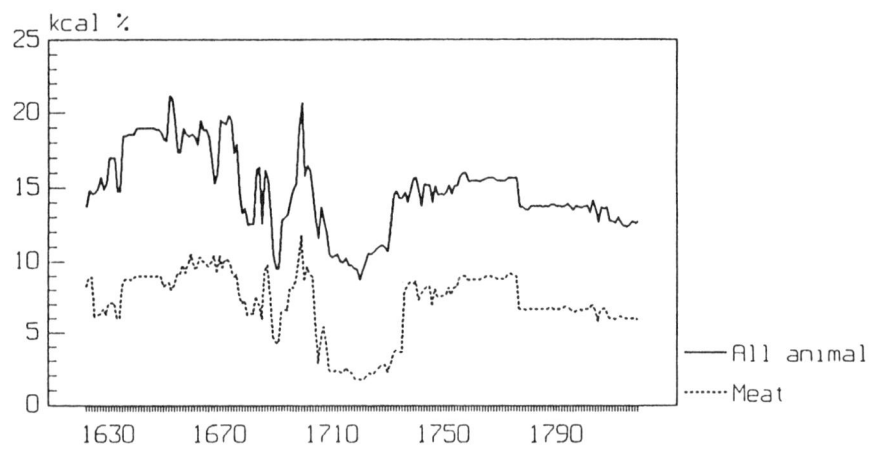

A general conclusion about diet at the hospitals is that it undoubtedly must have been less appreciated in the 18th and the first part of the 19th centuries than in the 17th century.

Iron-work labourers

As with the hospital inmates, the diet of iron-work labourers consisted mainly of rye bread, porridge, malt and Baltic herring, but in larger quantities, and this situation

Nutritional needs and social esteem: two aspects of diet in Sweden 273

Figure 15.18 Forgemen of Forsmarks bruk, 1730–1880: percentage share of energy intake provided by animal products
Source: Essemyr (1988), p. 141.

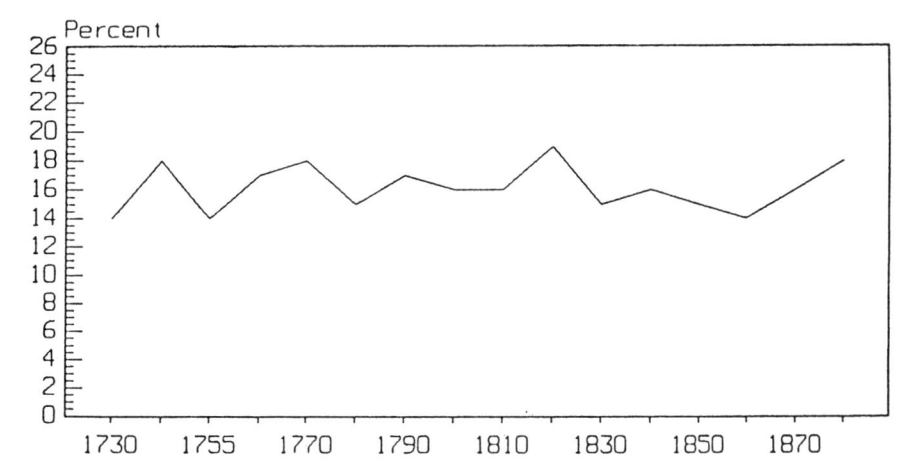

persisted well up to the eve of the 18th century. In contrast to the hospital inmates, the workers had legal access to small pieces of land and some fodder, thus guaranteeing them a permanent stock of animal food items. Also, from the 1820s potatoes became a staple product within their diet. However, it did not expand at the expense of cereals. Rather it merely followed tougher root crops, like turnips and swedes, that had been cultivated by the forgemen for centuries.

As the iron-work labourers were strong enough to guard successfully their diet of bread, meat and dairy products, the share of energy intake provided by animal products was not only high but also quite stable during the period (Figure 15.18). However, an increase in the consumption of cereals relative to other food items caused a downward trend during the first part of the 19th century.

Sawmill workers

Unlike the iron-work labourers, the sawmill workers' diet seems to have been rather poor in the second part of the 19th century. Up to the 1890s it mainly consisted of potatoes, flour and Baltic herring. Only small quantities of meat and dairy products were consumed. The figures available suggest that at the end of the 18th century protein contributed less than 10% of the total energy intake.

20th century

Micro-studies for the interwar period show that a remarkable increase in the consumption of animal food items had occurred during the first two decades of the

20th century. Meat, pork and especially milk were regularly available even to ordinary people. Animal products now accounted for 35–40% of total energy intake.[18]

Towards a synthesis

So far, three important circumstances in the development of food consumption from the 17th to the 20th centuries have been pointed out. First, on the macro level we can see a gradual increase in food demand between the mid-18th century and the late 19th century, reaching its peak in the 1820s and 1830s. The stagnation of population in the 17th century turned into a long-term growth that did not slacken until the final decades of the 19th century.

Second, despite the growth in demand the standard of nutrition did not show any significant declining trend below the level of nutritional needs. Those with low consumption, such as hospital inmates, as well as those with high consumption, such as iron-work labourers and sawmill workers, were quite well nourished as far as energy and protein are concerned.

Third, we find some evidence of a gradual decline in the consumption of animal food items relative to vegetable ones from the first part of the 18th century and up to the last decades of the 19th century. After the industrial breakthrough, the share of energy intake from animal products seems to have reached a higher level.

Of course, many factors have to be considered in any attempt to explain this development. It seems clear, though, that in feeding people under the conditions of population growth and low-productivity agriculture more emphasis will have to be put on the arithmetic of calories than on serving popular food items. When the limits of reclamation are reached, the only solution will be to seek alternative uses of land in order to produce as much of the essential nutritional elements as possible. In this context cultivation surpasses cattle-breeding by far.[19] Within cultivation the relation between the content of nutritional elements and the seed-to-yield ratio is more favourable for potatoes than for cereals. The essential point is that despite the lower energy content per unit weight of potatoes compared to rye, for example, its higher yield will produce a higher total energy output per unit area.

I would like to interpret developments in Sweden using this framework. As population growth was limited in the 17th century, much of the land could be used for pasture and cattle-breeding. As a consequence, the diet contained many animal products.

From the 1720s, when the population began to grow, the increase in demand was met first by reclamation, and later – when only marginal land was available – with a gradual transition from pasture to cereal cultivation. Hence, diet now became much more dominated by vegetable food items, especially bread.

The very strong population growth in the first part of the 18th century was matched by the rapid spread of the potato. Together with rye bread it now became the staple product for numerous groups of people.

The late 18th century became a watershed. Although population growth slowed down, the absolute number of people was higher than ever before. But now it could be supported by using high-productivity agriculture and imports, and hence much more emphasis could be put on serving more prestigious food items. As mentioned earlier, the growing use of artificial fertilizers and fodder crops, together with a growth in imports, loosened the bonds between the two forms of agricultural production. From the interwar period it became possible to expand the production and consumption of meat and dairy products, and thus to increase the social esteem attached to the diet to levels that had not been reached since the 17th century.

Some remarks about methods and sources

There are quite a few methodological problems involved in the historical analysis of food consumption. I will discuss some of the most important.

1. Finding relevant sources. In finding sources, it is necessary to look for populations whose food supply or food consumption was of particular interest to authorities, employers, and so on. Up to the end of the 19th century agricultural workers and iron-work labourers mainly received payment in kind, of which the greater part consisted of food provisions. As a result there are numerous sources on food supply among the working class in early Swedish industry. In hospitals communal feeding was strictly regulated and supervised by authorities, thus providing sources on actual individual allocations for each meal. At the sawmills, the credit system gives information about workers' spending in local shops.

2. Do the sources cover the total food supply? Concerning the iron-work labourers and the sawmill workers, payments in kind and money payments did not cover the total amount of foodstuffs available. Closer analysis revealed a substantial domestic food production. By using maps and probate inventories it became possible to quantify the contribution from the domestic sector.

3. Do the sources refer to households or individuals? As far as the inmates and the agricultural workers are concerned, the sources refer to individual consumption. For the workers, however, the food supply was meant to support the worker's household. In order to decide individual consumption, it is necessary to decide the structure and size of the household. By using the ecclesiastical population records which are available from the mid-18th century, this became possible. Also the size of households has been measured in terms of consumption units, which refer to differences in consumption according to age and sex.

4. Converting the food stock into nutritional elements. There are numerous tables describing the nutritional content in different food items. Most of them are modern ones. However, we do not know much about the difference in quality between earlier and modern foodstuffs. By using the oldest available Swedish food table, published in 1889, we have tried to get around this problem.

5. How much of the food supply was wasted? Not all of the gross quantities were consumed. Different forms of waste appeared as a result of refinement and cooking and during meals. By relating numerous ethnological references on refinement and cooking in earlier ages with modern tests of the loss of nutrients, we have been able to compensate for this. In some cases, the reductions were significant. Not less than 22% of the rye and barley available to the iron-work labourers was lost as a result of taxes, grinding and storage.

References

1. Braudel (1982), pp. 67ff.
2. Pollard (1981), p. 3.
3. Shammas (1984), p. 1.
4. Jonsson (1984), pp. 223ff.
5. Fridholm et al. (1976).
6. Isacson (1979), pp. 112–33; Hannerberg (1941).
7. Hannerberg (1971), pp. 91–6.
8. Fridlizius (1957).
9. Utterström (1943).
10. *Historical Statistics of Sweden* (1969), Table 2 and 3.
11. Eidlitz (1971).
12. Utterström (1943), pp.4–8; Thompson (1981), p. 348.
13. Abel (1980); Jörberg (1972).
14. Bentzel (1957), pp. 27–70.
15. This section refers to Morell (1987).
16. This section refers to Essemyr (1988).
17. Morell (1987), p. 180.
18. Essemyr (1983), p. 8.
19. Braudel (1982), pp. 88ff.

Literature

Abel, Wilhelm, *Agricultural Fluctuations in Europe. From the Thirteenth to the Twentieth Centuries* (London, 1980).

Bentzel, Ragnar, *Den privata konsumtionen i Sverige 1931-1965 [Private Consumption in Sweden 1931–1965]* (Stockholm, 1957).

Braudel, Fernand, *Vardagslivets strukturer [The Structure of Everyday Life]* (Malmö, 1982).

Cornell, Lars, *Sundsvallsdistriktets sågverksarbetare 1860–1890 [The Sawmill Workers of the Sundsvall District 1860–1890]* (Gothenburg, 1982).

Eidlitz, Kerstin, *Food and Emergency Food* (Kristianstad, 1971).

Essemyr, Mats, 'Food consumption and standard of living. Studies on food consumption among different strata of the Swedish population', *Uppsala Papers in Economic History*, 2(1983), pp. 7–30.

Essemyr, Mats, *Bruksarbetarnas livsmedelskonsumtion. Forsmarks bruk 1730–1880 [The Food Consumption of Iron-Work Labourers. Forsmarks bruk 1730–1880]* (Uppsala, 1988).

Fjellström, C., *Kostvanor och livsmedels konsumtion hos sågverksarbetarfamiljer på Stocka sågverk, Hälsingland kring sekkelskiftet* [*Diet and Food Consumption among Households at Stocka Sawmill at the Turn of the Century*] (Uppsala, 1986).

Fridholm, Merike, Maths Isacson and Lars Magnusson, *Industrialismens rötter* [*The Genesis of Industrial Change*] (Uppsala, 1976)

Fridlizius, Gunnar, *Swedish Corn Export in the Free Trade Era* (Lund, 1957).

Hannerberg, David, *Närkes landsbygd. Folkmängd och befolkningsrörelse. Åkerbruk och spannmålsproduktion (Rural Närke)* (Gothenburg, 1941).

Hannerberg, David, *Svenskt agrarsamhälle under 1200 år* [*1200 Years of Agricultural Society in Sweden*] (Stockholm, 1971).

Hirdman, Yvonne, *Magfrågan* [*The Food Question*] (Kristianstad, 1983).

Historical Statistics of Sweden, ed. National Central Bureau of Statistics, Part 1: Population (Stockholm, 1969).

Isacson, Maths, *Ekonomisk tillväxt och social differentiering 1680–1860* [*Economic Growth and Social Stratification 1680–1860*] (Uppsala, 1979).

Jörberg, Lennart, *A History of Prices in Sweden* (Lund, 1972).

Jonsson, Ulf, 'Population growth and agrarian economic and social structure: some Swedish examples', in Tommy Bengtsson, Gunnar Fridlizius and Rolf Olsson (eds), *Pre-Industrial Population Change* (Lund, 1984), pp. 223–4.

Morell, Mats, 'Eli F. Heckscher, Utspisningsstaterna och den svenska livsmedelskonsumtionen från 1500-talet till 1800-talet [Eli F. Heckscher, Food budgets and the Swedish food consumption from the 16th to the 19th Centuries]', *Uppsala Papers in Economic History*, 11(1986), 34–89.

Morell, Mats, *Studier i den svenska livsmedelskonsumtionens historia. Hospitalshjonens livsmedelskonsumtion 1621–1872* [*Studies in the History of Swedish Food Consumption. Food Consumption among Institutionally Supported Paupers 1621–1872*] (Uppsala, 1987).

Pollard, Sidney, *Peaceful Conquest* (Oxford, 1981).

Shammas, Carole, 'The eighteenth-century English diet and economic change', *Explorations in Economic History*, 43(1984), no. 1, pp. 24–39.

Thompson, Edward P., *The Making of the English Working Class* (London, 1943; repr. 1981).

Utterström, Gustaf, 'Potatisodlingen i Sverige under frihetstiden [Potato Cultivation in Sweden during the 18th Century]', *Swedish Historical Review*, (1943), pp. 1–40.

16 Divergences and convergences in the development of culinary cultures

Stephen Mennell

What is a 'culinary culture'? As Karl Popper says, definitions should be read from right to left, not from left to right: I use 'culinary culture' only as a shorthand expression for a whole complex of matters relating to food. By 'culture' I mean what anthropologists normally mean: everything that in human societies is 'learned, shared and transmitted', as Talcott Parsons phrased it. Culinary culture, by extension, includes everything that we mean by the 'cuisine' of society or social group, but a lot more besides. It refers not just to what foods are eaten and how they are cooked – whether simply or by increasingly elaborate methods – but also to the attitudes that are brought to cooking and eating. Those attitudes include the place of cooking and eating in people's patterns of sociability (eating out, in company, or in private); people's enthusiasm or lack of it towards food; their feelings, conversely, of repugnance towards certain foods or methods of preparation; the place of food, cooking and eating in a group or a society's sense of collective identity, and so on.

In short, we are here concerned with all the apparently 'subjective' components of what we often call 'taste'. But that is 'taste' in the collective sense, not as an individual, psychological matter. Taste in this sense is an aspect of what Pierre Bourdieu calls 'social habitus'.[1] By that he means those aspects of a person's individual make-up which are shared in common with a larger or smaller category of other people. The easiest way of making more precise what that means is to quote a dictum of Clyde Kluckhohn and Henry Murray:

> Every man is in certain respects
> (a) like all other men
> (b) like some other men
> (c) like no other men.[2]

The study of social habitus is concerned with level (b), and that is what is my concern when trying to compare different culinary cultures – whether the comparison is between quite different countries, or between different regions or different social classes within the same country. Note that this approach does not deny that there exist personal idiosyncracies in culinary taste (level (c)), nor that there are basic nutritional requirements (and possibly a few basic predispositions such as liking for sweetness) that are common to all humans (level (a)). But the focus, for present purposes, is on level (b).

The investigation of culinary cultures is more concerned with the aesthetic side of eating than the strictly nutritional. I agree with Mary Douglas when she writes:

> Nutritionists know that the palate is trained, that taste and smell are subject to cultural control. Yet, for lack of other hypotheses, the notion persists that what makes an item of food acceptable is some quality inherent in the thing itself. Present research into palatability tends to concentrate on individual reactions to individual items. It seeks to screen out cultural effects as so much interference. Whereas ... the cultural controls on perceptions are precisely what needs to be analysed.[3]

On the other hand, as I have argued elsewhere,[4] the structuralist approach associated with Douglas and with Claude Lévi-Strauss, Roland Barthes and others does not press its explanations far enough. It helps to reveal how interesting cultural patterns arose. Because culture is 'learned, shared and transmitted', in my view we can only understand the 'cultural controls on perception' by studying how they develop and are trans-mitted over time. An anthropology or sociology of food must also be a history of food.

A cultural history of food and diet

A history of culinary cultures is more a 'demand-side' history than a 'supply-side' history. A fairly high proportion of research in food history until recent years has been concerned with the supply side. Examples are works in the history of famines and fluctuations in output,[5] the history of particular foodstuffs (such as Salaman's classic *The History and Social Influence of the Potato*),[6] or the study of trends in the nutritional value of diets in the past (the widespread application of modern nutritional knowledge to historical data). My own interest lies more in what we can call the demand side – that is, in the study of social influences shaping people's tastes in food. That is not in any way to suggest that demand-side studies can take the place of, or are more important than, supply-side studies. Both are equally essential. Indeed, the distinction is even a little artificial because, especially when we look at these matters historically, we have to recognize that supply creates demand, as well as vice versa. This is especially well demonstrated, for example, in Sidney Mintz's *Sweetness and Power*,[7] which shows how the growth of sugar plantations in the West Indies was linked to the creation of a demand for sugar on a historically unprecedented scale in 18th- and 19th-century Britain, the USA and the Netherlands. All the same, even if supply- and demand-side considerations cannot be treated as entirely separate, the distinction still serves some purpose.

Obviously, in the first instance the availability of basic foodstuffs does play a part in the formation of culinary cultures. Staple foods[8] form the material basis on which cultural elaboration takes place, or does not take place. In many ways a culinary culture based on rice as the staple food will be different from one based on potatoes, or on bread and wheat, or on sorghum. But, in the modern world, and for the richer countries at least, that is now less important – given the availability there, at a price, of virtually any foodstuff from any part of the world. Perhaps we can see the beginnings of the globalization of culinary culture, as one aspect of the now widely discussed globalization of human society.[9]

What is meant by 'cultural elaboration'? Its absence can best be detected in the (possibly apocryphal) story of the African tribe whose staple food was boiled millet, and who, when offered anything different to eat, tended to reflect for a moment and then comment, 'Well, it's OK, but it's not as nice as boiled millet'. We find the story funny because this attitude is so very different from what we are familiar with in the rich West. In a more throughgoing anthropological comparison of the cuisines of Europe and Africa, Jack Goody[10] has shown that socially egalitarian, unhierarchical, relatively undifferentiated societies have rather plain, undifferentiated, socially homogenous cuisines; and that *hautes cuisines* only develop in highly stratified, highly differentiated, socially unequal, complex societies. In detail, Goody's book is excellent, a stimulating introduction to and critique of anthropologists's views on diet; but stated so baldly, its main thesis is perhaps a little over-obvious. In the advanced industrial societies we are familiar with the idea that there will not only be a vast variety of foodstuffs, and that tastes in food are highly charged with connotations of class and subcultural membership,[11] but that there will also be a complex elaboration of methods of preparation, generating an infinite variety of dishes. An elaborate cuisine involves, if we may echo the title of Piero Sraffa's famous contribution to modern economic theory, the production of commodities by means of commodities. The process or preparation of the most elaborate dishes involves indirect production through long sequences in which many intermediate products are first made. These characteristics, once the preserve of the *haute cuisine* of the grandest kitchens, are now shared by the food manufacturing industries whose products are less socially exclusive.

Now that these trends are so widespread throughout the world, it seems to me – although Jack Goody disagrees – that to explain why complex differentiated societies produce complex differentiated cuisines is a less difficult task than to explain why complex differentiated societies have produced culinary cultures with perceptibly different culinary cultures. That was why, in my book *All Manners of Food*,[12] I set out to compare the development of culinary taste in England and France. These are two countries which, from a world perspective, are actually rather similar; whose pattern of long-term development differs subtly in detail but is rather similar in broad terms. How, then, did their somewhat different culinary cultures take shape?

Divergences: The case of England and France, 14th–18th centuries

Caricature is a serious danger in this field. What people eat is universally a potent ingredient of national and social stereotyping. This applies both to the formation of people's 'we-images' of their own group and of their 'they-images' of outsider groups.[13] Food has long played a prominent part in the sense of national identity of both the English and French, and it is very risky to accept their reciprocal stereotypes of each other's cuisine at face value. At the very least, one must not fall into the trap of comparing say the food of Paul Bocuse with that served at some British transport café, or French professional cuisine with English domestic cookery. Yet, after a good deal of detailed work I came to the conclusion that the stereotypes really did have a kernel of truth in them, particularly in relation to underlying attitudes.

My investigation took as its baseline the late Middle Ages. I did not claim to have conducted any original research on this early period, but relied on the work of specialists, notably Stouff's outstanding monograph on late medieval Provence.[14] The picture which emerges from such studies can be briefly summarized.[15] First, the national differences in cuisine that we take for granted were as yet very little developed in medieval Europe. Members of the same estate of society ate in strikingly similar fashion throughout western Europe. Before Columbus, many of the vegetables now seen as typically Mediterranean were unknown, so that, for example, the humble cabbage was as prominent an item in Provence as in Northumberland. Second, however, the differences in consumption were possibly more striking than differences in quality (with an exception registered for a very small elite in really major courts). Stouff depicted graphically the increase in sheer quantity of food consumed as one progressed up the social ranks. Before the Black Death this was especially marked in the case of meat, though subsequently meat was relatively abundant for the lower ranks, too. The famous Gargantuan banquets thrown by kings and nobles to mark particular occasions were notable for their vast scale rather than the subtlety of the cooking; their motivation and social function resembled that of the Potlatch among the Kwakiutl Indians. Only in the greatest princely courts, and even there probably only for the more special occasions, was the famous courtly cuisine with its elaborate mixtures and proliferation of spices to be found. The recipes found in the manuscripts, whether from France, Italy, or England, are strikingly similar.[16]

Although the evidence from the Middle Ages is too sparse to be reliable, the best guess is that the pace of change in matters culinary was then very slow in all strata of society. From the time of the Renaissance onwards, however, the pace of change perceptibly quickened in these as in so many other aspects of everyday life,[17] at first among the secular upper classes and then very gradually among lower strata, too. We must be careful: the history of eating is a prime instance of what Elias has called 'the polyphony of history'. Marc Bloch contended that only in the nineteenth century was it possible to see 'the beginning of a trend towards greater uniformity in food – speaking in very relative terms – from the top to the bottom of the social ladder'.[18] Until then, the food and the cookery of the peasants in the countryside seems to have changed only extremely slowly over the centuries. It was something to be studied in the perspective of the *longue durée*. From the advent of the printed book, however, it is possible to trace a gradually accelerating pattern of change in the cookery of the upper and upper middle classes. If changes in technique and fashion never quite attain the pace of *histoire événementielle* – although the gastronomic myth-makers delight in representing the invention of new dishes as unique creations of great men on unique occasions[19] – it could fairly be portrayed as *histoire des conjonctures*.

The first elaborate cuisines representing a definite change from medieval traditions are to be found in the secular and religious courts of Renaissance Italy, but the leadership of Europe in culinary as in so many other facets of culture soon passed to France. Very detailed work by Jean-Louis Flandrin and his associates in Paris may be interpreted to show that French leadership goes back further, but from the appearance of La Varenne's famous book *Le Cuisinier françois* in 1651, it does not require in-depth research to see that something recognizable to later eyes as a distinctively French style of cuisine has emerged. From then on, the cookery-books are more numerous, and not only can advances in cookery techniques be seen but it is quite clear that contemporaries were conscious of the rapid pace of change, and of the importance of food as an aspect of fashion in courtly circles. By the 1740s, the first gastronomic controversies were being fought out in Paris between minor courtiers.[20] Although by then cookery-books were being directed specifically at the bourgeoisie, and some differentiation between courtly *haute cuisine* and domestic cookery was being codified, the models still clearly stemmed from courtly circles. One of the important consequences of this was that the spirit of thrift and economy in the kitchen, which was very marked from an early date in England, was much less in evidence even in French cookery-books, and something of the courtly functions of luxurious display heedless of the cost[21] lived on until the present day in the French kitchen.

In England, the cookery-books from the late 16th century onwards depict a more rustic, 'country housewife' style of cookery. They were still directed at readers among the nobility and gentry – this is not the food of the peasants – but they reflect their readers' greater continuing involvement in country life and pursuits than that of their French counterparts. There was, for a time, a line of English courtly cookery-books, too, but that tradition lost its vitality in England after the civil wars of the mid-17th century, and from the early 18th century it is eclipsed by the resurgence of the 'country housewife' style of book, written mainly by women, unlike those of the French and courtly traditions. The spirit of thrift and economy, often linked with an overt hostility to French extravagance, is strongly expressed.

This is a very compressed summary of only part of the evidence for differences in culinary culture between England and France. To counteract the necessary oversimplification, it needs to be emphasized that when speaking of 'English cookery' and 'French cookery', we are not dealing with two entirely separate things; French cookery had an early and continuing influence on English cookery, particularly through English cooks having worked in France and French cooks working for the very wealthiest English families. Yet there is a valid contrast. The food of the English gentry and prosperous farmers, depicted in the English cookery-books, enjoyed a prestige of its own to which there was no equivalent at that time in France. From the technical point of view there are also clear differences. The French developed a 'cuisine of impregnation', replacing the antique 'cuisine of mixtures'. The proliferation of sauces (a process carried still further in France in the 19th century) was precisely not the foundation of English cookery. In England, continuities from the past were much more in evidence. The old pies and joints of meat remained the centre of the English meal, whereas in France the focus of attention shifted to the ever-increasing variety of delicate little 'made dishes'.

What explanations can be offered for the rather different courses of development observed in the taste in food of the two countries? One explanation has been so often repeated that it has the force of conventional wisdom. This is that meat (and other raw materials) were so abundant and of such superior quality in England that it was not necessary to cook them with great skill, disguise their flavour, or eke them out in made dishes. I do not believe this explanation holds water. For one thing, the superiority and abundance of English raw materials is highly questionable. For another, this popular explanation rests on the implicit proposition that all human beings 'really', even innately, prefer the 'natural' taste of foods, transformed as little as possible by the culinary arts, which are thus seen as little more than a forced adaption to circumstance. There is no serious evidence to support this proposition.

I contend that three more explicitly 'social' strands of explanation bear closer examination. These are, first, the possible influence of Puritanism, or other religious differences between England and France; second, the role and influence of the court society, and more generally differences in the distribution of power and social stratification; and, third, the differing relationship between town and country on either side of the Channel.

The influence of religion on eating is certainly very strong and familiar in many of the world's cultures. But the contention that 'Puritanism' blighted the English kitchen needs to be treated with some scepticism. For one thing, it is not clear that the English Puritans of the mid-17th century were at all the general killjoys of later stereotype; they certainly do not have much to say against enjoying one's food. Later, perhaps, as dissenters, their outlook narrows, but by then they were not in the prominent positions in society from which they might once have commanded taste-setting power. Moreover, it is often overlooked that, besides the sizeable Huguenot community, 17th-century France also saw an influential Jansenist current within Catholicism, and the Jansenist outlook had many points of similarity with Calvinism. Yet no one has ever suggested that Jansenism permanently damaged French taste-buds.

As for the royal and princely courts, I have already argued that their direct influence on the authors of French cookery-books is plain to see. In the light particularly of Norbert Elias's account of the place of 'luxury' and display in French court society,[22] it is highly likely that competition between courtiers would be acted out through their kitchens and their tables as in many other aspects of culture. An essential link in the argument is that the French nobility, having emerged on the losing side from a series of struggles with the king, became deracinated and defunctionalized – deprived of their roots in a rural way of life, deprived in particular of their relatively independent power base and governmental functions in the provinces. This did not happen to the same extent in England. The power shifts which were the outcome of the civil wars, the Glorious Revolution of 1688, and the Hanoverian succession in 1714, nipped in the bud the growth of an absolutist monarchy and court society on the French model. The royal court in 18th-century England was more *primus inter pares*; noble houses and the gentry retained a relatively independent power and governmental function in the provinces; and the pressures towards competition through virtuosity in consumption were relatively less intense.

That connects with a third consideration. The relationship between town and country in England was rather different to that in France. It was not that England was a more rural country than France. Quite the contrary. London in the 18th century was much bigger than Paris, and her population still larger as a proportion of the nation as a whole. It is estimated that as many as one in six people in that period spent some part of their lives in London. Nevertheless, the prestige of the country way of life remained much higher in England than it did in France, and London and country society remained more closely interlocked than those of Paris and France. A larger proportion of English noblemen and gentlemen spent a larger proportion of the year living on their country estates and largely eating the seasonal products of their lands than was the case in France. Rustication from court was the ultimate punishment for a French courtier. Besides, it should not be forgotten that in a pre-industrial economy the range of available foods was generally more limited in the country than in the markets of major cities. The very diversity of the products to be found in the principal markets of great cities is a prerequisite for the creation of a great diversity of made dishes. *Haute cuisine* is a characteristic of urban life.

Convergences: Postscript on the 19th and 20th centuries

After the Napoleonic Wars, the divergence between English and French cuisines appeared to widen. What was actually happening was something rather more complicated. Certainly, French professional cuisine, founded in the aristocratic kitchens of the *ancien regime*, was raised to new heights through competition between the restaurants of nineteenth-century Paris. And there is a good deal of evidence that, especially in the latter half of the century, the rather fine English country cooking tradition declined and became coarsened. What I think happened was that French culinary hegemony in the higher circles of English society became far more firmly established than in the eighteenth century, when only a few of the greatest grandees had employed French chefs. French culinary colonialism now extended further down into the highest reaches of the middle class. Besides, the sheer number of families involved in London 'Society' was growing very rapidly,[23] and the intense competition created by this social inflation mimicked in some degree the competitive display found among French courtiers a century earlier.

It was not, however, likely that these conditions would favour the emergence of a separate and distinctive English *haute cuisine*. Something like 'dependency theory' or 'world-systems' theory applies to culinary colonialism as well as to colonialism proper. French cookery having already reached great heights, its techniques, recipes, rules and vocabulary were there to be adopted by the colonized, just as, at about the same time, the advanced state of many English sports led to the adoption of the games and their English vocabulary in many parts of the world.

The coarsening of the English 'country housewife' tradition of cookery in the 19th century may have been due not just to the defection of the social model-setting circles to French cuisine but also, lower down the social scale, to the disruptive effects of very rapid urbanization and population growth on the transmission of traditional knowledge from mother to daughter. Urbanization took place in England far earlier and far more rapidly than in France. By the time the corresponding movement to the towns took place in France, largely during the twentieth century, the popular press and other mass media may to some extent have provided alternative channels for the maintenance of traditional knowledge.

That is to some extent speculative, and requires deeper investigation. What is quite clear, however, is that by the 1960s forces leading to convergence between the culinary cultures of France and England were dominant over the forces of divergence. That was to be seen quite clearly in the further diffusion of French influence down the English social scale through cookery columns in women's magazines and cookery programmes on television. But far more important was the enormous growth of the food-processing industry and its impact on the domestic kitchen in both countries and indeed throughout the developed world. That, and the growth of the fast-food industry, have become very powerful agents for the internationalization of food, and that has involved contrary yet interlinked trends to cosmopolitan culinary culture. That applies not just to the actual dishes which come out of domestic and commercial kitchens, but also – in the richer countries – to social contrasts in eating. Both have been marked, in Elias's phrase, by 'diminishing contrasts and increasing varieties'.

An aside: What about other countries in Europe?

Although I have not conducted research into the culinary cultures of any other European countries in as much depth as I have given to England and France, it is difficult to resist speculating how the suggestions I have made might apply to the cuisines of other European countries.

Belgium and the Netherlands offer a most striking parallel to France and England.[24] It is not just that Belgian cookery is more like French and Dutch cookery is more like English in the overall stylistic impression they make, but the underlying attitudes the people of the two countries bring to their enjoyment of food also seem to differ in a similar way to Anglo-French difference. In this case, given that religious conflicts are historically the most salient reason for these being politically two separate states, it is even more tempting to appeal to Protestantism and Catholicism in explaining the differences, such as they are, in culinary culture. However, it must also be remembered that in the Austrian Netherlands court society remained a powerful cultural influence throughout the 17th and 18th centuries, while in the

Dutch Republic the French-influenced court circles around the Stadhouders in The Hague and Leeuwarden were small and less powerful as model-setting centres than the Regenten class of Amsterdam and Rotterdam. Anneke van Otterloo's investigation[25] of differences in the development of culinary cultures in the mainly Protestant North and the mainly Catholic South also fails to find much evidence for the independent causal influence of religion, even though it intermingled in a more local way with other elements.

Germany, like England, failed to develop any separate *haute cuisine* of its own. Its aristocratic courts were until the late 18th century centres of francophilia. The political fragmentation of the country, with its proliferation of small noble courts, was probably favourable to the strong persistence of regional specialities to the present day: Eva Barlösius has looked in more detail into the development of German culinary culture.[26]

Italy cries out for a similar comparative study. After leading the stylistic break with the common European medieval *haute cuisine*, Italy went on to develop one of the earliest very distinctive national cuisines. It did so at the price of no longer having wide influence on the rest of Europe, at least until the present day.

Conclusion

It is clear from anthropological and historical evidence that, world-wide, the three most powerful influences on what and how people eat are religion, class and nationality. In western Europe, in the absence of firmer evidence, I am not convinced that the formative influence of religious differences on differences in culinary culture was as strong as that of class and nation. These latter two, certainly in the cases of England and France which I have studied in most detail, interwove in a very complex way over time as ways of eating acquired connotations both of social superiority or inferiority and of patriotism or cosmopolitanism. Social competition appears to be the most powerful engine of change in culinary traditions, and the royal and princely courts of *ancien régime* Europe were particularly intensive forcing houses for culinary differentiation whose cultural influence has left its mark to the present day – even though most people may be largely unaware of it. Some support for this hypothesis seems to come tangentially from other historical civilizations such as India, where court society was also associated with the development of *hautes cuisines*. Of course, beneath all this, the impact of new raw materials such as all those which came from the New World is not to be ignored. But the diffusion of foods, like the diffusion of social customs, as anthropologists have long been aware, is never an adequate explanation of change in itself: we always need also to explain why one product, one custom, one taste, was formed or adopted rather than another.

References

1. Bourdieu (1984).
2. Kluckhohn and Murray (1948), p. 35.
3. Douglas (1978), p. 59.
4. Mennell (1985), pp. 6–15.
5. Curschmann (1900); Abel (1980); *Hunger and History* (1983).
6. Salaman (1985).
7. Mintz (1985).
8. See *Staple Foods* (1990).
9. See the special issue of *Theory, Culture and Society* (1990) devoted to the question of the globalization of human society; and, for a brief discussion, Giddens (1989), pp. 519–50.
10. Goody (1982).
11. See the discussions of food, class and social habitus, based on extensive survey data from France in Bourdieu (1984).
12. Mennell (1985).
13. These terms are borrowed from Norbert Elias. See Elias and Scotson (1965); Mennell (1989a), pp. 115–39.
14. Stouff (1970).
15. For more detail here and in the rest of this section, see Mennell (1985), especially chs 3,4 and 5.
16. This remark requires some qualification in the light of recent work by Bruno Laurioux and other members of Jean-Louis Flandrin's seminar at the École des Hautes Études en Sciences Sociales, Paris. They have demonstrated that there were regional differences in the use of particular spices, for example. The problem is that such evidence can trigger debates analogous to the question of whether a glass of water is best described as half full or as half empty. Differences of emphasis there may have been, but the similarities in broad style and indeed the evidence of transmitted influence from court to court across Europe still seem to me to remain unchallenged.
17. Elias (1982).
18. Bloch (1954), p.232.
19. See Mennell (1985), ch. 10.
20. *Lettre d'un pattisier* (1981).
21. Cf. Elias (1983).
22. Elias (1983).
23. Davidoff (1973).
24. Mennell (1989b).
25. Otterloo (1986).
26. Barlösius (1988).

Literature

Abel, Wilhelm, *Agricultural Fluctuations in Europe from the Thirteenth to the Twentieth Centuries* (3rd edn, London, 1980).
Barlösius, Eva, 'Soziale und historische Aspekte der deutschen Küche', in Stephen Mennell, *Die Kultivierung des Appetits* (Frankfurt am Main, 1988), pp. 423–44.
Bloch, Marc, 'Les Aliments de l'ancienne France', in Jean-Jacques Hémardinquer (ed.) *Pour*

une histoire de l'alimentation (Paris, 1954), pp. 231–35.
Bourdieu, Pierre, *Distinction: A Social Critique of the Judgement of Taste* (London, 1984).
Curschmann, Fritz, *Hungersnöte im Mittelalter* (Leipzig, 1900).
Davidoff, Leonore, *The Best Circles: Society, Etiquette and the Season* (London, 1973).
Douglas, Mary, 'Culture', in *Annual Report 1977–78 of the Russell Sage Foundation* (New York, 1978), pp. 55–81.
Elias, Norbert and John L. Scotson, *The Established and the Outsiders* (London, 1965).
Elias, Norbert, *The Civilising Process*, vol I: *The History of Manners* (Oxford, 1978); vol II: *State Formation and Civilisation* (Oxford, 1982).
Elias, Norbert, *The Court Society* (Oxford, 1983).
Giddens, Anthony, *Sociology* (Oxford, 1989).
Goody, Jack, *Cooking, Cuisine and Class* (Cambridge, 1982).
Hunger and History: The Impact of Changing Food Production and Consumption Patterns on Society, ed. Robert I. Rothberg and Theodore K. Rabb (Cambridge, Mass., 1983).
Kluckhohn, Clyde and Henry A. Murray (eds.), *Personality in Nature, Society and Culture* (New York, 1948).
Lettre d'un pâtissier anglois et autres contribution à une polémique gastronomique du XVIIIe siècle, ed. Stephen Mennell (Exeter, 1981).
Mennell, Stephen, *All Manners of Food: Eating and Taste in England and France from the Middle Ages to the Present* (Oxford, 1985).
Mennell, Stephen, *Norbert Elias: Civilisation and the Human Self-Image* (Oxford, 1989a).
Mennell, Stephen, Voorspel: 'Eten in de Lage Lande', in *Smaken verschillen* (Amsterdam, 1989b), pp. 15–29.
Mintz, Sidney W., *Sweetness and Power: The Place of Sugar in Modern History*, (New York, 1985).
Otterloo, Anneke van, 'Over culinare culturen in noord en zuid: enkele opmerkingen bij de sociogenese van nationale stijl en regionale variaties in Nederland', *Groniek: Gronings Historisch Tijdschrift*, 95(1986), pp. 36–55.
Salaman, Redcliffe Nathan, *The History and Social Influence of the Potato* (2nd edn, Cambridge, 1985).
Staple Foods. Proceedings of the 1989 Oxford Cookery Symposium, ed. Harlan Walker (London, 1990).
Stouff, Louis, *Ravitaillement et alimentation en Provence aux XIVe et XVe siècles* (Paris, 1970).

Subject index

Abattoir 14, 15
Account book, see household budget
Advertisement, see marketing
Agriculture, see food production
Alcohol 12, 14, 21–2, 46, 48, 50, 57–8, 63, 72, 93, 131, 149, 151–5, 157, 174, 204–5, 214–7
Ale, see beer
Amsterdam 62
Annales School 61, 75, 79, 90, 98, 113–5, 209
Antwerp 76, 81–4
Appetizer 110
Asparagus 51

Baby food 173
Bacon 29, 31, 33, 46, 49, 53, 151, 215–7
Baking (bakery, baking industry) 20, 51–2, 130
Banquet, see meals
Barley 48, 153, 204, 215, 219, 257, 270
Barm 51
Beans 57, 151
Beer 20, 22, 48, 50, 51, 67, 131, 148, 150, 154, 160, 173, 174, 200, 204–5, 214–7, 219, 220, 242, 257
Beets 151, 153, 173
Berne 78, 106
Biscuits 33
Black markets 156, 158
Bread 11, 19–20, 29, 31, 33, 49–52, 62, 64, 67, 75, 77–8, 93,. 113, 129, 148, 150–3, 155–9, 173, 176, 178, 201, 202, 204–206, 215–7, 240–2, 270, 272, 280
Breakfast, see mealtimes
Brewing, brewing industry, see beer
Brussels 74–6, 78, 83–4
Budapest 77
Butter 4, 15, 20, 23, 29–30, 45, 48–50, 52, 75, 84, 130, 135, 148, 153, 159–60, 208, 215–7, 219, 242–3, 270

Cabbage 151, 281
Cafeteria, see coffee

Cakes 51
Calories 12–3, 92, 96, 115–6, 152–3, 155–60, 200, 202–3, 213, 215–7, 238, 242–3, 259–74
Calory budget, see calories
Canned foods, see food preservation
Canteens 7, 159
Catering 132
Cattle 169–72, 174, 178, 199, 219, 257–8, 274
Cereals 11, 46–9, 51, 53, 75, 92–94, 114, 129, 133–135, 148, 153–4, 157–8, 169–73, 175–76, 178, 200–2, 204–5, 215–7, 240, 242–3, 257–9, 270, 272–4
Champagne 15
Cheese (-making, -monger) 19–20, 33, 50, 75, 84, 131–2, 148, 150, 153–4, 157, 160, 168–170, 172–4, 178, 215–7, 219, 242
Chicory 8
Child mortality, see infant mortality
Chocolate 15, 84, 113, 154, 159, 173–4, 177, 204–5
Cholesterol 57, 65
Cider 48
City, see towns
Cocoa, see chocolate
Coffee (-houses) 8, 14, 62, 73, 77, 113, 115, 149–52, 154, 157, 178
Commercialisation 48, 51, 67, 77–8
Conservation, see food conservation
Consumer co-operatives 77, 80, 82, 152, 169, 176–7
Consumption, see food consumption
Contamination, see food adulteration
Cookery-books 10, 13, 32, 50, 62, 84, 135, 175, 178–9, 206, 231, 236–7, 241, 282–35
Cooking (cook, cookery, cooking techniques) 9, 51, 206, 226, 280–2, 284–5
Cork 50
Corpulence (fatness) 160–1
Cost of living, see standard of living
Cost sheets, see household budgets
Country (countryside) 148, 152, 158, 160,

170–3, 176, 179–80, 237–9, 244
Cuisine 161, 168, 228, 236, 280–2, 285
Cuisine, national differences 281–2, 284, 286
Cuisine, rural 284
Culinary arts 109, 135, 230, 283

Dairies 23, 47, 52, 77, 79, 131, 134, 170–5, 180, 273, 275
Dessert 51, 110
Diet revolution 1, 256
Dining room (-hall) 9, 110, 120
Dinner, *see* mealtimes
Dishes 66, 135, 205, 218, 229, 280, 283, 285
Domestic sciences, *see* home economics
Drinks, alcoholic, *see* alcohol
Drinks, non-alcoholic (soft) 19, 21, 30, 67, 73, 75, 77, 95, 110, 112–20, 225
Dublin 47–8, 50, 52

Eating customs (-habits) 1–2, 4–5, 11, 16–7, 60–4, 66, 71, 76–7, 79, 85, 109, 111, 113, 131, 133, 200–2, 206–8, 224–9, 230–1, 259, 277
Eating prohibitions 225
Eating utensils 13, 120, 208, 224–5, 227–31
Eggs 30, 47, 49, 75, 148, 153–5, 157–8, 160, 176, 204–5, 215
Employees 149–50, 158–9, 178
Endive 151
Energy intake, *see* calories
Epidemics 115, 117
Evening supper, *see* mealtimes

Family budget, *see* household budget
Famine (hunger) 1, 10, 16, 45, 48, 52–3, 72, 92, 95, 114, 117, 133, 153, 156, 160–1, 170, 179, 218, 279
Fast food 146, 285
Fasting 208, 225–6, 237
Fats 14, 23, 57, 62, 93, 132, 134, 153–4, 157–60, 180, 201–2, 204–5, 207–8, 214–7, 220–30
Fatness, *see* corpulence

Feasts (feasting fares, festive days, feast meals) 9, 50–1, 109, 115, 135, 147, 160, 206, 213, 218, 220, 225–6, 229, 230, 237, 240

Feeding, communal
Fireplaces, *see* kitchen
Fish 50–1, 67, 75, 93, 132, 148, 154, 157, 160, 172, 202, 204–5, 208, 215–7, 228, 270, 272
Flour (-milling) 20, 47, 51, 130, 153, 155–6, 158–60, 204, 242, 273
Food adulteration 14, 57, 72
Food chain 169, 174
Food choice 213
Food conservation 4, 7, 11, 15
Food consumption 1–2, 4, 11, 17, 19–25, 46, 50–1, 57–9, 61, 72–85, 93, 95, 112, 114, 117, 147–60, 169, 171–5, 177–81, 199–202, 205–6, 208, 213–8, 220–1, 239–43, 257, 259–61, 266–70, 274, 279, 281
Food control, governmental
Food conservation 114, 131, 146, 150, 169, 181
Food crisis 16, 155, 159, 170, 173, 175, 266, 269
Food distribution 6, 28–9, 62
Food ethnology 199, 205, 208, 224, 225–7, 259
Food expenditure 29–31
Food habits, *see* eating customs
Food hygiene 7, 63, 238
Food in monasteries 214
Food in schools 214
Food in workhouses, *see* workhouse diet
Food industry 13, 46, 48, 64, 71, 114, 150, 168–9, 172–4, 177–8, 203, 206, 231, 245, 285
Food innovations 51, 64, 66, 71, 119, 136, 170–1, 203, 206, 208–9, 231
Food law 112, 173–174
Food maps 230
Food of agricultural workers 199, 201–2, 220, 260–1, 270, 274–5
Food of domestic servants 226, 260
Food of industrial workers 29, 34, 149–59, 173, 176–8, 180, 199–200, 227–8, 231, 238, 241–2, 260–1, 266–9, 272–5
Food of the gentry (nobility, aristocratic meals) 134, 206, 215–6, 281–2, 226
Food of the partisans 134, 206
Food of the peasants 134, 149, 171, 175, 177,

Subject index

208, 216–8, 220, 226–8, 230–1, 237, 239–40, 261, 281
Food of the poor 132, 199
Food policy 20, 62, 71–2, 80, 135, 175
Food production 2, 7, 8, 14, 46, 48, 61–2, 129–131, 133–7, 147, 157, 159, 169–73, 176–81, 199, 200–3, 213, 218–9, 220–1, 237, 239–40, 244, 257–8, 273–5
Food quality 14, 72, 281
Food riots 114
Food sciences, *see* nutritional sciences
Food statistics, *see* statistics
Food supply, *see* food consumption
Food surrogates (substitutes) 8, 14, 153, 158–9, 238
Food systems, alternative 60
Food taxes 80
Food technology 20, 66, 112, 129–33
Food trade 13, 20, 75, 84, 131, 134–5, 169, 171–4, 176, 229, 231
Food tradition 51–2, 203, 207–8
Food, artificial
Food, types of 270–5
Food-canning, *see* preservation
Food-manufacturing, *see* food industry
Foods, high-status, *see* nutritional status
Fork, *see* eating utensils
Fowl 47
Fruit 20, 29–30, 53–5, 57–60, 63, 73, 77, 153–5, 157–160, 176, 178, 204–5, 242
Funeral meals, *see* feast meals

Galway 51
Gardening 135
Gastronomy 4, 10, 51, 71, 109, 135, 147, 152, 176, 179, 231
Ghent 75–6, 79, 81–3
Gin, *see* alcohol
Goulash 207
Grain, *see* cereals
Griddle 51
Groceries 11, 73, 77, 152
Gruel, *see* porridge

Health reform movement 7
Health reports 61
Health, public 56, 65–6
Height of the body 46, 59, 61

Herbs 151
Herrings, *see* fish
Hoarding 156
Home economics (domestic sciences) 63
Honey 113, 130–1, 160
Hospitality 135
Hospital diet 50, 109, 179, 200, 214, 240–2, 261–7, 270–2, 274–5
Hotels *see* gastronomy
Household 148–52, 154–5, 157–9, 176–7, 237, 239–41
Household budgets 11–2, 15, 26, 30–1, 49, 58, 61, 72–8, 80, 112, 149–50, 155, 176–8, 202–3, 205, 215, 218, 231, 239
Household literature 10, 231
Household surveys 269
Hunger, *see* famine

Ice cream 67
Income (family income, per-capita income, wages) 1, 10–1, 16, 29, 46, 48, 50–1, 53, 63, 71, 75, 77, 148–52, 155, 159, 177, 200, 206, 219–20, 259
Infant mortality 26, 58, 62
Inn, *see* gastronomy
Inn, fare of the, *see* gastronomy
Instant meals, *see* fast food
Instinct

Jam 152, 154

Kale 33
Kitchen (kitchen utensils) 3, 18, 32, 51, 110–1, 120, 132, 152, 225, 227–31, 236, 240, 242, 244–5, 280, 282, 284

Lard 152, 155, 157, 159, 204
Leftovers 9
Legumes 148, 153–5, 160
Leuven (Louvain) 73–5, 78
Liquor, *see* alcohol
Living standard, *see* standard of living
Lunch, *see* mealtimes
Luxuries 4, 11, 14, 109, 147–8, 150–1, 155, 157–9, 203, 206

Magazines, Women's 13, 65–6
Main course, *see* meals

Maize 52–3, 204, 206
Malnutrition 47, 56, 58, 72, 78, 115, 155, 178–9, 180
Margarine 15, 23, 65, 73, 77, 135, 159, 173
Markets (local, weekly, national) 9, 13, 15, 28
Marketing 49, 61, 62–6
Marshall Plan 156
Meals (composition, courses, meal patterns, meal order inc. seating plans) 2–4, 6, 33, 47, 49, 51, 63–4, 111, 115, 117, 133, 146–7, 149–50, 152, 157, 161, 179–80, 203, 205–8, 213, 224–9, 231, 236–8, 240–2, 244–5, 283
Meals, festive, *see* feasts
Meals, ritual 225–6, 229–31
Mealtimes 32–4, 49–50, 71, 79, 110, 146, 150 152, 161, 208
Meat (meat trade) 12, 14, 20, 23, 29–31, 46, 50–1, 57, 59, 62, 67, 72, 75, 77–9, 82, 84, 93, 110, 112, 130, 147–8, 150–5, 157–8, 160, 169, 172, 176–80, 200–5, 207–8, 215–7, 220, 225, 228, 230, 242–3, 270–1, 273–5, 281, 283
Medical topography 206
Metabolism 2, 11
Military diet (food of the army, soldiers) 50, 132, 200, 204–6
Milk (-products, -trade) 7, 20, 33, 48, 50, 67, 75, 84, 130–4, 148, 153–5, 157–60, 172–3, 176, 178, 203–5, 214, 270, 274
Milk, mother's 7
Mills (milling) 173, 237, 240
Mineral water (table water) 174
Minerals 30, 93, 132
Ministry of Food and Agriculture, *see* food policy
Mushrooms 178
Mutton 50

Navy diet 214
Neo-Malthusians 16
Noodles 149, 207–8
Nutrients 17, 203
Nutrition chain 8
Nutritional diseases 2
Nutritional physiology 14, 129, 132, 199–200, 203, 205
Nutritional sciences 2, 50, 56, 60, 129, 173

Nutritional knowledge 64
Nutritional status 25–6, 150
Nutritional value calculations (balances) 200, 201, 203, 205, 279
Nutritives 132, 200, 201–3, 203–5, 214

Oat 47–48, 51, 153, 172, 204
Offal 155
Oil 157, 159–160, 180, 202, 216–7, 219–30
Oral history 62, 203
Outdoor eating, *see* gastronomy
Overweight (overnutrition) 1, 4, 56, 59–60

Paprika 206
Peas 202, 215–7
Population growth 94, 114, 257–8, 274–5, 285
Pork 46, 48, 50
Porridge 14, 33, 49–51, 110
Potatoes 4, 16, 29–30, 33, 45–50, 52–3, 57, 71–2, 75, 77, 130, 132, 136, 148, 151, 153–5, 158–60, 170, 177–8, 204–6, 257, 259, 273–4, 279
Poultry 148, 242
Poverty 1, 47, 49, 57, 241–2
Preparation of meals 4, 7, 9, 16–7, 63, 130, 146, 150, 152, 169, 175, 179–81, 238, 240
Preservation, *see* food conservation
Prices of foodstuff 9, 11, 16, 75, 94, 114, 117, 151, 157–9, 172–4, 176–7, 179–80, 203, 239–40, 259
Processing 130, 133, 134, 168–70, 172–5, 178, 181

Ration (-cards, -system) 78, 132, 153, 156–7, 180, 200, 201–3, 304, 306
Ration, of the army, *see* military diet
Recipe book, *see* cookery-books
Recipes 50, 62–3, 72, 84, 120, 132, 231, 281, 284
Regional differences of food habits 62, 75, 130–6, 136, 201, 203, 206, 208, 228, 230–1, 234
Religion (religious symbols) 115, 208, 230, 231
Restaurant, *see* gastronomy
Rice 73, 77, 92, 148, 154–5, 160, 205, 279

Subject index

Roughage 13
Rye 71, 77, 92, 204–5, 257, 270, 272, 274

Saccharin 8
Salt 134, 154, 169, 172, 175–6, 242–3
Sandwiches 33, 159
Sausages 150–3, 157, 178
Seating plans, *see* meals
Sexuality 115, 119
Shortages 153, 156, 179, 258–9, 266
Snacks 33, 152, 208
Social differentiation in eating and drinking 31–3, 114, 118, 132–5, 202–3, 205–6, 214–8, 221, 226–7, 229
Soup 4, 14, 149–51, 173, 178, 180, 207–8
Spices 133, 135, 218, 242, 281
Spirits, *see* alcohol
Standard of living (living standards) 1, 4, 12, 30, 61, 65, 73–4, 76, 78, 80, 147, 149, 169, 171, 176–80, 203, 240
Starch 57
Starvation, *see* famine
Statistics of food consumption 11, 13, 80, 117, 148–50, 168, 172, 176, 180, 199, 202–5, 215, 238–9, 242
Storage 11, 131, 224, 230–1
Stores (shops) 229
Sugar (beet sugar, cane sugar) 4, 8, 15, 23, 29–30, 52, 57, 73, 112–3, 133–4, 148–50, 152–5, 157–60, 173–4, 203–205, 206
Sunday dinner, *see* mealtimes
Supper, *see* mealtimes
Supply of food, *see* food supply
Surrogates of footstuff 153, 158–9, 238
Sweetener 4, 8
Sweets 67, 84, 159
Syrup 8

Table decoration (-design) 13, 110
Table manners, *see* eating customs
Tableware, *see* eating utensils

Taboos 17
Taste 18, 62, 65, 231, 277, 280, 283
Tea (tea industry) 14, 29–31, 33, 47–8, 51–2, 62, 113, 152, 154, 161, 204–5, 207–8
Temperance movement 180
Tobacco 48, 73, 77, 149, 155
Tomatoes 71
Towns 132, 134, 147–8, 153, 158, 171, 175, 177, 179, 200, 203, 205–6, 226, 228, 231, 236–7, 244
Trace elements 13
Trade, *see* food trade
Transport 9, 28
Turnips 273

Undernourishment, *see* malnutrition
Urbanization 118, 146, 148, 150, 175, 178–9, 231, 285
Utrecht 57–58, 61

Vegetables 23, 29, 48, 51, 63, 112, 117, 129, 133, 135, 150–1, 153–5, 157–60, 176, 178, 201–2, 204–5, 242, 270, 274
Vegetarians 161
Vitamins 13, 30, 52, 58, 65, 78, 93, 115, 132, 170

Wages, *see* income
Wars 31, 53, 72, 74, 78, 82, 113–4, 133, 153, 156, 158–9, 168, 171–5, 178, 180, 203, 237–8, 258, 266, 282, 284
Water 176, 178
Wedding meal, *see* feasts
Wheat 30, 92, 47, 50, 67, 73, 77, 199, 204–5, 280
Whisky (whiskey) 47
Wine 131, 148, 154, 160, 172, 178–9, 200–2, 204–5
Work productivity and food 1
Workhouse diet 52, 214
Working-class diet, *see* food of the industrial workers

Name index

Abel, Wilhelm 94–6, 117–8
Alexander, David 29
Andersen, Age Jørgen Christian 23
Aron, Jean-Paul 98
Ashley, William 21
Ashton, Thomas Southcliffe 26
Atkin, Peter J. 21, 23
Aykroyd, Wallace Rudell 23
Aymard, Maurice 61, 93, 95, 97, 115

Barker, Theodor Cardwell 19, 24
Barnett, Louise Margaret 20
Barthes, Roland 91, 98, 279
Battersby, Roy John 23
Bauters, Daniel 79
Bear, William E. 21, 23
Beaver, M. W. 26
Beeton, Isabella 32
Below, Georg von 111
Berzelius, Jöns Jakob v. 57
Biedermann, Karl 110, 112
Blackman, Janet 20–1, 28
Bloch, Marc 90, 92, 94, 281
Blomme, Jan 78
Blumroeder, Gustav 109
Böhmert, Victor 180
Booth, Alan 26
Booth, Charles 24, 30
Bourdeau, L. 94
Bourdieu, Pierre 98, 277
Braudel, Fernand 90–2, 94, 96, 114, 214, 256
Bresc, H. 97
Briffault, Eugène 93
Brillat-Savarin, Jean-Anthelme 93, 109
Broadley, H. 20
Brockway, Fenner 25
Buchanan, Ian 26
Bynum, W. F. 26

Calvin, Jean 171
Canetti, Elias 160
Capie, Forrest 23
Chaloner, William Henry 19

Cheke, Valerie 21
Clarkson, Leslie A. 24, 26, 52
Cobbett, Williiam 20, 31
Cohen, Ruth Louisa 21
Collin, Edward John T. 21
Conrad, Johannes 112
Corley, Thomas Anthony Buchanan 21
Corran, Harry Stanley 22
Crawford, Margaret 26, 52
Crawford, William 20
Critchell, James Troubridge 23
Cutting, Charles Lathan 22

Daiches, David 22
Davies, David 25
Davies, Maude 32
Deer, Noel 23
Denis, Hector 74
Devine, T. M. 45
Dewey, Peter E. 20
Donnachie, Ian 22
Douglas, Mary 60, 279
Driver, Christopher 33
Drummond, Jake Cecil 20, 24
Ducpétiaux, Edouard 12, 72, 74
Dupriez, Léon H. 73, 75, 82

Eden, Frederick Morton 25
Eeckhout, Patricia van den 76
Elias, Norbert 63, 119, 281, 283
Engel, Ernst 12, 72, 74, 155
Erixon, Sigurd 118

Febvre, Lucien 90
Fenton, Alexander 26
Figl, Leopold 156
Flandrin, Jean-Louis 95, 98–9, 116
Floud, Roderick C. 26
Fogel, Robert W. 26
Forrest, Dennis Mostyn 22
Fraser, H. 21
Freeman, E. J. 26
Freytag, Gustav 110

Name index

Fussell, George Edwin 21

Gledion, Siegfried 32
Glen, Isabel A. 22
Goldstrom, Joachim Max 24
Goodman, C. 21
Goossens, Martine 78
Gotthelf, Jeremias 174, 180
Gottschalk, Alfred 93
Gottschalk, Max 74
Griffiths, Percival Joseph 22
Grimm, Jacob and Wilhelm 111
Grimod de la Reyniére, Alexandre 93
Gruber, Ignaz 149
Guégan, Bertrand 93
Guyer, Jacob 171

Häpke, Rudolf 113
Harrison, Brian 19, 22
Hartley, Dorothy 22
Hémardinquer, Jean-Jacques 95–6
Henry, Albert 72
Herbert, Dorothea 51
Heyne, Moriz 111
Hintze, Kurt 94
Hobsbawm, Eric 45
Hoffmann, Johann Gottfried 111
Honegger, Claudia 92, 94
Hopkins, F. G. 58
Hume, J. R. 22
Hyman, Mary and Phillipp 99

Imhof, Arthur E. 115
Inama-Sternegg, Karl von 149

Jahoda, Marie 155
Janssen, Johannes 110
Jefferey, James 29
Jobse-van Putten, Jozien 63
Johnston, James P. 21
Julin, Armand 74
Justi, Johann Heinrich Gottlieb von 111

Kafka, Franz 161
Keller, Gottfried 180
Kennedy, Liam 24
Klemm, Gustav Friedrich 110
Komlos, I. 16

Kriegk, Georg Ludwig 110

Labrousse Ernest 94–5
Lamprecht, Karl 110
Lane, Frederic C. 97
Laverty, Maura 51
Lavoisier, Antoine Laurent 93
Lazarsfeld, Paul Felix 155
Le Play, Frédéric 12, 74, 149
Le Roy Ladurie, Emanuel 94, 96
Leichter, Käthe 152
Levenstein, Harvey 27
Levi, Leone 30
Lévi-Strauss, Claude 60, 91, 98, 279
Lewin, Kurt 60
Lichtenfelt, Alfred 94
Lippmann, Edmund O. von 112–3
Lis, Catharina 76
List, Friedrich 111
Longmate, Norman 22
Lucas, Anthony T. 45, 52
Lucassen, Jan 61
Lynch, Patrick 22
Lysaght, Patricia 52

MacDonagh, Oliver 22
Maggi, Julius 180
Malthus, Thomas Robert 49
Mandrou, Robert 94
Mannhardt, Wilhelm 110–1
Mathias, Peter 22, 29
Maurizio, Adam 94, 112
Mayhew, Henry 28
Mazarin, Cardinal 97
McCance, Robert Alexander 25
McKenzie, John Crawford 24–5
McKeown, Thomas 26, 115
Mead, Margaret 60
Miller, Derek S. 21
Mitchell, Margaret 25–6
Mitchison, R. 24
Mohl, Robert 111
Mokyr, Joel 22, 24, 45
Monckton, Herbert 22
Montbret, Coquebert de 47, 51
Morineau, Michel 46
Moss, Michael Stanley 22
Moulin, Léon 79

Mulder, Gerrit Jan 57

Neild, William 29
Neirynck, Michel 74
Newton, E. 21
Nicolai, Friedrich 147

Ó Gráda, Cormac 45
O'Neill, T. P. 52
O'Sullivan, Humphrey 48, 51
Ogburn, William F. 120
Orr, John Boyd 25, 28, 30
Otterloo, Anneke H. van 63

Parsons, Talcott 277
Peel, Constance S. 32
Pekelharing, A. C. 58
Perren, Richard 23
Philippe, Robert 91–3, 96
Philippovich, Eugen 149
Plattner, Felix 179
Popper, Karl 277
Post, John Dexter 26
Pyke, Magnus 57

Quetelet, Adolphe Lambert 12, 72

Rabb, Theodore K. 115
Raymond, J. 23
Reeves, Pember 39
Reich, Eduard 109–10
Rettigová, M. D. 237
Revel, Jacques 95
Richards, Audrey 60
Roberts, E. 24
Roebuck, P. 24
Roscher, Wilhelm 111, 117
Rotberg, Robert I. 115
Rousseau, Jean-Jacques 7
Rowntree, Benjamin Seebohm, 24, 30
Rumohr, Carl Friedrich von 109

Salaman, Redcliffe Nathan 22, 45
Salzman, Catherine 64
Scherr, Johannes 110
Schmidl, Adolf 148
Schmoller, Gustav 94–6, 111–2, 117
Schofield, E. M. 24

Schröder, Wilhelm von 160
Schuler, Fridolin 180
Scola, Roger 20, 29
Sering, Max 111
Severin, Pavel 236
Shelton, Walter James 26
Sheppard, Ronald 21
Sigsworth, Eric Milton 22
Simon, André 19
Simoons, Frederick 60
Smith, Edward 24–5, 27, 29
Soly, Hugo 76
Soyer, Alexis 109
Spooner, Frank, 93, 96
Spree, Reinhard 115
Stein, Lorenz von 111
Stern, Walter Marcell 21
Steven, Maisie 20
Stevenson, John 26
Stifter, Adalbert 161
Stokar, Walter von 113
Stouff, Louis 90, 96
Stuyvenberg, J. H. van 23
Sutton, David C. 19

Tannahill, Reay 20, 33
Thünen, Johann Heinrich von 111
Tighe, William 49
Trienekens, Gerard 61–2
Turner, Ernest 22

Vaerst, Eugen Baron 109
Vaizey, John 22
Vandenbroeke, Christiaan 75–6
Vogelsang, Freiherr von 149

Wachter, K. W. 26
Wähler, Martin 111
Walter, J. 26
Waser, Johann Heinrich 176
Watt, James 26
Webber, Ronald 23
Webster, Charles 25
Wecker, Anna 179
Wee, Herman van der 78
Weir, Donald B. 22
Whetham, Edith Holt 21
Widdowson, E. M. 25

Name index

Wiegelmann, Günther 117–8
Wilbraham 24
Wilbraham, A. 20
William, P. N. 23
Williams, Dale Edwards 26
Wilson, Anne 20
Wilson, Charles 23
Wilson, George Bailey 22
Woodham-Smith, Cecil 24

Wright, Lawrence 32
Wrightson, Keith 26

Young, Arthur 47, 49
Yudkin, John 23–4

Zeisel, Hans 155
Zwingli, Huldrich 178